Sir Robert Macintosh's
Lumbar Puncture and Spir
INTRADURAL AND EXTRADURAL

Sir Robert Macintosh's

Lumbar Puncture and Spinal Analgesia:
INTRADURAL AND EXTRADURAL

J. Alfred Lee
FFA RCS Hon.FFA RCS(I) DA
Honorary Consulting Anaesthetist to the Southend-on-Sea Hospital

R. S. Atkinson
MA MB BChir FFA RCS
Consultant Anaesthetist to the Southend-on-Sea Hospital

Margaret J. Watt
MB BS FFA RCS DA DRCOG
Consultant Anaesthetist to the Southend-on-Sea Hospital

FIFTH EDITION

CHURCHILL LIVINGSTONE
EDINBURGH LONDON MELBOURNE AND NEW YORK 1985

CHURCHILL LIVINGSTONE
Medical Division of Longman Group Limited

Distributed in the United States of America by
Churchill Livingstone Inc., 1560 Broadway, New York,
N.Y. 10036, and by associated companies, branches and
representatives throughout the world.

© E & S Livingstone Limited 1951, 1957

© Longman Group Limited 1973, 1978, 1985

All rights reserved. No part of this publication may be
reproduced, stored in a retrieval system, or transmitted
in any form or by any means, electronic, mechanical,
photocopying, recording or otherwise, without the prior
permission of the publishers (Churchill Livingstone,
Robert Stevenson House, 1–3 Baxter's Place, Leith
Walk, Edinburgh EH1 3AF).

Sir Robert Macintosh
  First Edition 1951
    German Edition 1953
    Spanish Edition 1953
  Second Edition 1957
Sir Robert Macintosh and J. Alfred Lee
  Third Edition 1973
J. Alfred Lee and R. S. Atkinson
  Fourth Edition 1978
  French Edition 1979
  German Edition 1981
  Spanish Edition 1981
J. Alfred Lee, R. S. Atkinson and Margaret J. Watt
  Fifth Edition 1985

ISBN 0 443 02671 8

British Library Cataloguing in Publication Data
Macintosh, *Sir*, Robert
  Sir Robert Macintosh's lumbar puncture and
  spinal analgesia. — 5th ed.
  1. Cerebrospinal fluid — Examination 2. Spine
  — Puncture 3. Spinal anesthesia
  I. Title II. Lee, J. Alfred
  III. Atkinson, R. S. IV. Margaret J.
  616.07′54   RB55

Library of Congress Cataloging in Publication Data
Macintosh, R. R. (Robert Reynolds), Sir, 1897–
  Sir Robert Macintosh's Lumbar puncture and spinal
analgesia.
  Includes bibliographical references and index.
  1. Spinal anesthesia. 2. Spine — Puncture.
I. Lee, J. Alfred (John Alfred) II. Atkinson, R. S.
(Richard Stuart) III. Watt, Margaret J. IV. Title.
V. Title: Lumbar puncture and spinal analgesia.
[DNLM: 1. Anesthesia, Spinal. 2. Spinal Puncture.
WO 305 M152L]
RD85.S7M2   1985   617′.964   84–7094

Printed in Hong Kong by Wing King Tong Company Limited

Preface to the Fifth Edition

Since the last edition of this book was published in 1978, a number of changes have taken place in the theory and practice of both intradural and extradural block. Recent work has challenged many of the long-established and traditional views relating to the mode of spread of local analgesic solutions within the intradural space, while the discovery of the fact that narcotic analgesic drugs relieve pain when injected into close proximity to the spinal cord has opened up new avenues for theoretical study and clinical practice. Although the practice and technique of central neural blockade have been used for 86 years, a period longer than that of any other method commonly employed today, there is room for further study, understanding and improvement, as it must be admitted that the clinical anaesthetist cannot always explain the occasional capricious behaviour of the solutions he is using for spinal block.

In recent years the increasing interest in spinal techniques has led to a number of clinical investigations and reports, so that hardly an issue of any of the major anaesthetic journals is without some comment on these methods. This has required much reading and sifting of the literature before making alterations on almost every page. To help them with their work the authors of the fourth edition have asked a colleague, Dr Margaret Watt, to join them in the preparation of the present book. She brings to her task a wide experience of the practice of the techniques described in it, as well as the outlook of a younger anaesthetist who is also familiar with the literature of the subject.

Like the edition it replaces, this book is essentially a practical one directed at the working anaesthetist. The safety of the patient both during and after the employment of the techniques described has been our constant concern, and we believe that the advice it contains and the methods discussed, if put into practice, will not harm any patient. We would, nevertheless, continue to emphasise that the greatest care is necessary when central neural blockade is employed;

care in observation of the patient; care in sterility of equipment; and care in judgement as to the safe indications for its use.

A number of changes have taken place in the format of the present volume. The sections on physiology and pharmacology have been expanded and much of the chapter on intradural analgesia has been rewritten to take account of current work. The chapter on spinal analgesia in obstetrics has been enlarged and there is an entirely new chapter relating to narcotic analgesic drugs in the intradural and the extradural space. The authors have little practical experience of central neural blockade deliberately extended to the thorax or neck, so that these aspects of technique are not dealt with in this small book. For those who are interested in high block, and in all aspects of extradural blockade, we refer them to the definitive work *Epidural Anesthesia* by P. R. Bromage (1978), Philadelphia and London: Saunders.

The authors wish to thank the publishers for their help, but regret that, because of the cost involved, they have not found it possible to reproduce the plates again in three colours, as was done in the first edition. A number of illustrations have been added and for some of these they would like to express their thanks to Professor R. J. Last who has given them his permission to use several figures from his book *Regional Anatomy*. The authors are indebted to Mr John Wood of the Photographic Department of the Southend Hospital for his help, as well as to others who have kindly allowed reproduction of their own work. For secretarial assistance they are grateful to Mrs Betty Bradbury and Mrs Penny McLagan.

Southend-on-Sea,　　　　　　　　　　　　　　　　　　　　J.A.L.
1985　　　　　　　　　　　　　　　　　　　　　　　　　　　R.S.A.
　　　　　　　　　　　　　　　　　　　　　　　　　　　　　M.J.W.

Preface to the First Edition

The literature on lumbar puncture and spinal analgesia is abundant enough to make an explanation necessary for any addition to it. The reasons for another book on this subject are various. Although lumbar puncture is often entrusted to the newly-qualified house doctor, it is seldom that he has had any instruction on how to carry it out. It is difficult to find a concise exposition of the technique to which he can refer; and the result is that early attempts are frequently and unnecessarily bungled. That is why I have included in this book the things I should have liked to have readily available for myself when setting out on my first lumbar punctures and spinal anaesthetics. A road-map is often a useful thing to have when one is exploring an unfamiliar locality.

The second reason is that some surgeons, encouraged by the fact that they are expert at lumbar puncture, have been tempted to take the further step of giving their own spinal anaesthetics: in which case, not infrequently, their lack of knowledge of basic principles leads them into difficulties. 'The apparent simplicity of the manoeuvre constitutes its greatest danger in the hands of the tyro' (Editorial, 1900). 'The factor most contributory to its tragic history is the ease with which it can be performed by anyone' (Greene, 1949). Forty-nine years intervened between the writing of the last two sentences. The quip that Pentothal is fatally easy to give, still has its counterpart in spinal anaesthetics. A patient under a spinal anaesthetic should be looked after by a trained anaesthetist. But if for one reason or another, the surgeon has both to operate and to keep an eye on the general condition of the patient, he should at any rate know something about the essentials of the subject and what to do if things go wrong.

A third reason for this book is that members of this Department have thrown light on certain obscure aspects of spinal analgesia, and I feel that the points cleared up will be of interest to others too.

My fourth reason is my desire to take advantage of the collaboration of Miss McLarty, which I have the good fortune to enjoy. Certainly I should not have embarked on this work without her help: for I believe that views on what is largely a technical subject can be conveyed more quickly and, what is more important, with greater accuracy by a few good illustrations than by pages of script. There is much to be said for Corning's observation in 1900: 'I advise those who contemplate practising spinal anaesthesia to take a look at the skeleton, especially the relations of the lumbar vertebrae. An intelligent glance of that sort is worth many words' (Corning, 1900). I have spent many unattractive but profitable hours working in the post-mortem room and, for the facilities provided, I am grateful to Dr A. H. Robb-Smith. If a dissection has been fruitful, Miss McLarty has recorded it clearly and with decision: and I am sure that these illustrations will be helpful to those who have no opportunity for dissecting this unfamiliar region. I am indebted, too, to Miss A. Arnott for other valuable illustrations. Some of the pictures may appear almost duplicates, but I include them deliberately where they are likely to help the reader to form a clear mental picture of the structures through which the needle passes on its way to the vertebral canal, and of the obstacles which are likely to be impeding it when it is off course; as well as of what happens to an anaesthetic solution deposited within the dura.

I do not intend to extol the virtues of spinal analgesia. The benefits of any method of pain relief, general or local, have to be paid for in terms of morbidity, and the price exacted to the patient in this respect depends little on the choice of method or agent, but very much on the care, skill and experience of the anaesthetist himself. From a purely selfish point of view, the consequences to the anaesthetist of carelessness or inexperience are much less serious with a general than with a spinal anaesthetic. Even in the event of death, a sympathetic pathologist has only to stress the unhealthy state of some organ; then everyone, including the anaesthetist himself, if he is complacent enough, will believe the coroner's finding that no one was to blame; and so the incident is soon forgotten. But a grave mistake with a spinal anaesthetic is quite another matter. A paralysed patient wheeled about in a bath-chair is a constant reproach, and does nothing to enhance the reputation of surgeon and anaesthetist concerned. Moreover, in some cases heavy damages have been awarded, although anomalously there would not have been the slightest prospect of this if the patient had been killed outright by a general anaesthetic badly given.

I have to thank my erstwhile Registrar, Dr A. Crampton Smith, now happily a Consultant, for his skill and care in cutting the bony vertebral sections and for his help in dissecting the specimens from which a number of the drawings were made. Even though the typescript is not extensive I am conscious of, and grateful for, the guidance extended to me by experts in allied subjects, especially Professor T. B. Johnston, Dr H. G. Epstein, Dr Grita Weiler and Mr Lionel Salt. Their help on doubtful points has been a source of considerable comfort.

I have only to add that although at first I intended to confine the scope of this book strictly to practical aspects of lumbar puncture and spinal analgesia, I have extended certain sections to include a few academic points likely to be of interest to the examination candidate.

Nuffield Department of Anaesthetics   R. R. Macintosh
University of Oxford, 1951

REFERENCES

Corning, J. L. (1900) *Medical Record (NY)*, **58**, 601–604; cf. p. 602.
Editorial (1900) *Medical Record (NY)*, **58**, 577.
Greene, B. A. (1949) Critical appraisal of spinal analgesia and anesthesia for obstetrics. In Greenhill, J. P. (ed) *The Yearbook of Obstetrics and Gynecology*, pp. 160–162. Chicago.

Contents

Introduction
1. History 4
2. Anatomy 38
3. Cerebrospinal fluid 88
4. Physiology of central neural blockade 98
5. Pharmacology 118
6. Equipment 151
7. Technique of lumbar puncture 159
8. Intradural analgesia (subarachnoid block) 188
9. Extradural analgesia 208
10. Management of the patient during the operation 242
11. Indications and contraindications 247
12. Intradural and extradural spinal analgesia in obstetrics 256
13. Complications and sequelae 278
14. Spinal analgesia and intractable pain 302
15. Narcotic analgesic drugs in the extradural and intradural space 306
16. Do's, don'ts and doubtfuls 314
Index 318

Introduction

There is no doubt that spinal analgesia, having gone through a period of loss of popularity, is being employed more extensively in recent years. The reasons for loss of enthusiasm are not hard to enumerate. The phenomenal muscular relaxation central neural blockade provides has for many years been matched by the use of curare, more easily administered. There is no doubt that the shadow of litigation discourages the use of spinal analgesia even in the patient's best interests. From a purely selfish point of view, the consequences to the anaesthetist of carelessness or inexperience are much less serious with a general than with a spinal anaesthetic. Cynical in the extreme, but true, is the opinion expressed by a colleague that in anaesthetics it is less expensive to kill than to maim.

Cogent arguments against the use of intradural spinal analgesia have appeared in medical journals from 1906 onwards: (Kennedy et al, 1950; Cope, 1954; Koenig, recorded by Greene, 1961). While in no way belittling the calamity of a post-spinal neurological lesion, the probability of faulty technique must be borne in mind. Seldom are details given of the training, skill and experience of the anaesthetist concerned. To get these tragedies into perspective, consideration must be given to the large number of less publicised silent witnesses, in the graveyards, of general anaesthesia incompetently administered. Moreover, major neurological lesions are not confined to intradural and extradural spinal analgesia (Pisetsky, 1945; Ciliberti, 1948; Zweighaft, 1949; Thomas and Dwyer, 1950; Sinclair, 1954; Norman, 1955; Lett, 1964); and paraplegia has been reported after spinal analgesia, but otherwise unrelated to it (Leatherdale, 1959).

We concur in the view that postoperative complications are no more common after both forms of spinal analgesia than after general anaesthesia (King, 1933; Dripps and Deming, 1946; Urbach et al, 1964) and we believe the safety of well-conducted spinal analgesia is attested by the reports of thousands of carefully followed-up cases by recognised authorities (Dripps and Vandam, 1954; Vandam and Dripps, 1955, 1956; Lake, 1958; Wilkinson, 1963; Moore and Bridenbaugh, 1966; Phillips et al, 1969). The results bear comparison with those of any other similar series given general anaesthetics. Our belief is reinforced by a publication (Gordh, 1969) which states that in the 24 years up to 1969, 50 000 intradural spinal anaesthetics had been administered in the Department of Anaesthetics of the Karolinska Hospital in Stockholm without any serious neurological sequelae, while from Canada comes a review of over 78 000 cases from teaching hospitals with no serious sequelae (Noble and Murray, 1971).

Although the first three editions of this small book dealt primarily with spinal or intradural analgesia, much of what we have written can be applied to the slightly more difficult technique of extradural block, which was incorporated in the fourth edition. The widespread interest in narcotic analgesic drugs injected into the extradural or intradural space has necessitated an additional chapter in this fifth edition. We hope that the increasing number of anaesthetists who employ these techniques will find the new edition useful.

REFERENCES

Ciliberti, B. J. (1948) Paraplegia following inhalation anaesthesia for sub-total gastrectomy. *Anesthesiology*, **9**, 439.
Cope, R. W. (1954) The Woolley and Roe case. Woolley and Rowe v. the Ministry of Health and others. *Anaesthesia*, **9**, 249.
Dripps, R. D. & Deming, M. V. (1946) Postoperative atelectasis and pneumonia. *Annals of Surgery*, **124**, 94.
Dripps, R. D. & Vandam, L. D. (1954) Long-term follow-up of patients who received 10 098 spinal anesthetics: failure to discover any neurological sequelae. *Journal of the American Medical Association*, **156**, 1486.
Gordh, T. (1969) *Illustrated Handbook of Local Anaesthesia*. Edited by Ericksson, E., p. 120. London: Lloyd-Luke.
Kennedy, F. G., Effron, A. S. & Perry, G. (1950) The grave spinal cord paralyses caused by spinal anesthesia. *Surgery, Gynecology and Obstetrics*, **91**, 385.
King, D. S. (1933) Postoperative pulmonary complications; the part played by anesthesia. *Anesthesia and Analgesia, Current Researches*, **12**, 243.
Koenig, recorded by Greene, N. M. (1961) Neurological sequelae of spinal anesthesia. *Anesthesiology*, **22**, 682.
Lake, N. (1958) Spinal anaesthesia: the present position. *Lancet*, **1**, 387.
Leatherdale, R. A. L. (1959) Spinal analgesia and unrelated paraplegia. *Anaesthesia*, **14**, 274.
Lett, Z. (1964) Two thousand spinal anaesthetics. *British Journal of Anaesthesia*, **36**, 266.
Moore, D. C. & Bridenbaugh, L. D. (1966) Spinal (subarachnoid) block; a review of 11 574 cases. *Journal of the American Medical Association*, **195**, 907.

Noble, A. B. & Murray, J. J. (1971) A review of complications in spinal anaesthesia with experience in Canadian teaching hospitals. *Canadian Anaesthetists' Society Journal*, **18**, 5.

Norman, J. E. (1955) (a letter). Nerve palsy following general anaesthesia. *Anaesthesia*, **10**, 87.

Phillips, O. C., Ebner, H., Nelson, A. T. & Black, M. H. (1969) Neurological complications following spinal anesthesia with lidocaine: a prospective study of 21 000 cases. *Anesthesiology*, **30**, 284.

Pisetsky, J. E. (1945) Hemiplegia following ether anesthesia. *Anesthesiology*, **6**, 522.

Sinclair, R. N. (1954) Ascending spinal paralysis following hysterectomy under general anaesthesia. *Anaesthesia*, **9**, 286.

Thomas, P. & Dwyer, C.(1950) Postoperative flaccid paraplegia: a case report, *Anesthesiology*, **11**, 635.

Urbach, K. F., Lee, W. R. & Sheely, L. L. (1964) Spinal or general anesthesia for inguinal hernia repair: a comparison of certain complications in a controlled series. *Journal of the American Medical Association*, **190**, 25.

Vandam, L. D. & Dripps, R. D. (1955) A long-term follow-up of 10 098 spinal anesthetics — II. Incidence and analysis of minor sensory neurological defects. *Surgery* (St Louis), **38**, 463.

Vandam, L. D. & Dripps, R. D. (1956) Long-term follow-up of patients who received 10 098 spinal anesthetics. *Journal of the American Medical Association*, **161**, 586.

Wilkinson, W. M. (1963) Two thousand spinal anaesthetics. *British Journal of Anaesthesia*, **35**, 711.

Zweighaft, J. F. (1949) Hemiplegia following tonsillectomy. *Anesthesiology*, **11**, 729.

1

History

Intradural analgesia

The introduction of the hollow needle and a conveniently sized glass syringe by Alexander Wood (1817–1884) (Wood, 1855) in 1853 and the clinical demonstration of the local analgesic properties of cocaine by Koller (1858–1944) (Koller, 1884a) in 1884 were direct steps leading to spinal analgesia. Corning (1855–1923), a neurologist, who wrote the first textbook on local anaesthesia, *Local Anesthesia in General Medicine and Surgery* (New York, 1886) was the first to inject cocaine into the region of the spinal cord (whether intra- or extra-durally, is not quite certain), but it is not surprising that this work passed unacclaimed by contemporary workers. It was in 1885 that he injected cocaine into the subarachnoid space, but he did so unintentionally and without recognising what he had done. The result was indeed dramatic, but it is certain that it could not be reproduced at will, either by Corning himself or by anyone else carrying out the technique he described. Corning's experiment was based on faulty physiological and anatomical premises: for he believed that cocaine injected into the region between two spinous processes would be absorbed by veins and 'transferred to the substance of the cord, and give rise to anaesthesia of the sensory and perhaps motor tracts of the same' (Corning, 1885a). The fact that morphine and other narcotic analgesics can act at sites distal to the brain, is one of the most interesting discoveries of recent years (Snyder, 1977; Behar et al, 1979).

At this time the aim of any injection was to deposit the drug as near as possible to the site on which it was desired to act. Thus Wood (Wood, 1855; Howard-Jones, 1947) believed that the main virtue of the hollow needle was that it deposited morphine in close contact with painful nerves, and for many years physicians continued to consider morphine effective only if injected actually into the painful lesion. Corning was in a dilemma. He wished to deposit the cocaine reasonably close to the cord, and yet avoid the risk of injuring it by puncture. He performed a preliminary experiment on a dog, injecting, at an unstated depth, 20 minims of 2 per cent cocaine 'into the space situated between the spinous processes of two of the inferior dorsal vertebrae'. This was followed by loss of sensation, and incoordination of the hind legs. The fact that the effect had not spread to the forelegs was attributed to 'the lethargy of the circulation at this point'.

After this he carried out his now well-known experiment on man. He had noted that in the lower thoracic region the transverse processes of the vertebrae lie at the same depth as the laminae which form the posterior boundary of the vertebral canal. He therefore first inserted the needle lateral to the mid-line until the point touched the transverse process, and adjusted the marker on the shaft of the needle to skin level (Fig. 1.1). The needle was then reinserted, this time in the mid-line between two spines, but as a guarantee against injury to the cord, not quite up to the marker (Fig. 1.2). He now injected — with what object it is not clear — 60 minims of 3 per cent cocaine 'into the space situated between the spinous process of the 11th and 12th dorsal vertebrae' of a man who suffered from

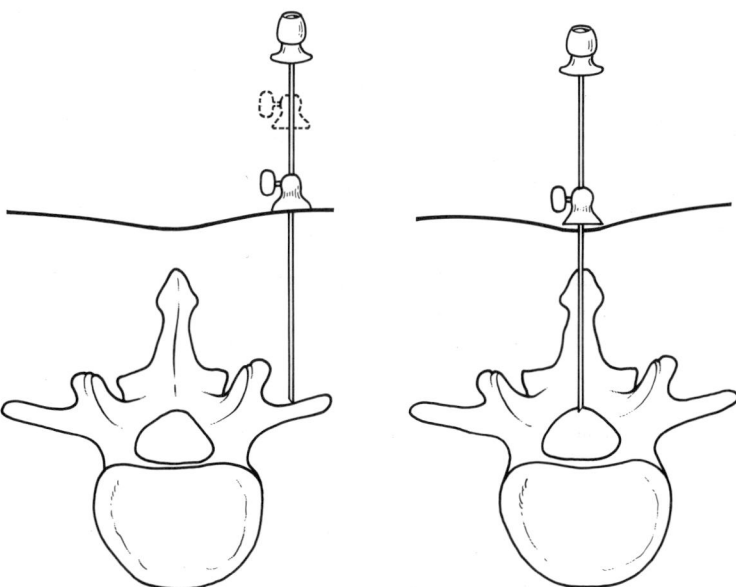

Fig. 1.1   Fig. 1.2

'spinal weakness and seminal incontinence'. Ten minutes later the legs felt sleepy, and later still there was complete analgesia of legs and perineum. If these directions are followed, the tip of the needle will lie roughly at the depth of the ligamentum flavum, and in the hands of a cautious contemporary investigator trying to corroborate Corning's findings, well proximal to it. Corning does not mention the ligamentum flavum nor the dura mater: yet such anatomical boundaries are of the greatest significance when considering the spread of injected fluid. If the tip of the needle lies superficial to the ligamentum flavum, the effect of the injection is nil. Even if the tip penetrates the ligament and lies within the extradural space, the effect of 3 to 4 ml of 3 per cent cocaine is negligible. If, inadvertently, the needle happens to have been inserted a fraction of an inch further on, the dura is pierced and the wide spread of the injected fluid in the cerebrospinal fluid gives striking results. The dripping of cerebrospinal fluid through the needle, the sure sign that the dura has been entered, was denied to Corning because, as his article makes clear, he introduced his needle with a charged syringe already attached.

In 1894 this prolific writer published another book of essays (Corning, 1894), some rehashes of previous articles, others of mixed value, so that it is not surprising that two arresting paragraphs passed unnoticed at the time even by his own countrymen. Under the heading 'The irrigation of the cauda equina with medicinal fluids', he wrote '... I became impressed with the desirability of introducing remedies directly into the spinal canal with a view to producing still more powerful impressions on the cord, and more especially on its lower segment.' He introduced a small director about half an inch long between the spines of L. 2–3 and through this passed a fine needle deliberately to perform lumbar puncture, but this was three years after the technique of lumbar puncture had been described in detail by Quincke (1842–1922) (Quincke, 1891a and b) and by Essex Wynter (1891). Into the first of his two patients Corning injected a mixture of aconite and cocaine to medicate the cord because of 'spinal irritation' 10 days after an operation on the urethra. Five to eight minutes after the puncture subjective feelings were experienced, and in a quarter of an hour all pain had gone; and when it did come back some hours afterwards, it was less than before. In the second case, 'the injection was made with the hope of relieving the severe vesical and abdominal pains' which are a peculiarly distressing feature of caisson disease, then common because of the building of the tunnel under the Hudson

River. As well as in these two cases, he had 'occasionally resorted to the procedure in properly selected cases'.

In 1885, Corning finished his article describing the patient to whom he had introduced cocaine unwittingly and unknowingly into the subarachnoid space with the following dramatic passage: 'Whether the method will ever find an application as a substitution for etherisation in genito-urinary or other branches of surgery, further experience alone can show. Be the destiny of the observation what it may, it has seemed to me, on the whole, worth recording.' These two sentences have often been taken incorrectly from their context to give Corning credit for the introduction of spinal analgesia. It is strange that in 1894, when he purposefully introduced mixtures containing cocaine into the subarachnoid space, he did not realise that the case he reported in 1885 was one of inadvertent spinal analgesia, and that there was now a more dependable method of achieving this which would allow certain surgical operations to be performed without general anaesthesia.

There was, however, a defect in Corning's technique which made it not nearly as reliable as it would at first appear. The needle, before it was introduced through the skin, was screwed on to the nozzle of the syringe already charged with solution. It was then a matter of hit or miss, with the latter a strong probability. The needle was inserted and the solution injected; and such a procedure would necessarily lead to a percentage of failures high enough to be discouraging. Present-day spinal analgesia would soon be abandoned if, before injection, the anaesthetist did not confirm that the point of the needle lay within the dural sac. Even after spinal analgesia for surgery had been generally accepted, such blind shots appear to have been commonplace, for many writers found it necessary to stress that the solution should not be injected until cerebrospinal fluid was seen to issue from the needle (Lusk, 1911). On one occasion the anaesthetist, having introduced his needle, accepted a shooting pain down the leg as his clue to inject (Trantenroth, 1906). A glance at Figure 7.18 suffices to explain why the resultant analgesia was restricted.

Corning appears to have regarded his intentional intradural injection only as a means of alleviating existing pain. He overlooked its possibilities in surgery. One is reminded of the part played by Humphry Davy (1778–1829) (Davy, 1800) in the discovery of general anaesthetics. He recorded when inhaling nitrous oxide experimentally that the pain caused by an erupting wisdom tooth was relieved; but he did nothing further about the matter and his observation had no direct bearing on the introduction of general anaesthetics some 46 years afterwards. Similarly, Corning's writings attracted no attention at the time, and it is certain that they had no influence upon the ultimate adoption of spinal analgesia in surgery (see also Little, 1979).

In 1891, Essex Wynter (1860–1945) (Wynter, 1891), physician to the Middlesex Hospital in London, briefly described four cases in which he had performed lumbar puncture with Southey's tubes (used in the treatment of dropsy and ascites) to allow continuous drainage of cerebrospinal fluid, in an attempt to relieve increased intracranial pressure associated with tuberculous meningitis. A few months later, Quincke (1842–1922) (Quincke, 1891a), acknowledging Wynter's work, described the technique of lumbar puncture, essentially the same as that practised today, and showed how the cerebrospinal fluid pressure could be relieved by simple puncture. The practice of present-day spinal analgesia is a direct consequence of this admirable article. The withdrawal of fluid proved disappointing as a therapeutic procedure: but soon hope was transferred from simple withdrawal to replacement of the fluid by a solution which would come into contact with the region which it was desired to treat. Ziemssen (von Ziemssen, 1893) suggested this after injecting methylene blue intrathecally into corpses, and Sicard (1872–1929) (Sicard, 1898, 1899), after preliminary work on animals, injected antitetanus serum by the same route into a patient with tetanus.

The first two publications on spinal analgesia for surgical operations were made in 1899. At the time of their investigations neither author knew of the work of the other, but both acknowledged their indebtedness to Quincke. The article by Bier (1861–1949) (Bier, 1899) (who worked at the same hospital as Quincke at Kiel) preceded that of Tuffier (1857–1929) (Tuffier, 1899) by a few months, and in it he described six patients to whom he had given 10 to 20 mg cocaine intradurally for operations on the lower limb, the first receiving his injection on 16th August 1898. The question of sterility is not mentioned, and since he used tap water to dissolve the cocaine crystals (Sebrechts, personal communication) and placed his finger over the hub of the needle to lose as little cerebrospinal fluid as possible, it is not surprising that headache and vomiting were marked features of convalescence. These unpleasant after-effects were described as being as bad as those after chloroform and ether, with the added disadvantage that they sometimes lasted longer. In order to investigate their causation,

Bier asked that a spinal analgesic should be given to him. Lumbar puncture was performed one week later, but as the syringe would not fit the needle, 'much cerebrospinal fluid was lost, and the major part of the cocaine came out of the side'. His assistant, Hildenbradt, offered himself as a substitute, and that 5 mg cocaine eliminated pain is clear from the exacting tests which included pulling the pubic hair, hard pressure on and pulling of the testes, and a sharp blow with an iron hammer on the shin! These experiments, which started at 7.30 in the evening were followed by dinner, wine and cigars. Both volunteers were in poor shape for a few days afterwards. Bier's symptoms of headache and dizziness, relieved when he lay down, could easily be attributed to leakage of cerebrospinal fluid, and those of Hildenbradt, which included vomiting, suggest that the cause was meningeal irritation.

Bier's article includes some pertinent observations resulting from his own experience, and ends by saying that he does not feel justified in continuing his work on humans without carrying out animal experiments with a view to eliminating vomiting. Further communications by Bier followed (Bier, 1900, 1901) but, unlike the wholly enthusiastic reports from American and French sources, his observations continued to sound a note of caution and he expressed dissatisfaction with the drug cocaine, the sole local analgesic agent then available . Only after the discovery of Stovaine by Fourneau (1872–1949) (Fourneau, 1904) did the method achieve any real popularity (Chaput, 1904). By 1904, writing with Dönitz (Bier and Dönitz, 1904) he felt justified in stating 'after many disappointments we believe now that we can recommend spinal anaesthesia', and then qualified this by adding, 'although it is still capable of and needs plenty of improvement'.

Tuffier (Tuffier, 1899) first tried cocaine intrathecally to relieve the pain of sarcoma of the leg in a young man on whom morphine was losing its effect. Even if only temporary, 'the results were truly remarkable'. He then gave a similar injection to a young woman with painful recurrent sarcoma of the thigh, and to his great surprise was able to remove the tumour without causing any discomfort. He operated rapidly, but remarked that haste was unnecessary as analgesia lasted more than an hour. It was only after this that he heard of Bier's publication. Tuffier's short paper pointed out that spinal analgesia was satisfactory for vaginal hysterectomy, but not for abdominal operations. By the time of his much more extensive contribution in January 1901 (Tuffier, 1901), he had improved his own technique by vigorous attention to asepsis, by altering the height of puncture, and by putting the patient in different positions immediately the injection had been carried out. In this way he had extended the field of operation from the perineum to the abdominal cavity and higher, as his list of organs operated on included kidney, stomach and breast. The article has a particularly good section on technique. He discusses headache fully, acknowledges an incidence of 40 per cent, points out that beyond causing discomfort to the patient the complication is not serious, and adds 'the explanation of it will come later'. He is the first to record a follow-up examination of patients operated on under spinal analgesia; in 60 operated on between six and 13 months previously, he found no complications attributable to the anaesthetic.

For some years, most of the work on spinal analgesia came from the Continent, and this was probably accounted for by the poor standard of general anaesthesia prevailing there. The first mention of spinal analgesia in the British literature was an annotation in *The Lancet* (1899), 2, 1536. In 1909, a leading article in *The Lancet* (4th Dec.) stated that 'spinal anaesthesia does not appear to be welcomed so warmly in Great Britain as in some of the continental countries, and we believe that the main reason is that there is less cause to be dissatisfied with the use of general anaesthetics here than abroad.' Nevertheless, by this time the *British Medical Journal* had already published what is probably the most painstaking and helpful study of the subject ever written. Barker (1850–1916), Professor of Surgery at London's University College Hospital, was no innovator and was aware that Bier had already given 1000 spinal injections and Tuffier 2000, both using Stovaine (Barker, 1907). But he was renowned for the thoroughness of his clinical research and for the attention he paid to practical details which can make the difference between success and failure. He had studied at Bonn, was fluent in German and acknowledged the contributions of Bier and others, but was concerned about the lack of uniformity in the results of spinal analgesia. His three articles (Barker, 1907, 1908a, 1908b) written 77 years ago each record 100 carefully studied cases. In them he advocated general principles many of which, though temporarily forgotten, are in current use. He took pains to prepare an isotonic solution of glucose — Stovaine, holding that all fluids injected into the tissues of the body should possess the same osmotic tension as the blood serum, and demonstrated with a 'glass spine' how this solution, heavy relative to cerebrospinal fluid, could be made to flow to involve the required nerve roots. He pierced the theca below the termination of the cord, and stressed that the point of the needle (or of his specially devised blunt cannula inserted through the needle) should lie wholly within the theca, or some of the solution would be discharged into the extradural space, and advocated a mid-line approach. He insisted that his syringes and needles should be kept exclusively for spinal analgesia and that alkaline contamination must be avoided. He noted that in order to prolong anaesthesia 'adrenalin chloride' was added to the injected solution 'almost as a routine by others' (Dönitz, 1903; Bier, 1905) but he decided against this after injecting the mixture, which made him speculate '... whether some of the undesirable sequelae recorded in a few cases of spinal analgesia might not have been due to the adrenal compounds'. The last sentence of his first article runs 'It is not for casual use by the inexperienced', a sentiment which had been expressed before (*New York Medical Journal*, Editorial, 1900). 'The factor most contributory to the tragic history, is the ease with which it can be performed by anyone' (*Year Book of Obstetrics*, 1949).

Barker, however, was not the first in Britain to report on spinal analgesia. Robert Jones (1858–1933) the Liverpool orthopaedic surgeon did so in 1904 (Brownlee, 1911) and Dean, surgeon to the London Hospital and the first to treat a perforated peptic ulcer surgically (Dean, 1894), saw merit in its use in abdominal emergencies (Dean, 1906). Dean's article, which finishes 'It seems, however, definitely proved that whatever the danger may be the mortality is by no means so large as with general anaesthetics', includes the first account of infusion during spinal analgesia which we have found. A man gravely ill from intestinal obstruction and peritonitis collapsed during the course of the operation and had to be given artificial respiration. The pulse at the wrist could just be felt. 'We then transfused into the internal saphenous vein three pints of normal salt solution in the usual way, and to the fourth pint we added an ounce of brandy. Quick improvement was noted and finally in about an hour the patient was breathing well with all the intercostal muscles acting and the pulse very much better than it was before the operation.'

It is an interesting fact that although spinal analgesia is seldom employed in children today, this was not always so. Among other workers, Tyrrell Gray, a distinguished surgeon working at the Hospital for Sick Children in London, was an early pioneer and warm advocate of what was then a new technique, both in children and in adults (Gray, 1909, 1910, 1911). It was a commonly held view in the early years of the century, a view supported by Crile of Cleveland whose influence was strong (Crile, 1899), and many other surgeons, that surgical shock was due in large part to the bombardment of the brain by noxious afferent impulses from the site of the operation. These were of course blocked by the analgesic technique and this fact was one of the main reasons for its employment. American surgeons were also early in the field of paediatric spinal analgesia, W. S. Bainbridge reporting his first successful cases in 1900 (Bainbridge, 1900). In the following year he was able to report over 40 successful operations under spinal analgesia, the youngest in an infant aged 3 months (Bainbridge, 1901).

Spinal analgesia was used for Caesarean section soon after it was employed in general surgery (Kreis, 1900).

In the USA it appears that the first patient deliberately to be given a spinal analgesic was a man from whose tibia a piece of bone was excised in October 1899, by Frederick Dudley Tait (1862–1918) and Guido Caglieri (1871–1951) in San Francisco. The account of this operation was not published until the following year (Tait and Caglieri, 1900), and in the meantime Rudolf Matas (1860–1957) of New Orleans had both used the procedure for haemorrhoidectomy and published the fact (Matas, 1899). Later, another warm supporter of the method was W. W. Babcock (1872–1963) of Philadelphia, who included alcohol in the injection in order to make it lighter than cerebrospinal fluid (Babcock, 1913).

During the time that spinal analgesia has been in use it has gone through alternating periods of enthusiastic acceptance and relative unpopularity. One who championed the procedure was Gaston Labat (1872–1934). His book dealing with the subject soon attained rapid popularity and remains a classic (Labat, 1922). Labat's technique was to aspirate a predetermined volume of cerebrospinal fluid and in this dissolve an ampoule of Neocaine (procaine crystals) (Einhorn, 1899) conveniently available in different weights. For high blocks, Labat employed barbotage, a technique first described by his fellow countryman Le Filliatre (Le Filliatre, 1921). He was an advocate of the Trendelenburg position because of its beneficial effects on the cardiovascular system and on the blood supply to the brain, thus differing from Barker who preferred the head to be well raised, both during and after the operation. But not so impressive to us was his faith in 'stimulants' such as adrenaline, strychnine and caffeine.

Basic work in the pharmacology of local analgesics was little in evidence during these early years, but W. E. Dixon (1891–1931) the Cambridge pharmacologist, showed that sensory fibres are less resistant than motor fibres, an observation still known as Dixon's law (Dixon, 1905). Barker himself did some experiments which showed that stovaine remained in the theca after spinal analgesia for some two days (Barker, 1909). Förster's classical work on sensory innervation appeared in 1933 (Förster, 1933).

In 1927 George Pitkin of New Jersey gave a fresh impetus to the method by combining superb technical ability with an attractive modicum of showmanship. His message was controllability and to this end used Spinocaine (hypobaric) or Gravocaine (hyperbaric), both basically solutions of procaine (Einhorn (1856–1917), 1899 and 1905) but neither attained any lasting popularity. He was on firm ground when he stressed the importance of using a fine bore needle with a short bevel (Pitkin, 1927).

A valuable advance was the introduction of the long-acting local analgesic Percaine, later to be known as Nupercaine, cinchocaine and dibucaine (Uhlmann, 1929). Techniques employing a weak (1:1500) hypobaric solution were described by Howard Jones (Jones, 1930), anaesthetist, of London and by Etherington Wilson (Wilson, 1934) and Lake (Lake, 1938), surgeons of the same city. Continental surgeons who developed special techniques using Nupercaine were Kirschner (1879–1942) (Kirschner, 1932) of Heidelberg, and Sebrechts (Sebrechts, 1934) of Bruges. The first use of a heavy solution of the drug in 0.5 per cent concentration in 6 per cent glucose was described by Keyes and McClelland in 1930 (Keyes and McClelland, 1930).

Fresh attention was drawn to spinal analgesia when Lemmon of Philadelphia wrote of his method of continuous administration to get over the limitation of time imposed by the single shot injection (Lemmon, 1940; Lee, 1943, 1944). He used a special mattress with a segment cut out to correspond with the patient's lumbar vertebrae. This was to accommodate the lumbar puncture needle which was connected by means of rubber tubing (there was no plastic tubing at that time) to a syringe containing local analgesic solution, injections being given as required. It is interesting that a somewhat similar technique had been described by Dean 34 years before (Dean, 1906). Tuohy modified Lemmon's technique by substituting for the indwelling needle a plastic catheter which could be threaded through Tuohy's ingenious needle (Tuohy, 1945).

Deliberate total spinal analgesia has fallen into desuetude but the following references show that the possibilities of widespread analgesia have been explored sporadically. As early as 1901 the American surgeon Morton wrote (Morton, 1901), 'I think I have a safe and reliable analgesic in the subarachnoid injection of cocaine for the performance of any surgery in any position of the body.' In 1907 the Frenchman, M. Chaput (1857–1904) in an article entitled 'Total spinal analgesia' reported enthusiastically on his results after 17 operations 'without incident' on breast, arm, parotid, and cervical glands (Chaput, 1907.) In 1909 the Roumanian surgeon, Jonnesco (1860–1926) (Jonnesco, 1909) described his technique of cervical dural puncture which he had used in over 80 operations on the skull, face and throat. He also gave a demonstration in London at which McGavin was sufficiently impressed to give the method a trial. The following year McGavin published his own results of 18 cases (McGavin, 1910) some of which — on the arm, mastoid, malignant glands of the neck and cranium — were spectacularly successful. For instance, the trephine case — 'Analgesia was complete from the crown of the head to the umbilicus. The patient chatted of various subjects throughout the operation ... there was no alteration whatever in pulse or respiration ... after the operation he expressed his thanks, and walked back to his bed saying he felt none the worse for his experience.' But some of the remaining cases were so far from being uneventful that he did 'not feel justified in employing it further for the present'. Relevant correspondence followed (Madden, 1910).

Le Filliatre was no less enthusiastic than Jonnesco about spinal analgesia, but he held firmly to the view that whatever the operation, spinal puncture should be restricted to the lumbar region. At the International Medical Congress in London in 1913 he reported on his 12 years' experience of 2837 cases *toujours sans accident*. His list included 29 operations on the head and neck, amongst these a total laryngectomy and enucleation of the eye (Le Filliatre, 1913). This work is set out more fully in his book, published in 1921 (Le Filliatre, 1921). In more recent times, Koster used spinal analgesia as a routine, and one of the authors witnessed in New York the brilliant way he exploited the advantages afforded by widespread spinal block. Before his tragic death from a riding accident he wrote extensively on the subject (Koster, 1928). Round about this time, Dickson Wright (Wright, 1931) described the attractions which high spinal analgesia held out to him, and Vehrs (Vehrs, 1934) described his method of attaining 'massive spinal analgesia'. It is noteworthy that all three insisted that the patient should be tilted head downwards.

It is not surprising that total spinal analgesia never achieved general acceptance. The alarmingly low blood-pressure inevitably associated with total sympathetic paralysis was a main deterrent.

Sympathetic blockade was shown to be the main cause of hypotension, experimentally, in the cat in 1915 (Smith and Porter, 1915). From Edinburgh two workers (Griffiths and Gillies, 1948) however, capitalised this very feature when they were faced with the problem of anaesthetising hypertensive patients for the then popular operation of thoraco-abdominal splanchnicectomy performed by Professor Sir James Learmonth, where excessive bleeding militated against success. They were not interested in widespread skin analgesia, but after reading the above works, felt justified in giving intradural procaine high enough to paralyse the sympathetic outflow from the cord. Their excellent article, a landmark in the history of hypotension (Griffiths and Gillies, 1948), states that at times 'no pressure readings could be recorded from the brachial artery and no arterial pulse could be palpated at the wrist' ... a state of affairs which would not have supported life unless the table had been sloped slightly head downwards. Spontaneous respiration was maintained as it was a valuable indication of the relative integrity of the cerebral circulation. The technique of Lincoln Sise of the Lahey Clinic in Boston has been widely used in the US. He employed amethocaine hydrochloride made hyperbaric with glucose (Sise, 1935).

The use of spinal analgesia was greatly encouraged by the introduction of the use of ephedrine to combat hypotension in 1927 by Ockerblad and Dillon (1927) of the University of Kansas School of Medicine, and by Rudolf and Graham (1927). This was a great advance. The active principle of the herb ma huang, known to Chinese medicine for millennia, ephedrine was isolated in a pure state and named by Nagai in 1887 (Nagai, 1887) and introduced into Western medicine by Chen and Carl F. Schmidt (1926), Professor of Pharmacology at the School of Medicine of the University of Pennsylvania, following a visit to China in 1926. Schmidt should also be remembered as a warm friend to anaesthetists in the days when they were showing signs of developing into a reputable speciality. At this time, intravenous infusions were rarely employed and the only pressor drugs available were adrenaline with its evanescent action and methyl guanidine, a relatively toxic agent with a too positive and prolonged effect. Since then many pressor amines have come and gone, but ephedrine has stayed the course and is still today considered by many workers to be the preferred drug to combat low blood-pressure associated with both intra- and extradural block, should the rapid infusion of a plasma volume expander prove inadequate (Cain and Hamilton, 1966; Rolbin et al, 1982). Curare, which became popular in the 1940s, could so safely and easily produce muscular relaxation but did little to encourage the spread of spinal analgesia.

An unusual sidetrack in the pharmacology of intradural block, which so far has led nowhere, was the demonstration by S. J. Meltzer, whose name is known for his pioneering efforts during the early development of tracheal intubation (Meltzer and Auer, 1909) of the use of magnesium sulphate. He found that if he injected 1 ml of 25 per cent solution of magnesium sulphate per 12 kg, paralysis and analgesia came on three or four hours afterwards and produced good operating conditions. At the end of the procedure, he suggested that the theca should be irrigated to get rid of the salt (Meltzer, 1906).

We feel that a Roumanian gentleman by the name of Tzaicou merits a paragraph in the history of spinal analgesia. At the age of 26, while preparing his postgraduate doctoral thesis on the subject, he decided to have his inguinal hernia repaired. How better could he demonstrate his good faith in his choice of subject than by submitting himself to this form of pain relief. As he wrote (Tzaicou, 1911), 'We should be prepared to have ourselves what we recommend to others in similar circumstances ... moreover I would have a chance of submitting the procedure to "auto-observation",

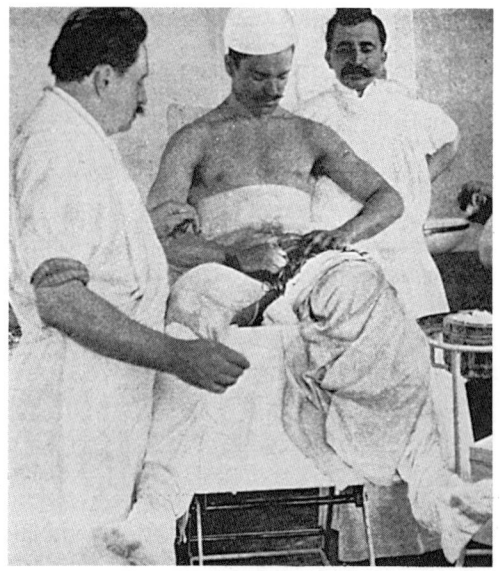

Fig. 1.3

much more valuable to medicine than "objective observation".' Nothing unusual so far as one of the authors can testify. But he went a step further when he decided to operate on himself to demonstrate that Jonnesco's technique (Jonnesco, 1909) could provide the necessary analgesia, yet leave the brain and arms unimpaired, and was safe enough to allow him to remain seated throughout the operation (Fig. 1.3). Moreover, the undertaking would give him a chance to study the causes of pain, if any, during herniotomy. The outcome justified his faith for 'I suffered no disagreeable phenomenon even though I operated on myself, that I had to remain in a sitting position, make the movements necessary to reach the instruments and to wash my hands red with blood, and to make all the other movements necessary to carry out the operation'. Postoperative sequelae worthy of note were insomnia and cephalalgia.

Attention has recently been directed to the use of bupivacaine for intradural block and experience with 0.5 per cent solution has been satisfactory. It has been used both in its isobaric state and made hyperbaric by the addition of glucose.

Extradural analgesia

Extradural block is a development from intradural block, its main attractions over the older method being that it never causes headache. The German surgeon Heile suggested that the lumbar extradural space could be entered by a needle introduced through an intervertebral foramen (Heile, 1913) but the method never became popular, perhaps because of its technical difficulty. Some years later the lumbar approach to the extradural space was described by the Spaniard, Fidel Pagés in 1921 (Pagés, 1921) but was largely forgotten owing to his death on active service soon after the publication of his paper. Ten years later the Italian surgeon A. M. Dogliotti, who was always interested in the subject of anaesthesia, rediscovered it, naming it peridural segmentary analgesia (Dogliotti, 1931). He employed it in his own patients, possibly because the standard of general anaesthesia in Italy at that time was not very high. The subatmospheric pressure in the extradural space was described by Jansen (1926). This technique, like all techniques of local analgesia was greatly benefited as to reliability and increased duration of effect by the substitution of lignocaine for procaine in 1948 (Gordh, 1948), a further advance being the employment of bupivacaine, with its long action, by Telivuo in 1963 (Telivuo, 1963).

Pioneers in the use and investigators into the effects of extradural block have included Aburel in Roumania (Aburel, 1931); C. J. Massey Dawkins in the UK (Dawkins, 1945); Odom (Odom, 1936); Lund (Lund, 1966); Moore (Moore, 1953); Bromage (Bromage, 1954) and Bonica with members of the Seattle school (Bonica, 1959) in the US. To a Cuban anaesthetist, M. M. Curbelo (Curbelo, 1949), must go the credit for being the first to insert a ureteric catheter into the extradural space following a visit to the Mayo Clinic where he saw Tuohy performing continuous intradural block (Tuohy, 1945). Curbelo gave his first continuous extradural block in Havana, Cuba on 13th January 1947. Some time later, Tuohy adapted his special needle, first used for continuous intradural analgesia, for extradural block, through which small bore plastic catheters could be passed when they became available (Tuohy, 1945).

The sacral approach to the extradural space was employed before the lumbar, its first exponents probably being the Frenchmen Cathelin and Sicard in 1901, (Cathelin, 1901; Sicard, 1901). Stoekel used it in gynaecology and Arthur Laewen in surgery some years later in Germany (Stoekel, 1909; Laewen, 1910). Gaston Labat popularised sacral block in 1923 (Labat, 1923), while John Lundy at the Mayo Clinic was a frequent user of the technique (Lundy, 1942). Its most influential exponent was R. A. Hingson (Hingson and Edwards, 1943) whose method of continuous caudal analgesia, and enthusiasm for it, attracted wide attention.

Waldo B. Edwards and Robert A. Hingson, working at the US Marine Hospital, Staten Island, New York, applied Walter Lemmon's technique of continuous spinal analgesia to sacral block in order to ensure a more prolonged effect than could be obtained by the 'one-shot' injection (Lemmon, 1940). Hingson was not only an enthusiastic salesman of the technique he described, but a highly competent practitioner of it at the bedside, both in the labour ward and the operating theatre. He advocated the use of the ester-linked agent piperocaine (Metycain) and travelled widely, advocating continuous caudal analgesia. He had received his early training at the Mayo Clinic and went on to hold appointments at Philadelphia, the Johns Hopkins Hospital in Baltimore and at Western Reserve University, Cleveland. His successful tour of anaesthetic centres in the UK in 1950, like that of George Pitkin before him, will be still remembered.

For the history of central neural blockade in obstetric practice see Chapter 12.

Caudal analgesia was first described in infants by Campbell in 1933 (Campbell, 1933).

Injection of the posterior divisions of the sacral nerves as they emerge from the sacrum, a technique originally described by Victor Pauchet of Paris, Labat's mentor, is termed trans-sacral block. Bilateral injection of S.1 and S.2 has been used to potentiate extradural sacral block.

Since the last edition of this book appeared in 1978, a totally new concept of both intradural and extradural analgesia has arisen, following the description of opiate receptors in the spinal cord (Pert and Snyder, 1973; Snyder, 1977). The first report of the use of narcotics injected into the extradural space came from Jerusalem (Behar et al, 1979) and since then a large amount of work from many countries has been reported. Inevitably, the initial enthusiasm for this very new procedure has been tempered in the light of increasing experience.

Biographies

James Leonard Corning (1855–1923)

Corning was born at Stamford, Conn., in 1855, nine years after Morton's ether demonstration in nearby Boston. As a medical student he spent much time in Germany and, as was common practice, studied at several universities including Heidelberg and Würzburg. On gaining his MD in 1878 he returned to the US and, developing an interest in neurology, settled in New York City. In 1885 he became interested in finding out the possible actions of drugs, including the new agent cocaine described by Koller in the previous year, on the spinal cord, and engaged in experiments to try to solve the problems. He injected cocaine into the vicinity of the veins of the extradural space, and hoped that its absorption into the bloodstream would lead to rapid and intense sensory and motor effects, a sort of temporary transverse myelitis. In a dog he injected 20 drops of 2 per cent cocaine and caused paralysis of the hind legs; he then injected 30 minims of 3 per cent solution into a patient between the 11th and 12th thoracic vertebral spines, followed eight minutes later by a second similar dose. This caused analgesia of the lower part of the body, so that when Corning passed a urethral sound, the patient experienced no pain and his knee-jerks were abolished. It will never be known for certain whether he deposited his cocaine into the extradural or the intradural space, but he ended the article describing this work (Corning, 1885a) with the well-known sentence.

> Whether the method will ever find an application as a substitute for etherisation in genito-urinary or other branches of surgery, further experience alone can show. Be the destiny of the observation what it may, it has seemed to me, on the whole, worth recording.

Corning's clinical curiosity extended more widely. He was the first to show that the effects of cocaine when injected subcutaneously could be prolonged by producing ischaemia in the anaesthetised area by elastic compression (Corning, 1885b); he wrote the first textbook on local anaesthesia (Corning, 1886); extended his investigations on medication of the cord (Corning, 1888) and was a pioneer of hyperbaric medicine. Unfortunately his work on clinical local analgesia attracted little attention and had no influence on clinical practice, but his investigations on cocainisation of the cord antedated Bier's classic and highly influential experiments by 18 years. Leonard Corning was an eccentric personality who had an extensive private practice as a neurologist and psychiatrist and was reputed to be a millionaire. He was much interested in music and musicians and was brother-in-law to the famous Wagnerian tenor, Heinrich Knote (1870–1953), who was a regular member of the Metropolitan Opera Company of New York until 1914. In his private house Corning had a hyperbaric chamber reminding one observer of something out of the imagination of E. T. A. Hoffman, and his music room contained four grand pianos. (See also Gustav Mahler, *Memories and Letters* (1973), edited by D. Mitchell, London: Murray.) Corning claimed to have invented spinal analgesia. He died in Morristown, New Jersey, just two years after lumbar extradural analgesia was placed on a secure clinical footing by Fidel Pagès; he was 68.

Carl Koller (1858–1944)

Carl Koller was the first worker to employ the analgesic properties of cocaine, already well known, to relieve the pain of surgical operations. He was born in 1858 in Scheuttenhofen in Bohemia, then in the Austro-Hungarian empire, the son of a Jewish businessman from Teplitz, Leopold Koller. When Carl was a young boy he lost his mother so his father moved with him to Vienna, the capital city. As the family was not orthodox he was educated at the local *academische gymnasium* by Jesuit fathers. On leaving school he decided that he wanted to become a doctor, but first he had to serve his term of two years as a conscript in the army. When he entered the medical school he soon began to show signs of a gift for scientific investigation and before graduation he did some creditable work in the experimental pathology laboratory of Salomon Stricker and published an original paper on the embryology of the mesoderm of the chick. In later life he always regarded this work as his most valuable contribution to science. He qualified as a doctor in 1882.

Koller soon developed an interest in ophthalmology and rapidly acquired skill and facility in operations on the eye. As a result of unhappy experience he quickly felt a profound disenchantment with the standard of anaesthesia prevailing in the great Viennese teaching hospital, the Allegemeine Krankenhaus. His anaesthetists were either medical students or very junior doctors without interest or skill in the administration of anaesthetics, and sometimes were not even medically qualified. He quickly realised that if he was to do justice to his patients undergoing operations on the eye he would require better methods of pain relief than were then available. He considered the usual postoperative restlessness, retching and vomiting as quite unacceptable and consequently was on the look-out for some substance which, if instilled into the conjunctival sac, would obliterate the pain inevitably caused by his surgery, and so save the patient from these undesirable sequelae of general anaesthesia. He experimented with all the sedatives then available and tried morphine, chloral hydrate and bromide, but of course failed in his purpose.

While these experiments were going on a young friend and fellow resident in the hospital was Sigmund Freud, 18 months his senior and a tyro neurologist and psychiatrist, ambitious to follow an academic career in the city so that he could be married to his fiancée. In the early months of 1884 Freud was particularly interested in a relatively new drug, cocaine, which 20 or 30 years previously had been brought back to Austria from the eastern slopes of the Andes, in Peru and Bolivia by members of a round-the-world scientific expedition. From the leaves of this exotic plant, known as coca, an alkaloid was isolated by Niemann, a chemist in Göttingen, who called it cocaine (Niemann, 1860). Niemann mentioned that it would cause numbness when injected under the skin or when painted on to mucous membranes. Several other workers (Schroff, 1867; Moreno y Miaz, 1868), including the Esthonian surgeon and pharmacologist von Anrep, then working in Würzburg, also noticed this unusual pharmacological effect (von Anrep, 1880). Freud, who was aware of the strange analgesic phenomenon, wrote a monograph on cocaine (Freud, 1884) and had high hopes that it might prove to be a useful nerve tonic in the treatment of his neurasthenic patients and in counteracting morphine addiction. Before starting off on a trip to Hamburg to see his fiancée, he suggested that Koller might investigate the effects of the drug, when taken by mouth, on the body's muscular power, using a dynomometer. He also asked another friend Leopold Konigstein, *privatdozent* in the eye department, if he would care to try the effect of cocaine in painful conditions of the eye. So with Freud happily enjoying his holiday, both Koller and Konigstein, quite independently, commenced their investigations on cocaine. Koller started by swallowing some of the drug himself and immediately noticed, afresh, its remarkable numbing effect on his lips and tongue and, in a flash of inspiration, realised that it might be the agent he had been looking for. He returned to Stricker's laboratory, tested it on lower animals, on his friends, on himself and on several of his patients, and soon came to realise that in cocaine he had found the local analgesic he had been searching for. Quite naturally he wanted to publish this important discovery as soon as possible and remembered that in a short time the annual Heidelberg meeting of the German Ophthalmological Society would be taking place. As he was temporarily short of funds he realised that he could not attend it himself as he could not afford the railway fare, so he asked the organisers at the last minute for permission for a colleague, Dr Brettauer from Trieste, whom he knew would be there, to read the paper for him. Permission was given and Brettauer read the paper on 15th September 1884 (Koller, 1884a). It created a sensation and this was reinforced when Brettauer gave a practical demonstration of the effects of the drug in the hospital eye clinic, using some of the 2 per cent solution entrusted to him by Koller. Koller himself read a fuller paper about his discovery before the Vienna Medical Society on 17th October in which he acknowledged the previous descriptions of the analgesic properties of cocaine made by Niemann, von Anrep and others, years previously (Koller, 1884b). He also mentioned that he had been introduced to the new agent by Freud. The paper was translated into English (Noyes, 1884). While all this was going on, Konigstein's investigations into the effects of cocaine on the eye led him to similar conclusions to Koller's, although they were reported several weeks later and with no mention of Koller (Konigstein, 1884). He too showed that it was a practical local analgesic agent and attempted to claim that the discovery was his. Eventually he was persuaded by his friends Freud and Wagner-Jauregg (who later introduced the treatment of general paralysis of the insane by malaria parasites) to acknowledge the primacy of Koller. Freud, although disappointed at not being associated with the work on local analgesia for surgery, which really was quite outside his main professional interest, readily agreed that the credit for the discovery should go to Koller. So Carl Koller, now recognised as the discoverer of the analgesic property of cocaine and its use in surgical operations, returned to the practice of ophthalmology and took no further part in its development. Within a few weeks of the reading of the cocaine paper at Heidelberg the drug was being investigated and employed, usually with success, in various anatomical situations and for surgical operations of many types throughout Europe and the US (Jellinek, 1884; Halsted, 1885).

Koller's subsequent history is interesting (Koller-Becker, 1963; Liljestrand, 1967). He was a forceful personality and suffered from fits of depression, being sometimes difficult to get along with. To increase his knowledge of ophthalmology further, he went to Utrecht to work under Cornelius Donders (1818–89) who was the first to use cylindrical lenses for astigmatism, and his son-in-law, Herman Snellen (1834–1908) who in 1862 invented the type still used for testing visual acuity. Koller thought of settling in Holland but instead returned to Vienna, still restless. One evening he was in the casualty department of the General Hospital and became involved in a slanging match with Theodor Billroth's house surgeon, in which anti-Semitism played a part. As he and his opponent were both reserve army officers he was challenged to a duel, and although no swordsman, accepted the challenge. He took hurried lessons in duelling with sabres and the contest took place in the grounds of a neighbouring barracks with army surgeons as seconds. After three 'thrusts' or rounds, Koller slightly winged his man who was removed to hospital. Duelling was of course strictly illegal in Vienna in 1885 and this fact, in spite of the creditable outcome of the contest, increased his feeling of discontent with the city and this was made worse by his failure to obtain an assistantship in the academic department of ophthalmology, which he had every right to expect. So he decided after consultation with his friends, including Freud, to emigrate to the US and set off in May 1888 for New York, travelling via London. He put up his plate and soon became established in New York City. He was elected on to the staff of several good hospitals including the Mount Sinai Hospital, and spent the remainder of his long life as an eye specialist with increasing reputation and success. As the years passed he received many honours, won many medals and was recognised by learned societies in several continents. He died, a greatly respected figure, as recently as 1944.

Koller's discovery in 1884 led to the whole theory and practice of local analgesia (Koller, 1928).

Walter Essex Wynter (1860–1945)

To Wynter and to Heinrich Quincke we are indebted for the introduction of lumbar puncture as a safe, practical and necessary part of a thorough neurological examination. Son of Andrew Wynter, one-time editor of the *British Medical Journal*, he was educated at Epsom, St Bartholomew's Hospital and the Middlesex Hospital. He qualified in 1887, and was later appointed physician and medical officer-in-charge of the Electrical Department of the Middlesex Hospital. He was the author of a minor classic, *Minor Medicine*, which appeared in 1907 and also of *A Manual of Clinical and Practical Pathology* (1890). His article on lumbar puncture entitled 'Four cases of tuberculous meningitis in which paracentesis of the theca vertebralis was performed for the relief of fluid pressure', appeared in *The Lancet* (1891), **1**, 981. He first employed a Southey tube and later asked a surgical colleague to remove the spinal laminae, for easier insertion. His first case was a boy, 3 years old, in February 1889, three years before Quincke's publication. He is said to have 'flung away ambition' and was a happy and charming physician who ambled through life, unhurried, unconcerned and unperturbed. He lived in a manor house in Newbury where he grew his own tobacco and brewed his own mead. In his will he left his beautiful home for the use of nurses from the Middlesex Hospital in their retirement.

Heinrich Irenaeus Quincke (1842–1922)

With Essex Wynter of London, Quincke introduced lumbar puncture in 1891. He was born at Frankfurt-an-der-Oder, the son of a distinguished physician. Educated at the Universities of Berlin, Würzburg and Heidelberg, he was appointed while still a young man to the chair of Internal Medicine at Bern, and in 1878 moved to Kiel where he became a colleague of August Bier. He died aged 80 at Frankfurt-am-Main in 1922. He described angioneurotic oedema (Quincke's Disease) in 1882 and made many original observations in the fields of neurology and internal medicine. He did experimental work which resulted in the discovery of lumbar puncture to relieve hydrocephalus in children (Quincke, 1891a), and later developed the technique in both neurological diagnosis and treatment. He recognised that paralysis of the 6th cranial nerve was an occasional sequel to withdrawal of cerebrospinal fluid. Bier had the foresight of uniting the pharmacological knowledge of Koller (cocaine) with the technology of Quincke (lumbar puncture) to produce intradural spinal analgesia in 1898. (See also *The Founders of Neurology* (1953), edited by W. Haymaker, Springfield: Thomas.)

August Bier (1861–1949)

Bier, one of the great figures of surgery on the continent of Europe during the first half of this century, was born near Waldeck in Germany in 1861. As is common in his country of origin he was educated at several universities and attended the medical schools at Berlin and Leipzig. He graduated in 1889 at Kiel and, deciding to devote his life to surgery, he became assistant to Professor Friedrich von Esmarch (1823–1908) at Kiel. While there he supervised the change-over from the antiseptic to the aseptic system in the operating theatres. He moved on to Griefswald and in 1903 became Professor of Surgery at Bonn. So high was his reputation that four years later Bier was appointed to succeed the great von Bergmann in the chair of Surgery in Berlin, which he occupied for the remainder of his life and which he adorned as a master surgeon and a fine lecturer. He retired in 1932. In outlook and tradition August Bier was a loyal Prussian, and this led to his refusal of the invitation to follow Theodor Billroth (1829–1894) in the chair of Surgery at Vienna. Bier had an original and penetrating intellect and, in addition to discovering spinal analgesia, he was the originator of passive hyperaemia with the Esmarch bandage in 1907, which enabled him to treat tuberculous bones and joints with success, and he made original contributions to the treatment of amputation stumps, to the study of blood transfusion, and to vascular surgery during the war of 1914–1918. In 1908, Bier described intravenous procaine analgesia, a method which produces analgesia of a limb when the local agent is injected into a vein distal to a compression bandage. This he called direct vein anaesthesia (Bier, 1908). He invented the steel helmet for German troops during the First World War. He was an accomplished classical scholar and did serious research on Hippocrates and on Heraclitus. In 1913, at the

International Medical Congress held in London, he was elected to the Fellowship of the Royal College of Surgeons of England (1913) and in his own country became a Privy Councillor with the title of *Geheimrat* and was held in the highest esteem. He was interested in the therapeutic value of athletic exercise and calisthenics.

In 1898 he became familiar with the work of a medical colleague in his hospital at Kiel, Heinrich Irenaeus Quincke (1842–1922) who established lumbar puncture as a safe investigation in routine neurological examination (Quincke, 1891b). Bier conceived the idea that by injecting the then new drug cocaine by Quincke's technique widespread analgesia might be produced. This proved to be true and the discovery of spinal analgesia was made in the University Hospital in Kiel in 1898 (Bier, 1899).

The story is well known how Bier, after successfully using the method in half a dozen patients, allowed his junior colleague Otto Hildenbrandt to inject into his theca 2 ml of 1 per cent cocaine solution and how, presumably because of the large size of the trocar used, he developed a severe headache and was nursed by his chief's wife, Frau von Esmarch. Chaput, one of the pioneers of the revival of interest in ether in France, first used Stovaine in spinal analgesia in 1905.

In later life, Bier deviated from the paths of orthodox science and came to be regarded by the younger generation as an eccentric has-been. He delved deeply into esoteric systems of philosophy and at the age of 70 he retired to the countryside there to devote his closing years to tree culture. August Karl Gustav Bier died on his farm in the Russian zone of Germany in 1949, aged 88.

Theodore Tuffier (1857–1929)

Tuffier was a surgeon working in Paris and in 1899 he was one of the earliest followers of August Bier in the development of spinal analgesia, recognising it as a method which, while providing admirable relaxation of the abdomen during the operation, left the patient afterwards in a reasonably fit condition (Tuffier, 1899). He sought to employ the new method for all operations below the diaphragm and became more of an enthusiast than Bier himself. He was a man of original views and this was not his only contribution to knowledge. With Hallion he was an early advocate of endotracheal insufflation anaesthesia and employed assisted respiration to overcome the ill effects of the open pneumothorax; this enabled him to do a partial resection of a lung in 1896. Two years later he massaged the heart of a patient who had died on the operating table but the effort was not successful and indeed the technique was not successfully accomplished until 1902, when Ernest Starling and Arbuthnot Lane reported the first case to be thus revived, at Guys Hospital, London. Tuffier had a reputation of being awkward and never became a full professor, remaining an *agrégé*. As a member of the staff of the British Hertford Hospital in Paris, he did not always get on well with some of his British colleagues, but attained fame and fortune and, especially in foreign countries, became one of France's best-known surgeons. He was an early advocate of blood transfusion directly from the radial artery into the saphenous vein of the recipient, effectively transplanted the ureter into the bowel following a total cystectomy in 1895, and was an early practitioner of cardiac surgery. Fernand Sicard was one of his pupils. He was awarded an honorary Fellowship of the Royal College of Surgeons of England in 1913, along with Bier, and was made an honorary KBE by King George V for his care of British troops during the 1914–1918 war. His advocacy of spinal analgesia did much to raise its status during the early years of the century.

Arthur Edward James Barker (1850–1916)

Intradural spinal analgesia became established in Britain largely owing to the foresight and enthusiasm of the surgeon Professor Arthur Barker. He was the son of a doctor, born and educated in Dublin. He qualified at the medical school of the Royal College of Surgeons in Ireland in 1870, and after resident appointments went to Bonn for further experience: Germany then led the world in surgery. He learnt, read, wrote and spoke French and German fluently and throughout his career was one of the chief bridges over which surgical ideas, originating in Germany, crossed into the English-speaking world; one of the most important of these ideas was spinal analgesia.

He returned to Dublin in 1875 and was soon appointed to the staff of the City of Dublin Hospital, and demonstrator of anatomy in its medical school. But London attracted him, and at the age of 25 he secured an appointment as assistant surgeon to University College Hospital, being one of the few surgeons to have secured such a position without a Fellowship in surgery. Later he took the Fellowship of the Royal College of Surgeons in Ireland and was awarded the FRCS England *ad eundem* in 1880. After 1880 Barker followed the aseptic system of von Bergmann and other German surgeons, believing it to be an improvement on Lister's antiseptic practice, and commenced to make surgical history. In 1886 he did the first successful gastroenterostomy in London for pyloric cancer and his patient lived for a year after it. He developed the specialty of otolaryngology, set up the first department for it in his hospital and became the first surgeon to diagnose, then to localise pus from a cerebral abscess secondary to middle ear disease, and finally to evacuate the pus. He became a leader in the early diagnosis and treatment of intussusception and the surgery of hernia. It is an interesting fact that the surgeons at his great teaching hospital opened the abdomen only seven times during the year 1886!

Barker was one of the earliest practitioners of local infiltration analgesia in Britain and finally recommended, after most careful preliminary investigation, a 0.2 per cent solution of beta eucaine in normal saline with 1: 100 000 adrenaline (Barker, 1899, 1903).

His work on intradural spinal analgesia has been influential from the time he started his investigations until the present day. His problem, then as now, was the accurate localisation of the solution of local analgesic within the intradural space. He was able to show, using a glass replica of the vertebral canal and different solutions of varying specific gravity, that a heavy solution would find its own level *vis-à-vis* the anatomical curves of the canal. He finally settled on a solution containing 5 per cent Stovaine in 5 per cent glucose. He wrote three papers which are classics and all of them repay reading today (Barker, 1907, 1908a, 1908b). He described a special lumbar puncture needle, too large by today's standards, but malleable, and took great care with the sterility of the whole of his set of instruments. He pioneered the use of rubber gloves for the surgical team during operations in Britain, a practice started by Halsted in Baltimore in 1890. Barker regarded the whole subject of spinal analgesia with great seriousness and realised that its practice was not for those lacking care and skill. He taught that the essence of the technique, which was of the greatest importance was 'to enter the lumbar dural sac effectually with the point of the needle and to discharge through this all the contemplated dose of the drug, directly and freely into the cerebrospinal fluid below the termination of the cord' (Barker, 1907).

He became full surgeon to his hospital in 1885 and was appointed Professor of Surgery in its medical school in 1893. When he retired in 1915 the First World War was a cause for concern to all surgeons and so he joined the Army Medical Service and, after preliminary work at Netley Hospital, was sent to Malta and then to Salonika. Here he died of pneumonia in 1916 (Barker, 1916).

For many years anaesthetists have followed Barker's advice as to the behaviour of hyperbaric solutions in the intradural space, but recent work (Wildsmith et al, 1981; Sinclair et al, 1982) has shown that, in a small series of cases, gravity may not play so important a role in the intrathecal distribution of hyperbaric solutions as Barker and those who copied him, over 70 years ago, imagined. (See also Lee, J. Alfred (1979) Arthur E. Barker 1850–1916. *Anaesthesia*, **34**, 885.)

Fernand Cathelin (1873–1945)

Fernand Cathelin was a urological surgeon in Paris, a founder of the Hospital for Urology there and a writer of many books and papers on his specialty. He was familiar with the work of Tuffier and Bier on intradural analgesia and had given such injections himself, but was not very happy with the after-effects. Following extensive work on animals he injected 1 and 2 per cent solutions of cocaine into the sacral canal of four patients about to undergo operations for hernia repair. The first was on 5th February 1901 in one of Dr Lejar's wards at the Tenon Hospital. He was able to produce relative analgesia, but not of sufficient intensity to allow the operations to proceed.

Jean-Athanase Sicard (1872–1929)

Dr Sicard was a neurologist working in Paris. He was on the staff of the Necker Hospital there and was interested in intradural analgesia as practised by Bier and his fellow countryman, Theodore Tuffier. Like Cathelin he was unhappy with the headaches which so frequently followed successful block, a frequency explained no doubt by the large lumbar puncture needles used and by technique which was not always bacteriologically satisfactory. So, independently of Cathelin and after experiments on dogs and cadavers, he described extradural sacral injection of cocaine solution as a form of treatment for sciatica and lumbago, and for the pains of tabes dorsalis. He himself did not use the new technique for the production of surgical anaesthesia, but recommended its possible employment for such a purpose to surgeons. He and Forestier pioneered the use of Lipiodol, a contrast medium in radiology

(Sicard and Forestier 1921), and he was the first to use sodium salicylate as a sclerosant in the treatment of varicose veins in 1922. He injected antitetanic serum intradurally to relieve the spasms of tetanus.

Fidel Pagés-Miravé (d.1924)

Fidel Pagés described what he called 'metameric anaesthesia' in a paper in 1921 which can be consulted in its English translation in *'Classical File' Survey of Anesthesiology* (1961), 5, 326 (Pagés, 1921). He was a graduate of the University of Zaragoza and became an experienced and fearless surgeon who was quite prepared to operate on the head and neck under intradural spinal analgesia, following the techniques of Le Filliatre and Jonnesco. In November 1920 at the General Hospital, Madrid, he 'had the idea of detaining the needle within the spinal canal before it pierced the dura mater and then blocking the roots outside the meningeal space'. He had already experimented with sacral extradural analgesia as described by Sicard in 1901, by Läwen in 1910, and Reclus. He injected 20 to 25 ml of 2 per cent procaine with adrenaline and was not averse to making his puncture in the cervical or lower thoracic region if necessary. To identify the extradural 'or extrameningeal' space he used tactile loss of resistance to the advancement of the needle together with the audible sound resulting from the needle point leaving the ligamentum flavum. In his paper Pagés described 43 cases of extradural block, 40 of them successful, and he stated that his results appeared sufficient to justify further investigation. Pagés was a captain in the medical corps of the Spanish army and in 1924 was killed on active service in North Africa. Thus he died before he was able to pursue the further investigation of extradural analgesia that he thought was necessary. After a lapse of 10 years this was undertaken by Dogliotti who was originally unaware of Pagés' pioneering work.

Achile Mario Dogliotti (1897–1966)

Dogliotti was born in Turin in northern Italy in 1897 and graduated in medicine there in 1920. He obtained his higher qualification in 1926 and this led to his appointment as Professor of Surgical Pathology at the University of Modena. He practised as an active surgeon both here and later in Catania in Sicily, and in 1943 he followed his old teacher, Uffreduzzi, in the chair of Surgery at

Turin. His work in Turin led to his becoming recognised as one of the leading surgeons in Europe and he was specially notable for his operations on the heart, inventing one of the earliest heart-lung machines. He was a great surgical innovator, a pioneer of the radiography of the biliary passages and the organiser of the first blood bank in Italy. He was also a great organiser of and attender at international surgical congresses and was a frequent visitor to the UK, where he lectured. He served a term as president of the International College of Surgeons.

Dogliotti soon developed an interest in anaesthesia, a relatively neglected subject in Italy during his early years. In 1931 he developed his method of peridural segmental analgesia and used it extensively on his patients. He described block of the posterior roots of the spinal nerves for the treatment of pain and wrote an excellent textbook on anaesthesia which was translated into English in 1939 (Dogliotti, 1939). With his family he survived the Second World War and visited the UK, where he again gave lectures, in the post-war years. He died in 1966 in Turin, after a long and painful illness.

Gaston Labat (1877–1934)

Gaston Labat was born on Mahe, the largest of the Seychelles islands. His parents, both of them French speaking, were born in Mauritius. When young Gaston was 6 years old his father was drowned some years after settling in business in the Seychelles, and his mother, with her three young children, returned to Mauritius. Gaston was sent to Durban to live with a maternal uncle and here he continued his education and became proficient in the English language. As a young man he seemed to be more interested in engineering than in medicine, but after changing jobs several times, returned to Mauritius and was taken on as a partner in a local pharmacy owned by his brother-in-law, R. Rochcouste, in 1912. Hard work and enterprise had its expected result so that the pharmacy flourished. Soon, however, the partners separated amicably. Labat went to Montpellier in 1912 to study medicine at the age of 37, while Rochcouste remained at home to 'mind the shop' which continued to do well. He was a leading citizen of his community and was mayor of Curepipe, the main city of Mauritius, in 1931. Meanwhile, after spending two years in Montpellier, Labat moved to Paris where he graduated in medicine. In the capital he soon became an associate of and anaesthetist to Victor Pauchet

(1869–1936) a leading surgeon and a pioneer of regional analgesia whose book entitled *L'Anaesthesie Regionale*, published by Dion, appeared in 1914 and became a classic. In the fourth edition (1921) Labat became part author with Pauchet. As one who spoke both English and French with equal facility Labat decided to emigrate to the US and was soon invited by Dr William J. Mayo to become special lecturer in regional analgesia at the Mayo Foundation of the University of Minnesota at Rochester. His years as teacher of regional analgesia and as a demonstrator of its practice at the Mayo Clinic in 1920–21 led to the publication in 1922 of one of the most influential books in our specialty, *Regional Anesthesia*. It was lavishly produced by its American publishers and contained a large number of excellent anatomical drawings with precise details of technique for the production of analgesia in various parts of the body. Its section on intradural block was outstanding and he advocated the injection of procaine powder dissolved in cerebrospinal fluid. To maintain adequate cerebral circulation he advised that the patient should be placed in the Trendelenburg position. The contents of this book showed that Pauchet's influence on his young colleague had been very important and many of Pauchet's illustrations were incorporated in it. It stimulated interest in all forms of regional analgesia, especially in spinal analgesia, in English-speaking countries.

After leaving the Mayo Clinic, Labat was appointed Clinical Professor of Surgery at New York University and Bellevue Hospital Medical College, and visiting Regional Anesthetist to the Presbyterian Hospital, New York. At these institutions his enthusiasm for regional analgesia had a great influence on the surgeon Dr Hippolyte Wertheim and the anesthetist E. A. Rovenstine and, after his death, these and other workers carried on the torch. Before Labat's time, the injection of local anaesthetics had been done by the surgeon, but after his work it became largely the province of the anaesthetist. He founded the American Society of Regional Anesthesia in 1923.

A third edition of Labat's book was edited and revised by John Adriani of New Orleans in 1967 (see Macintosh, 1978).

REFERENCES

Intradural

Babcock, W. W. (1913) Spinal anesthesia: a clinical study of 658 administrations. *New York Medical Journal*, **98**, 897.

Bainbridge, W. S. (1900) Analgesia in children by spinal injection with a report of a new method of sterilisation of the injection fluid. *Medical Record* (NY), **58**, 937.

Bainbridge, W. S. (1901) Report of twelve operations on infants and young children during spinal analgesia. *Archives of Paediatrics*, July.

Barker, A. E. (1899) A clinical lecture and demonstration on local anaesthesia. *Lancet*, **1**, 282.

Barker, A. E. (1903) Clinical remarks on some improvements in the method of local analgesia. *Lancet*, **2**, 203.

Barker, A. E. (1907) Clinical experiences with spinal analgesia in 100 cases. *British Medical Journal*, **1**, 665.

Barker, A. E. (1908a) A second report on clinical experiences with spinal analgesia with a second series of 100 cases. *British Medical Journal*, **1**, 264

Barker, A. E. (1908b) A third report on clinical experiences with spinal analgesia. *British Medical Journal*, **2**, 453

Barker, A. E. (1909) Elimination of stovaine after spinal analgesia. *British Medical Journal*, 18th Sept.

Barker, A. E. (1916) Obituary. *British Journal of Surgery*, **4**, 11; (see also Lee, J. Alfred (1979) *Anaesthesia*, **34**, 885).

Bier, A. (1899) Ver. über Cocainisierung des Rückenmark. *Deutsche Zeitschrift für Chirurgie*, **51**, 361. Translated in *'Classical File' Survey of Anesthesiology* (1962), **6**, 352.

Bier, A. (1900) *Münchener Medizinische Wochenschrift*, **47**, 1226.

Bier, A. (1901) *Münchener Medizinische Wochenschrift*, **48(i)**, 724.

Bier, A. (1905) *Verhandlungen der Deutschen Gesellschaft für Chirurgie*, **34**, 115.

Bier, A. (1908) Über einen neuen Weg Lokalanaesthesie an den Gliedmassen zu erzeugen. *Langenbecks Archiv für Klinische Chirurgie*, **86**, 1007.

Bier, A. & Dönitz, A. (1904) Rückenmarken Anaesthesie. *Langenbecks Archiv für Klinische Chirurgie*, **51(i)**, 593.

Brownlee, A. (1911) History of spinal anaesthesia. *Practitioner*, Feb., p. 214.

Cain, W. E. & Hamilton, W. K. (1966) Cerebral and peripheral oxygen saturation during spinal anesthesia. *Anesthesiology*, **27**, 209.

Chaput, H. (1904) *Bulletin de la Société de Chirurgie* (Paris), **30** (n.s.), 835.

Chaput, H. (1907) Total spinal analgesia. *Presse Médicale*, **94**, 753.

Chen, K. K. & Schmidt, C. F. (1926) The action and clinical uses of ephedrine. *Journal of the American Medical Association*, **87**, 836.

Corning, J. L. (1885a) Spinal anaesthesia and local medication of the cord. *New York Medical Journal*, **42**, 483. Reprinted in *'Classical File' Survey of Anesthesiology* (1960), **4**, 332.

Corning, J. L. (1885b) On the prolongation of the anaesthetic effects of the hydrochlorate of cocaine when subcutaneously injected. An experimental study. *New York State Journal of Medicine*, **42**, 317.

Corning, J. L. (1886) *Local Anesthesia*. New York: Appleton.

Corning, J.L. (1888) A further contribution on medication of the spinal cord with cases. *Medical Record* (NY), **33**, 291.

Corning, J. L. (1894) *Pain in its Neuropathological Relations*, p. 247. Philadelphia.

Crile, G. Washington (1899) *On Experimental Research into Surgical Shock*. Philadelphia: Lippincott.

Davy, H. (1800) *Researches Chemical and Philosophical*, p. 464. London.

Dean, H. P. (1894) Excision of chronic perforating ulcer of the duodenum *Lancet* **1**, 1191.

Dean, H. P. (1906) The importance of anaesthesia by lumbar injection in operations for acute abdominal diseases. *British Medical Journal*, **1**, 1086; (see also Akhtar, M. (1972) *Anaesthesia*, **27**, 330).

Dixon, W. E. (1905) The selective action of cocaine on nerve fibres. *Journal of Physiology* (London), **32**, 87.

Dogliotti, A. M. (1939) *Anesthesia: Narcosis; Local; Regional; Spinal.* Chicago: Debour.
Dönitz, A. (1903) *Münchener Medizinische Wochenschrift*, **50**, 1452.
Einhorn, A. (1899) *Münchener Medizinische Wochenschrift*, **46**, 1218.
Einhorn, A. (1905) Synthesised p-aminol-benzoyl-diethylamino-ethanol hydrochloride. *Deutsche Medizinische Wochenschrift*, **31**, 1668.
Förster, O. (1933) The dermatomes in man. *Brain*, **56**, 1.
Fourneau, E. (1904) Stovaine, anaesthetique locale. *Bulletin de la Société de Pharmacie* (Paris), **10**, 141.
Freud, S. (1884) Über Coca. *Zentralblatt für die Gesamte Therapie*, **2**, 209.
Gray, H. Tyrrell (1909) A study of spinal anaesthesia in children and infants. *Lancet*, **2**, 913.
Gray, H. Tyrrell (1910) A fresh study of spinal anaesthesia in children and infants. *Lancet*, **1**, 1611.
Gray, H. Tyrrell (1911) Indications for the employment of spinal anaesthesia in abdominal surgery. *British Medical Journal*, **2**, 497.
Griffiths, H. W. C. & Gillies, J. (1948) Thoracico-lumbar splanchnicectomy and sympathectomy: anaesthetic procedure. *Anaesthesia*, **3**, 134.
Halsted, W. S. (1885) Practical comments on the use and abuse of cocaine; suggested by its invariably successful employment in more than 1000 minor operations. *New York Medical Journal*, **42**, 294.
Hingson, R. A. and Edwards, W. B. (1942) Continuous caudal anesthesia during labor and delivery. *Anesthesia and Analgesia, Current Researches*, **21**, 301.
Howard-Jones, N. (1947) A critical study of the origins and early development of hypodermic medication. *Journal of the History of Medicine*, **2**, 201.
Jellinek, E. (1884) Das Cocaine als Anästheticum und Analgeticum für den Pharynx und Larynx. *Wiener Medizinische Wochenschrift*, **34**, 1334, 1364.
Jones, W. H. (1930) Spinal analgesia: a new method and a new drug, Percaine. *British Journal of Anaesthesia*, **7**, 99.
Jonnesco, T. (1909) Remarks on general spinal anaesthesia. *British Medical Journal*, **2**, 1396.
Keyes, E. L. & McClelland, A. M. (1930) Preliminary report on a new anesthetic; Percaine. *American Journal of Surgery*, **9**, 1. Reprinted in *'Classical File' Survey of Anesthesiology* (1978), **22**, 301.
Kirschner, M. (1932) Spinal zone anaesthesia. *Surgery, Gynecology and Obstetrics*, **55**, 317.
Koller, C. (1884a) Vorlaufige Mitteilung über lokale Anaesthesierung am Auge. Bericht über die 16 Versammlung der ophthalmologischen Gesselschaft. Heidelberg. *Beilageheft zu Klinische Monatsblatter für Augenkeilkunde*, **60**.
Koller, C. (1884b) Über die Verwendung des Cocain zur Anaesthesierung am Auge. *Wiener Medizinische Wochenschrift*, **34**, 1276, 1309.
Koller, C. (1928) Historical notes on the beginning of local anesthesia. *Journal of the American Medical Association*, **90**, 1742.
Koller-Becker, H. (1963) Carl Koller and Cocaine. *Psycho-analytical Quarterly*, **32**, 309.
Konigstein, L. (1884) Über das Cocainum muriaticum in seiner Anwendung in der Okulistik. *Wiener Medizinische Presse*, **25**, 1340, 1365.
Koster, H. (1928) Spinal analgesia with special reference to its use in surgery of the head, neck and thorax. *American Journal of Surgery*, **5**, 554. Reprinted in *'Classical File' Survey of Anesthesiology* (1978), **2**, 301.
Kreis, A. (1900) Über Medullarnarkose bei Gebärenden. *Zentralblatt für Gynäkologie* (1900, July) p. 742.
Labat, G. (1922) *Regional Anesthesia. Its Technique and Clinical Application.* Philadelphia: Saunders.
Lake, N. C. (1938) Precision in spinal anaesthesia. *Lancet*, **2**, 241.

Lee, J. Alfred (1943) Serial spinal analgesia. *Lancet*, 2, 156.
Lee, J. Alfred (1944) Serial spinal analgesia. *Anesthesia and Analgesia, Current Researches*, 23, 171.
Le Filliatre, G. (1913) Anaesthésie générale par rachicocainisation lumbo-sacrée. *17th International Congress on Medicine* (London), Subsection vii(b), p. 177.
Le Filliatre, G. (1921) *Précis de Rachianaesthésie Générale*. Paris: Libraire le François.
Lemmon, W. T. (1940) A method of continuous spinal anesthesia. *Annals of Surgery*, 111, 140.
Liljestrand, G. (1967) Carl Koller and the development of local anaesthesia. *Acta Physiologica Scandinavica* (suppl. 299), 3, 30.
Little, D. M. (1979) *'Classical File' Survey of Anesthesiology*, 23, 271.
Lusk, W. C. (1911) The anatomy of spinal puncture with some considerations on technic and paralytic sequels. *Annals of Surgery*, 54, 449.
Macintosh, R. R. (1978) The Gaston Labat award acceptance address. *Regional Anesthesia*, 3, 2.
Madden, F. (1910) Correspondence. *British Medical Journal*, 24th Sept.
Matas, R. (1899) Report on successful spinal anesthesia. *Journal of the American Medical Association*, 33, 1659.
McGavin, L. (1910) Remarks on eighteen cases of spinal analgesia by the Stovainestrychnine method of Jonnesco, including six cases of high dorsal puncture. *British Medical Journal*, 2, 733.
Meltzer, S. J. (1906). *Berliner Klinische Wochenschrift* 3, 73. (quoted by Gwathmey, J. T. in *Anesthesia* (1914) p. 770. New York: Appleton.
Meltzer, S. J. & Auer, J. (1909) Continuous respiration without respiratory movements. *Journal of Experimental Medicine*, 11, 622.
Moreno y Miaz (1868) Recherche chemique et physiologique sur l'Erythroxylum Coca du Perou. Thèse de Paris, p. 91.
Morton, A. W. (1901) The subarachnoid injection of cocaine for operations on all parts of the body. *American Medicine*, 3rd Aug.
Nagai, N. (1887) Ephedrine. *Pharmazeutische Zeitung*, 32, 700.
New York Medical Journal, (1900) Editorial. 58, 577.
Niemann, A. (1860) Cocaine. *Annals of Chemical Pharmacology*, 114, 216.
Noyes, H. D. (1884) The Ophthalmological Congress in Heidelberg. *Medical Record*, 26, 417.
Ockerblad, N. F. & Dillon, T. G. (1927) The use of ephedrine in spinal anesthesia. *Journal of the American Medical Association*, 88, 1135.
Pagés-Miravé, F. (1921) Segmental anaesthesia. *Revista de Sanidad Militar* (Madrid), 11, 351. Translated in *'Classical File' Survey of Anesthesiology* (1961), 5, 326.
Pert, C. B. & Snyder, S. H. (1973) Opiate receptors; demonstration in nervous tissue. *Science*, 179, 1011.
Pitkin, G. P. (1927) Controllable spinal anesthesia. *Journal of the Medical Society of New Jersey*, 24, 425.
Quincke, H. (1891a) *Deutsche Medizinische Wochenschrift*, 17, 809.
Quincke, H. (1891b) Die Lumbalpunction des Hydrocephalus. *Berliner Klinische Wochenschrift*, 28, 929.
Rudolf, R. D. & Graham, J. D. (1927) Notes on the sulfate of ephedrine. *American Journal of Medical Science*, 173, 399.
Schroff, C. D. (1867) Über Cocaine. *Woch. Zeit. ges. Artze*, 18, 233, 261.
Sebrechts, J. Personal communication.
Sebrechts, J. (1934) Spinal anaesthesia with regulation of dosage; author's technique. *British Journal of Anaesthesia*, 12, 4.
Sicard, A. (1898) *Comptes Rendus des Séances de la Société de Biologie* (Paris), 50, 472.
Sicard, A. (1899) *Comptes Rendus des Séances de la Société de Biologie (Paris)*, 51, 408.
Sicard, A. & Forestier, J. (1921) Mèthode radiographique de l'exploration de la cavité epidural par la Lipiodol. *Revue de Neurologie*, 28, 1264.

Sinclair, C. J., Scott, D. B. & Edstrom, H. H. (1982) Effect of Trendelenburg position on spinal anaesthesia with hyperbaric bupivacaine. *British Journal of Anaesthesia*, **54**, 497.

Sise, L. (1935) Pontocaine-glucose solution for spinal anesthesia. *Surgical Clinics of North America*, **55**, 1501.

Smith, G. S. & Porter, W. T. (1915) Spinal anesthesia in the cat. *American Journal of Physiology*, **38**, 108.

Snyder, S. H. (1977) Opiate receptors in the brain. *New England Journal of Medicine*, **296**, 266.

Tait, F. D. & Caglieri, G. (1900) Experimental and clinical notes on the subarachnoid space. Transactions of the Medical Society of California. (Abstract) *Journal of the American Medical Association*, **35**, 6.

Trantenroth, A. (1906) *Deutsche Medizinische Wochenschrift*, **32**, 253.

Tuffier, T. (1899) Analgesie chirurgicale par l'injection sous arachnoidienne lombaire de cocaine. *Comptes rendus des Séances de la Société de Biologie* (Paris), **51**, 882.

Tuffier, T. (1901) L'analgesie chirurgicale par voie rachidienne. *Oeuvre Médicale et Chirurgicale*, **24**.

Tuohy, E. B. (1945) Continuous spinal anesthesia; a new method utilising a ureteral catheter. *Surgical Clinics of North America*, **25**, 834.

Tzaicou, M. A. (1911) Auto-observation d'une auto-operation de hernie sous la rachstrychno-stovainisation. *Presse Médicale*, **19**, 105.

Uhlmann, T. (1929) *Narkose und Anaesthesie*, **6**, 168.

Vehrs, G. R. (1934) *Spinal Anesthetic Technique and Clinical Applications*. St Louis: Mosby.

von Anrep, B. (1880) Über die physiologische Wirkung des Cocaine. *Pflügers Archiv für die Gesamte Physiologie des Menschen und der Tiere*, **21**, 38.

von Ziemssen, H. (1893) *Berliner Klinische Wochenschrift*, **30**, 460.

Wildsmith, J. A. W., McClure, J. H, Brown, D. T. & Scott, D. B. (1981) Effect of posture on spread of isobaric and hyperbaric amethocaine. *British Journal of Anaesthesia*, **53**, 273.

Wilson, W. E. (1934) Intrathecal nerve rootlet block. *Proceedings of the Royal Society of Medicine*, **27**, 323.

Wood, A. (1855) A new method of treating neuralgia by direct application of opiates to painful joints. *Edinburgh Medical Journal*, **82**, 265.

Wright, A. D. (1931) *Proceedings of the Royal Society of Medicine*, **24**, 613.

Wynter, W. E. (1891) Four cases of meningitis in which paracentesis of the theca vertebralis was performed for the relief of fluid pressure. *Lancet*, **1**, 891.

Year Book of Obstetrics and Gynecology (1949) p. 161. Chicago: Year Book Medical Publishers.

Extradural

Aburel, E. (1931) L'anaesthésia locale continue (prolongée) en obstétrique. *Bulletin de la Société d'Obstétrie et de Gynaecologie*, **20**, 85.

Behar, M., Magora, P., Olshwane, D. & Davidson, J. T. (1979) Epidural morphine in the treatment of pain. *Lancet*, **1**, 527.

Bonica, J. J. (1959) *Clinical Applications of Diagnostic and Therapeutic Nerve Blocks*. Springfield: Thomas.

Bromage, P. R. (1954) *Spinal Epidural Analgesia*. Edinburgh: Livingstone.

Campbell, M. F. (1933) Caudal anesthesia in infants. *American Journal of Urology*, **30**, 245.

Cathelin, F. (1901) A new route of spinal injection; a method of epidural injections by way of the sacral canal. *Comptes Rendus des Séances de la Société de Biologie* (Paris), **53**, 452. Translated in *'Classical File' Survey of Anesthesiology* (1979), **23**, 271.

Curbelo, M. M. (1949) Continuous peridural segmental anesthesia by means of a ureteral catheter. *Anesthesia and Analgesia, Current Researches*, **28**, 12.

Dawkins, C. J. M. (1945) Discussion on extradural block. *Proceedings of the Royal Society of Medicine*, **38**, 299.
Dogliotti, A. M. (1933) A new method of block; segmental peridural spinal anesthesia. *American Journal of Surgery*, **20**, 107.
Gordh, T. (1948) Xylocaine; a new local analgesic. *Anaesthesia*, **4**, 4. Reprinted in *'Classical File' Survey of Anesthesiology* (1977), **21**, 314.
Heile, B. (1913) Der epidurale Raum. *Archiv für Klinische Chirurgie*, **101**, 845.
Hingson, R. A. & Edwards, W. B. (1943) Continuous caudal anesthesia in obstetrics. *Journal of the American Medical Association*, **121**, 225.
Jansen, E. (1926) Der negativevorschlag bei Lumbalpunktion. *Deutsche Zeitschrift für Nervenheilkunde*, **94**, 280.
Labat, G. (1923) *Regional Anesthesia*. Philadelphia: Saunders.
Laewen, A. (1910) The utilization of sacral anaesthesia in surgery. *Zentralblatt für Chirurgie*, **37**, 708.
Lund, P. C. (1966) *Peridural Anesthesia and Analgesia*. Springfield: Thomas.
Lundy, J. S. (1942) *Clinical Anesthesia*. Philadelphia: Saunders.
Moore, D. C. (1953) *Regional Block*. Springfield: Thomas.
Odom, C. B. (1936) Epidural anesthesia. *American Journal of Surgery*, **34**, 547.
Pagés-Miravé, F. (1921) Anesthesia matamerica. *Revista de Sanidad Militar* (Madrid), 11, 351.
Rolbin, S. N., Cole, A. F. D., Hew, E. M., Pollard, A. & Virgint, S. (1982) Prophylactic intramuscular ephedrine before epidural anaesthesia for Caesarean section. *Canadian Anaesthetists' Society Journal*, **29**, 148.
Sicard, A. (1901) Extradural injection of medication by way of the sacrococcygeal canal. *Comptes Rendus des Séances de la Société de Biologie* (Paris), **53**, 396. Translated in *'Classical File' Survey of Anesthesiology* (1979), **23**, 271.
Stoekel, W. (1909) Über sakrale Anaesthesie. *Zentralblatt für Chirurgie*, **33**, 1.
Telivuo, L. (1963) A new long-acting local anaesthetic solution for pain relief after thoracotomy. *Annales Chirurgiae et Gynaecologiae Fenniae*, **52**, 513.
Tuohy, E. B. (1945) The use of continuous spinal anesthesia — utilising the ureteral catheter technique. *Journal of the American Medical Association*, **128**, 262.

2

Anatomy

It is important that the anaesthetist should possess a good knowledge of the anatomy of the lumbar vertebrae, since it is in this region that a needle can be introduced into the vertebral canal most safely and easily. He must be familiar also with the disposition of the three membranes which envelop the central nervous system, with the anatomy of the extradural space, and with the anatomy of the thoracic vertebrae. In the vertebral canal these three tubular membranes enclose the cord in an elongated compartment, annular in cross section — the subarachnoid or intradural space (Fig. 2.18) — in which a local analgesic solution can be made to spread to any desired height after it has been introduced low down in the lumbar region.

Some useful surface markings

The spine of C.7 (vertebra prominens) is easily palpable.

The tip of the spine of T.3 is opposite the roots of the spine of the scapula with the arms to the sides.

The tip of the spine of T.7 is opposite the inferior angle of the scapula with the arms to the sides.

The highest points of the iliac crests are on a line crossing the spine of L.4 or the L.4/5 interspace.

The dimples overlying the posterior superior iliac spines are on a line crossing the 2nd posterior sacral foramina; the dural sac usually ends at this level in adults.

The lower end of the spinal cord is opposite the upper border of the body of the 2nd lumbar vertebra and sometimes extends a little below this.

Vertebral column

At birth the vertebral column has two curves concave anteriorly, the thoracic and the sacral. The cervical and the lumbar curve develop later and become obliterated when the spine is fully flexed. The 3rd lumbar vertebra is the highest point in the lumbar curve while the 5th thoracic is the lowest point in the thoracic curve when the patient is lying supine. Pathological deformities of the spine may alter these relationships and of course may well make lumbar puncture difficult. The spines of the cervical, the first two thoracic and the last four lumbar vertebrae are all more or less horizontal and are therefore opposite the bodies of their respective vertebrae. The remaining spinous processes are directed downwards, their tips being opposite the bodies of the vertebra next below. The 5th lumbar spine overhangs the lumbo-sacral interspace. The direction of the spinous processes determines the direction in which a spinal needle must be inserted when the mid-line approach is used. The vertebral column protects the spinal cord. A typical vertebra is made up of:

1. A body which bears and transmits weight, and forms the base for
2. An arch, composed of pedicles and laminae, which surround and protect the cord laterally and posteriorly.

There are seven projections from these vertebral or neural arches. They are:

(a) Three muscular processes — two transverse and one spinous — for the attachment of muscles and ligaments, and
(b) Four 'articular' processes — two upper and two lower — which in the lumbar region prevent rotation but allow limited flexion and extension between contiguous vertebrae.

A typical lumbar vertebra

A lumbar vertebra and its attachments should be studied to obtain a mental picture of the course the needle should take during lumbar puncture. The bone is a massive structure with the following notable features: the spine points almost straight backwards and viewed from the side is square, the vertebral foramen is triangular, the body is kidney shaped. A lumbar vertebra can be distinguished from any of the lower thoracic vertebrae, the only ones which approach it in size and with which it is likely to be confused, by the absence of articular facets for the ribs (Figs 2.1 to 2.4).

Each half of the neural arch is divided into two parts by the root of the transverse process. Anteriorly, the arch is formed by the powerful somewhat rounded pedicle or root, part of whose function is to transmit muscular stress; posteriorly it is completed by the thinner, flatter lamina whose function is mainly protective.

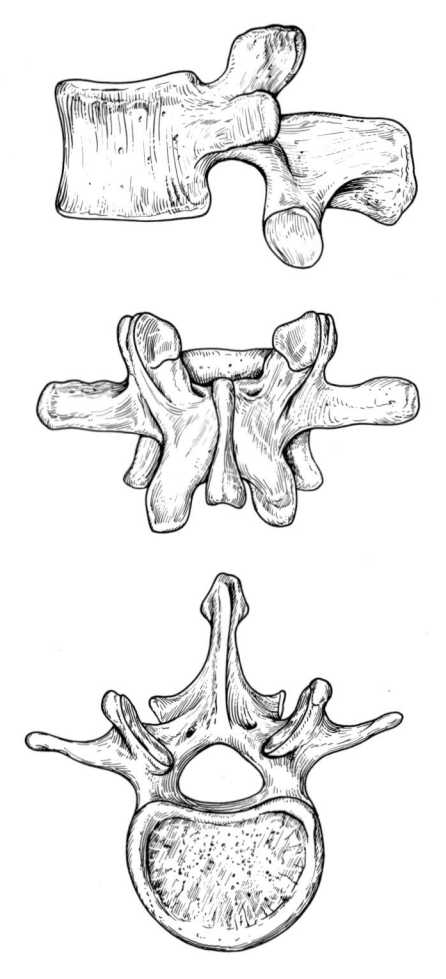

Fig. 2.1 Corning (Corning, 1900): 'I advise those who contemplate practising spinal anaesthesia to take a look at the skeleton, especially the relations of the lumbar vertebrae. An intelligent glance of this sort is worth many words.'

From the neural arches the four articular processes project, two upwards and two downwards, to articulate with processes on the arches of the two neighbouring vertebrae. The upper ones, like the transverse processes, spring from the junction of pedicles and laminae. They project upwards behind the pedicles and come to lie just above the level of the transverse processes; and the articular facets on their posterior surfaces face backwards and medially. The lower articular processes extend downwards from the infero-lateral

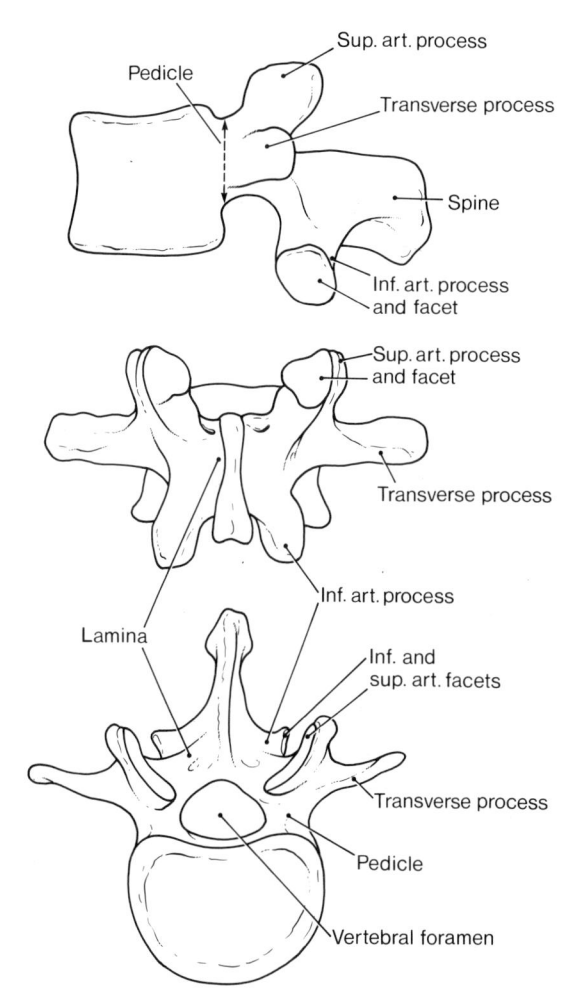

Fig. 2.2 A typical lumbar vertebra.

aspect of the laminae. They lie well below the level of the transverse processes, and the articular facets on their anterior surfaces face forwards and laterally, so that they accurately oppose the facets on the upper processes of the vertebra below.

The pedicles are noticeably less deep than the body of the vertebra to which they are attached. They arise more from the upper than the lower part of the postero-lateral surface of the body, so that of the two notches formed between body and pedicle the inferior is much the deeper. When two vertebrae articulate, the inferior notch of

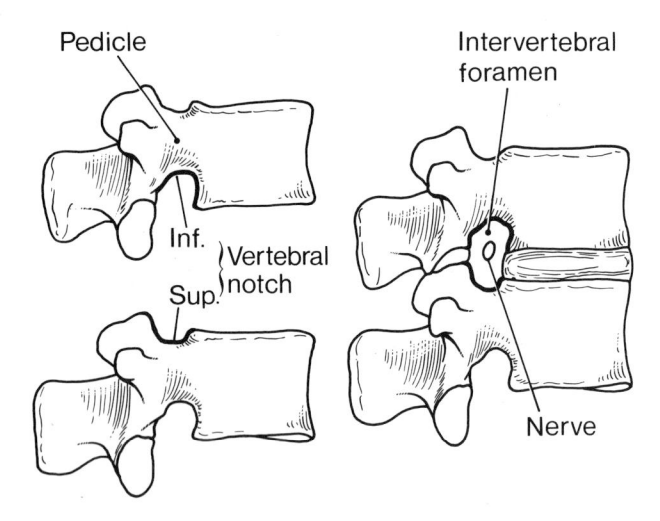

Fig. 2.3 Lateral view of lumbar vertebra

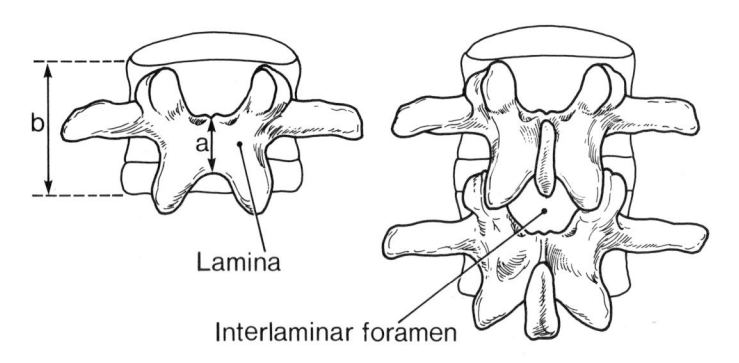

Fig. 2.4 An intervertebral foramen

one vertebra together with the superior notch of the vertebra below it, and the posterior aspect of the intervertebral disc, form a large intervertebral foramen through which the spinal nerve of that particular segment issues from the vertebral canal. The boundaries of an intervertebral foramen are superiorly and inferiorly the pedicles of adjoining vertebrae, posteriorly the capsule surrounding the articulating processes of adjoining vertebrae, and anteriorly an intervertebral disc and the lower part of the body above it (Fig. 2.3).

The posterior surface of the body and the neural arch together form the boundaries of the vertebral foramen (Fig. 2.2 bottom), and in the articulated column these foramina collectively form the

ANATOMY 43

vertebral canal which contains the spinal cord and its surrounding membranes.

The anterior boundary of the vertebral canal presents a

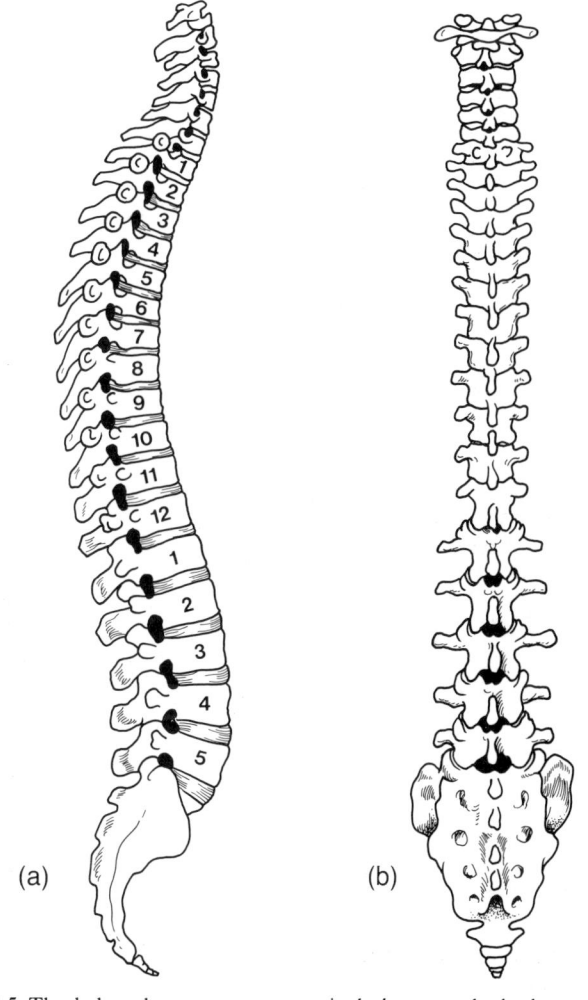

Fig. 2.5 The darkened areas represent gaps in the bony vertebral column which encloses the dura and the extradural space. On the left the intervertebral foramina are seen, and on the right the lumbar interlaminar spaces and the sacral hiatus. The interlaminar gaps between the thoracic vertebrae are concealed from view by the spines of the vertebrae above which overlap the laminae of the vertebrae below like tiles. The five sacral vertebrae are united so that here there are no interlaminar spaces, but failure of the laminae of S.5 to fuse in the mid-line results in the formation of the sacral hiatus. The spine of L.5 overhangs the lumbo-sacral interlaminar space making mid-line lumbar puncture difficult here (Taylor, 1940).

continous solid surface being composed of the posterior aspects of the vertebral bodies and intervertebral discs, covered by the posterior longitudinal ligament (Fig. 2.6). The lateral and the posterior walls, formed by the vertebral arches, however, are incomplete. In the articulated skeleton, it is seen that gaps occur:

1. Laterally (Fig. 2.5a). The formation of the intervertebral foramina in the sides of the column has just been described. Through these run the spinal nerves.

It is quite feasible to give a spinal analgesic by means of a needle inserted through an intervertebral foramen, the route used by Heile in 1913 in an early attempt at extradural blockade (Heile, 1913). The opening is large, and we have pierced the theca inadvertently, when attempting paravertebral block. However, if one tries deliberately to reach the subarachnoid space by this route, difficulties arise owing to the absence of a good landmark to locate with certainty the intervertebral foramen. Consequently this approach is unlikely to oust in popularity the conventional posterior interlaminar or interspinous approach.

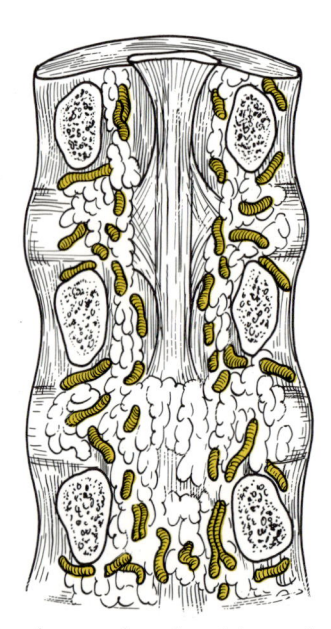

Fig. 2.6 The pedicles have been cut through, and the vertebral arches, meninges and spinal cord have been removed revealing the continuous anterior surface of the vertebral canal. In the upper part of the central portion the extradural fat and vessels have been cleared away to show the somewhat narrow posterior longitudinal ligament which broadens out opposite each intervertebral disc.

2. Posteriorly (Fig. 2.5b). In the lumbar region the gaps are conspicuous, as the depth of the central part of the laminae behind (Fig. 2.4a) is much less than the combined depths of the body and corresponding disc in front (Fig. 2.4b).

By taking the spine of the vertebra below as the bony landmark, the situation of an interlaminar foramen can be estimated with considerable accuracy, and advantage is taken of these openings in the bony posterior wall of the vertebral column to perform lumbar puncture.

In the lumbar region an interlaminar foramen is small and triangular in shape when the vertebral column is extended (Fig. 2.7 and 2.8). The base is formed by the upper borders of the laminae of the lower vertebra, and the sides by the medial aspects of the inferior articular processes of the vertebra above. During flexion the inferior articular processes slide upwards. The interlaminar foramen enlarges and becomes somewhat diamond shaped since now the medial borders of the upper articular processes of the vertebra below form the lower lateral boundaries of the aperture (Fig. 2.8).

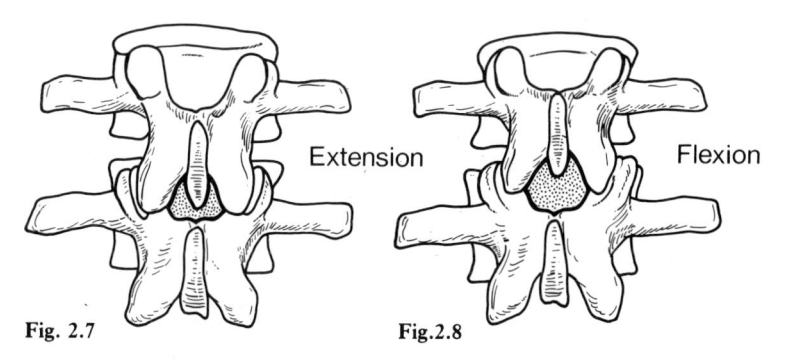

Fig. 2.7 Extension

Fig. 2.8 Flexion

Lumbar intervertebral joints

The fact that the vertebrae are separate units gives flexibility to the vertebral column. Although the sum total of movement is considerable and of great practical value to the individual, the movement between any two vertebrae is small and the articulations are designed more for stability or 'backbone'.

The joint between the bodies of two vertebrae is fibro-cartilaginous; the union between the arches is ligamentous. The joints between the articular processes are synovial in type. The articular surfaces on the processes effectively prevent rotation, but permit of free gliding movement in flexion and extension.

Bodies of vertebrae

The flat articular surfaces of a vertebral body are covered with hyaline cartilage and this is very firmly united to the fibro-cartilaginous intervertebral discs; and this union between the bodies is reinforced by anterior and posterior longitudinal ligamentous bands, which run the whole length of the vertebral column. The broad anterior longitudinal ligament (Fig. 2.27) is firmly attached to the intervertebral discs and more loosely to the anterior surfaces of the vertebral bodies. The posterior band (Fig. 2.6), necessarily narrrower since it lies within the vertebral canal, expands opposite each disc, and is similarly attached to the posterior surfaces of discs and bodies. It sends a few irregular slender fibres to join the anterior surface of the spinal dura mater. In this way the spinal cord is indirectly steadied, yet is little involved in any movement of the vertebral arches during flexion and extension.

Vertebral arches

The vertebral arches of neighbouring vertebrae are bound together by three ligaments which are of interest to the anaesthetist:
1. The ligamenta flava, which stretch between the laminae.
2. The interspinous ligaments which join the opposing borders of the spinous processes.
3. The supraspinous ligaments which unite the tips of the spinous processes.

A narrow vertebral arch will cause a narrow spinal canal. In the rare case when this abnormality exists slight haemorrhage, which might be harmless in a normal patient, may cause pressure on the cord and paraplegia (Chaudhari et al, 1978; Ballin, 1981; Critchley, 1982).

Ligamentum flavum

This ligament is composed almost entirely of elastic fibres, and as its name implies is yellow in colour. It runs from the anterior and inferior aspects of one lamina to the posterior and superior aspects of the lamina below (Fig. 2.9 to 2.11). Laterally it blends with the capsule of the joint between the articular processes and from here extends backwards and medially to meet its opposite number in the median plane. Here small foramina give passage to veins from the internal to the posterior external vertebral plexuses. Occasionally a

ANATOMY 47

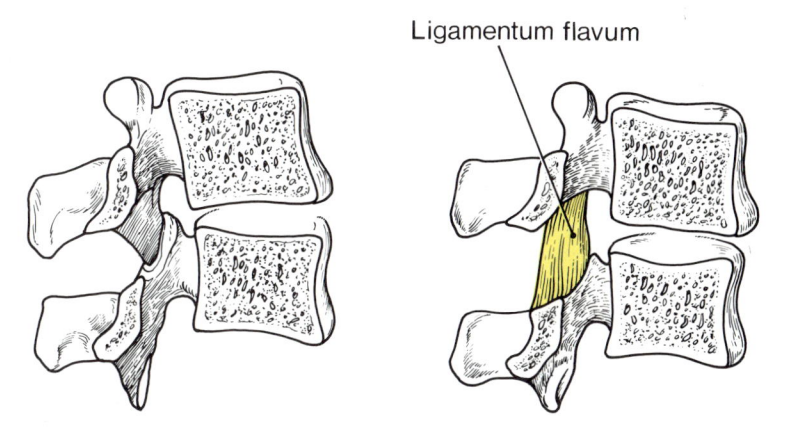

Fig. 2.9 and **Fig. 2.10** Attachments of the ligamentum flavum

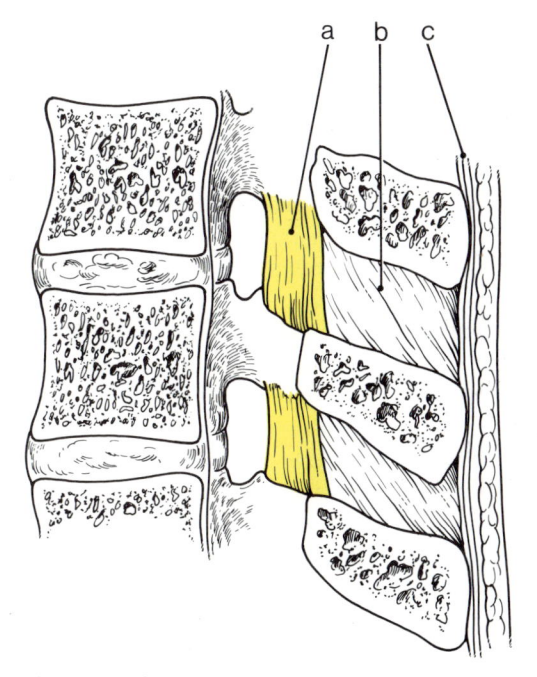

Fig. 2.11 The ligamentum flavum (*a*) and the interspinous (*b*) supraspinous (*c*) ligaments.

lumbar puncture needle punctures one of these. Just as the two vertebral laminae fuse to form the root of the spine, so the two ligamenta flava meet to become continuous with the deep fibres of the interspinous ligament (Fig. 2.30).

If the pedicles are cut across and the vertebral arches looked at from within, the ligamenta flava can be seen almost in their entirety (Fig. 2.27). They cover the capsules of the articular facets, the lower part of the upper laminae, and the interlaminar spaces.

From behind, the ligamenta flava cannot be seen at all throughout most of the thoracic region; for here the laminae and oblique spines, like overlapping tiles, effectively obscure the vertebral canal. In the lumbar region, however, the ligaments become apparent because of the shallowness of the laminae and the horizontal direction of the spines. But even here the ligaments are seen only where they fill the interlaminar spaces and where their lower attachments conceal a small amount of the upper part of the succeeding laminae. Whether viewed from in front or behind, then, part of the ligament is always hidden from view, whilst the portion of the ligament occupying the interlaminar gap is seen from both aspects.

The ligamenta flava constitute slightly more than half of the posterior wall of the vertebral canal. They are thickest and strongest in the lumbar region where powerful stresses and strains have to be countered. They act as muscle sparers in maintaining erect posture: they help to regulate flexion so as to prevent injury to the intervertebral discs, and they help to restore the body to the erect position after it has been flexed. In the dissections from which Figures 7.22 to 7.26 were drawn, the vertebrae were in extension; the ligamenta flava are therefore shown thicker than when encountered during lumbar puncture in life with the back well flexed and the ligaments stretched. Nevertheless, the ligamentum flavum is thicker than commonly imagined.

One often sees the anaesthetist correctly recognise the ligament by touch as the needle penetrates its dorsal aspect. As he pushes on through the thick ligament, another sudden alteration in resistance is sometimes encountered as the needle passes through the deep surface into the extradural space; and this slight jolt is often incorrectly interpreted as penetration of the dura mater. This double alteration in resistance together with the absence of flow of cerebrospinal fluid locates the point of the needle in the extradural space.

It is clear that a needle piercing the ligament at its lower margin may be prevented from reaching the theca by the upper edge of the lamina to which the ligament is attached. This point is of importance in helping the anaesthetist to visualise the state of affairs when he has sensed that the needle has penetrated the ligamentum flavum and is immediately afterwards held up by bone (see Fig. 7.26).

Interspinous ligament

This is a thin ligament, the fibres of which are attached along the lengths of the spinous processes, uniting the lower border of one with the upper border of its caudal neighbour; in the lumbar region, therefore, the ligament is rectangular in shape (Fig. 2.11). Anteriorly, at the level where the spines are formed by the fusion of the laminae, the interspinous ligament blends with the ligamenta flava; posteriorly, the interspinous fibres are continuous with those of the supraspinous ligament. Cyst formation in the interspinous ligament can occur, especially in elderly patients, and may confuse the anaesthetist as it can cause loss of resistance to the advancing needle at an unusually superficial level (Sharrock, 1979).

Supraspinous ligament

The fibres of this tough ligament unite the apices of the spines of the lumbar and thoracic vertebrae and continue above as the ligamentum nuchae. The ligament may be almost half an inch wide in the lumbar region to correspond with the spines which are broadest in this situation. In labourers and in old age, ossification from the spine may extend along the fibres of this tough ligament; the space then available in the median plane between two spines for the passage of a lumbar puncture needle is therefore less than a study of the dry bones would suggest. In fact in these cases it may be almost impossible to insert a needle in the median plane, but a needle inserted just lateral to the supraspinous ligament can be directed to the interlaminar space without meeting obstruction: the lateral, or paramedian approach.

Intervertebral disc

The intervertebral discs form at least one-quarter of the total length of the vertebral column. In the cervical and lumbar regions they are somewhat wedge shaped and thus contribute to the characteristic curves of the column. The discs are thickest in the lumbar region where weight bearing is maximal, and movement, except rotation, is considerable.

Each disc consists of a fibrous outer cover, the annulus fibrosus, which is attached to the hyaline cartilage covering the articular surfaces of the two vertebral bodies it connects. The annulus encloses a core of gelatinous material, the nucleus pulposus, which accommodates itself to the changes in shape of its covering during movement between the vertebrae. Intervertebral discs thus act as shock absorbers and give flexibility to the vertebral column.

As a result of weakness or strain the annulus may rupture, usually posteriorly where it is thinnest. The nucleus pulposus may then herniate through the deficiency, causing symptoms and signs which depend on the nerve or nerves involved (Mixter (1880–1958) and Barr (1900–1963), 1934) (Fig. 2.12). Protrusion of the nucleus pulposus — a 'prolapsed disc' — has been described following lumbar puncture, and it must be borne in mind that careless technique may be a contributing factor. The mechanics of such an injury are easy to visualise. The nucleus pulposus, through which passes the axis of flexion or extension of one vertebra on another, is situated somewhat posteriorly in the disc. The nucleus pulposus draws its fluid content from the spongiosa of the adjacent vertebrae by osmosis (Crisp, 1955) and even in normal circumstances is under

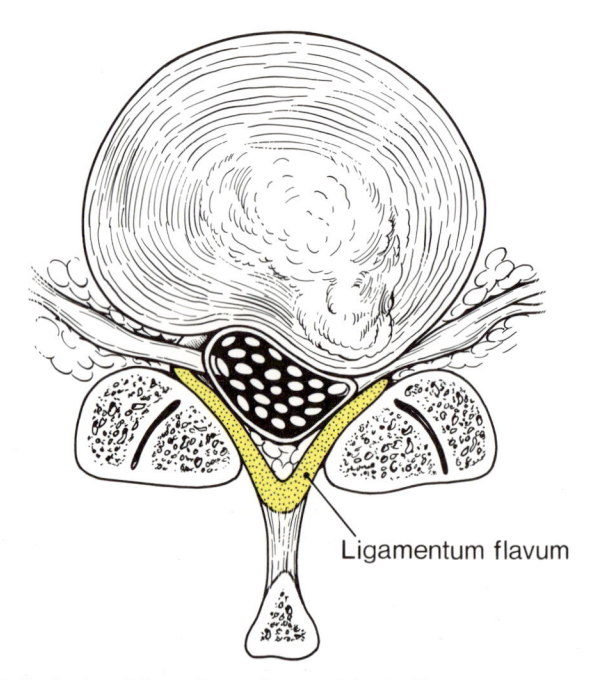

Fig. 2.12 Protrusion of the nucleus pulposus. (After Naffziger and Boldrey, 1946.) This disability has been reported frequently following lumbar puncture. On the right-hand side the nerve roots for that segment are compressed against the ligamentum flavum and articular processes.

considerable pressure. When the lumbar vertebrae are fully flexed, as during lumbar puncture, the nucleus pulposus is squeezed backwards, greatly increasing the strain on the annulus posteriorly where it is weakest. If, in these circumstances, a needle is inadvertently pushed through the subarachnoid space and the annulus is pierced, a prolapsed disc may result, while this accident is more likely to happen if the needle is blocked so that cerebrospinal fluid cannot issue when the tip is correctly placed.

Spinal cord and nerve roots

The spinal cord is a cylindrical mass of nervous tissue, 42 to 45 cm in length occupying the upper two-thirds of the vertebral canal. At its rostral end it is continuous with the medulla oblongata and extends to the superior border of the 2nd lumbar vertebra or sometimes to the 3rd. From the apex of the conical lower end, the conus medullaris, a delicate filament, the filum terminale, stretches downwards to be attached to the 1st segment of the coccyx. At birth the cord reaches to the level of the 3rd lumbar vertebra.

There is an anterior median fissure and a posterior median septum. The former extends for about 3 mm into the substance of the cord and contains small blood vessels beside which local analgesic solution can enter the substance of the cord. The posterior median sulcus contains a septum of neuroglia.

To the spinal cord are attached 31 pairs of spinal nerves, each arising from a ventral and a dorsal root. These anterior and posterior roots cross the subarachnoid space, pass through the dura and extradural space independently and unite in the intervertebral foramina to form spinal nerve trunks which soon divide into anterior and posterior primary divisions. These mixed nerves are blocked only secondarily in spinal analgesia; it is the block of the nerve roots which produces the typical effects. There is, however, evidence that, following its injection into the subarachnoid space, a solution of a local analgesic agent can travel along the mixed nerve trunks for as much as 2 cm beyond the intervertebral foramina as well as into the substance of the cord.

Local analgesic solutions act on autonomic, sensory and motor fibres, the autonomic being the most sensitive, the motor fibres the least sensitive. Fibres which block easily, hold the drug longest. For a given level of sensory block, following extradural injection, sympathetic block will extend about two segments higher, while motor block will be two or three segments lower.

The anterior roots, somatic and splanchnic, are made up of axons of cells in the anterior and lateral columns of the cord, and are efferent and transmit motor impulses. They also contain sympathetic preganglionic axons which arise from cells in the intermedio-lateral horn of the cord from the level of the 1st thoracic to the 2nd lumbar segments. These efferent fibres which are myelinated cross the intradural and the extradural spaces and then pass in the white rami communicantes to the ganglia of the paravertebral chain. In the ganglia, each pilomotor, sudomotor and vasomotor fibre synapses with a number of cells, and from the ganglia postganglionic fibres (unmyelinated), the grey rami communicantes, join the spinal nerves and pass to the effector organ. The preganglionic fibres conveying inhibitory motor fibres to the gut pass through the ganglia of the sympathetic chain and synapse with cells in the coeliac, superior mesenteric and other prevertebral plexuses from which postganglionic fibres originate. Each posterior or dorsal root has a small swelling, the spinal ganglion, in the intervertebral foramen, outside the dura, and contains largely afferent fibres (Bell-Magendie Law) arising from nerve cells in the corresponding spinal ganglion. These cells give off axons which soon divide; one entering the cord, the other passing peripherally in the mixed spinal nerve.

Visceral afferent fibres from the abdominal and thoracic viscera travel (1) with the efferent sympathetic nerves, pass through the paravertebral ganglia without synapsing and proceed in the white rami to the mixed spinal nerves and have their cell stations in the posterior root ganglia and (2) in the vagus, where they are unaffected by central neural blockade.

The spinal nerve roots have a dural covering which passes to the intervertebral foramina, at right angles higher up and obliquely lower down, and end by becoming attached to the distal portion of posterior root ganglion, where the two roots fuse to form the mixed spinal nerve. This attachment becomes more medial in the lumbar and sacral regions than in the cervical and thoracic regions. The roots vary both in size and thickness being larger in the cervical and lumbo-sacral enlargements than in the thoracic region. In old age, neurons become replaced by fibrous tissue. Large roots are more difficult to block than small ones (e.g. occasional difficulty with S.1.). Segmental innervation does not always run true to the average pattern and intersegmental communication occurs, disturbing the theoretical arrangement of cutaneous nerve supply.

Blood supply of the spinal cord

The spinal cord can function properly only if it receives an adequate blood supply, and one of the explanations advanced for the occasional catastrophe following spinal analgesia is interference with this flow due either to physical damage, hypotension and consequent ischaemia, or to prolonged vasoconstriction. The supply is from the anterior and posterior spinal arteries. Ischaemia for more than two to three minutes may result in permanent damage to the cord.

The anterior spinal artery is a single vessel lying in the pia mater in front of the anterior median fissure. It arises from the junction of two small arteries, one given off from each vertebral artery at the level of the foramen magnum. It descends along the whole length of the cord, receiving small communications from the intercostal and lumbar arteries. To provide the extra blood supply needed in the thoracic and lumbar enlargements, the communicating branches at the level of T.1 and T.2 are larger than the others (the arteries of Adamkiewicz). Thrombosis of the anterior spinal artery results in the syndrome in which there is paraplegia without involvement of the modalities subserved by the posterior columns, e.g. joint, position, touch and vibration sense (Wells, 1966).

The posterior spinal arteries are two or three in number on each side and originate in the posterior inferior cerebellar arteries at the base of the brain. They supply the posterior columns of the cord. There are no anastomoses between the anterior and posterior spinal arteries: in fact, the vascularisation of the cord comprises three independent territories, anterior and two posterior (Gilliatt, 1958; Djindjian, 1970). The blood supply of the cord has been reassessed recently (Costello and Fisher, 1983). Ischaemia of the cord can follow general anaesthesia, e.g. for aortic surgery, leading to paralysis.

The extradural veins

These have an important function and have an influence on both the spread of local analgesic solutions and on their absorption and hence their toxicity (Batson, 1940; Domisse, 1976). They form a plexus which is most dense in the antero-lateral compartment of the extradural space and this is one argument for inserting the needle in the median plane. The veins receive blood from the cord and from the vertebral canal and its contents and they communicate above with intracranial sinuses and below with tributaries of the inferior vena cava. They also communicate with the azygos system. Each nerve root is surrounded by a venous plexus and the main longitudinal channels are without valves (Batson, 1940). Thus there is a continuous vascular connection between the pelvis and the cranium, bypassing the vena cava. Changes in intra-abdominal and intrathoracic pressure due to swellings, coughing or straining may cause dilatation of the veins and so reduce the capacity of the extradural space. If the vena cava is partially obstructed as in late pregnancy, the venous plexus forms a second channel of drainage.

Meninges

The names of the enveloping meninges or membranes of the central nervous system are self-descriptive. The dura mater is tough, the arachnoid cobweb-like, and the pia mater tender and clinging.

Dura mater

The dura mater, although continuous, can be described in two parts, cranial and spinal. The cranial dura consists of two layers, endosteal and meningeal, closely united except where they enclose the great venous sinuses which drain the blood from the brain (Fig. 2.13). At the foramen magnum the endosteal layer which lines the skull becomes continuous with the periosteum on the outer surface of the bone. The meningeal layer invests the brain and folds inwards to form the tentorium cerebelli and falx cerebri which divide the cranial cavity into freely communicating compartments, and being taut 'prevent shifting of the cranial cargo' (Grant, 1952).

The outer or endosteal layer of the cranial dura mater is represented in the vertebral canal by the lining periosteum.

The spinal dura mater or theca, the loose outermost and by far the toughest of the three sheaths surrounding the spinal cord, is the continuation downwards of the inner or meningeal layer of the cranial dura mater. Above, it is firmly attached to the circumference of the foramen magnum of the occipital bone. Below, the dural enclosure ends at the lower border of the 2nd sacral vertebra (Fig. 2.14), where it is pierced by the filum terminale, the terminal thread of pia mater which runs from the end of the spinal cord to blend with the periosteum on the back of the coccyx. The filum terminale anchors cord and theca and the latter is further steadied, particularly in the lower end of the vertebral canal, by fibres from

ANATOMY 55

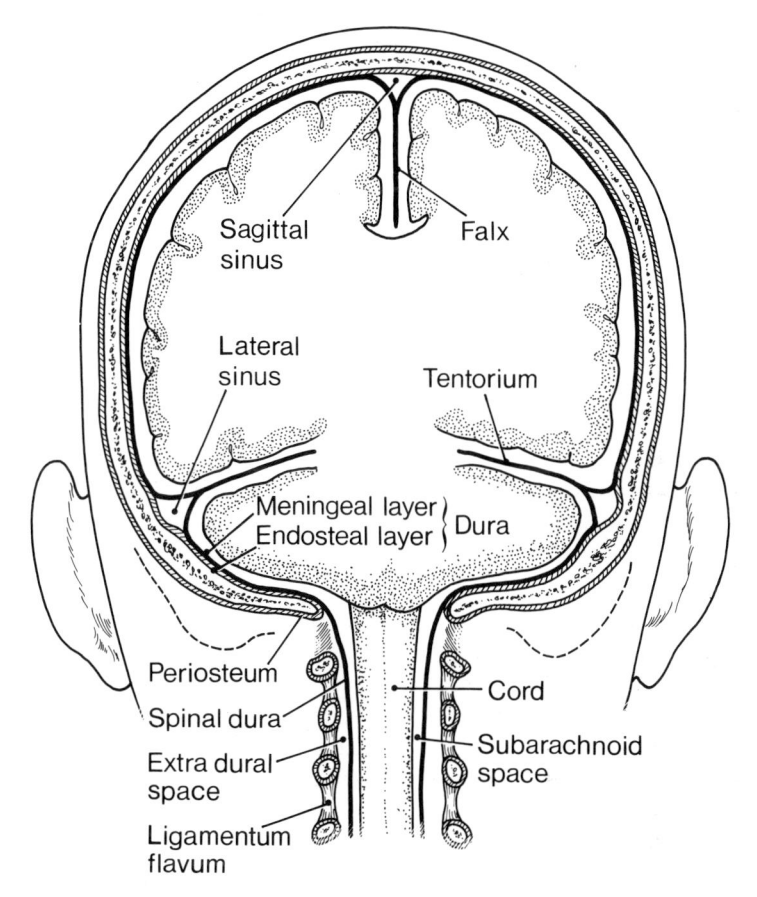

Fig. 2.13 The cranial meninges. See also Fig. 2.14.

the posterior longitudinal ligament. The dura invests the roots of the spinal nerves and also the mixed nerve as it leaves the intervertebral foramen. A congenital intra- or extradural mid-line diffusion barrier in both spaces may result in unilateral block (Bozeman and Chandra, 1980).

Arachnoid mater

The arachnoid is the middle of the three coverings of the brain and spinal cord. It is a delicate non-vascular membrane closely applied to the dura mater, and with it ends at the lower boder of the 2nd sacral vertebra (Fig. 2.14).

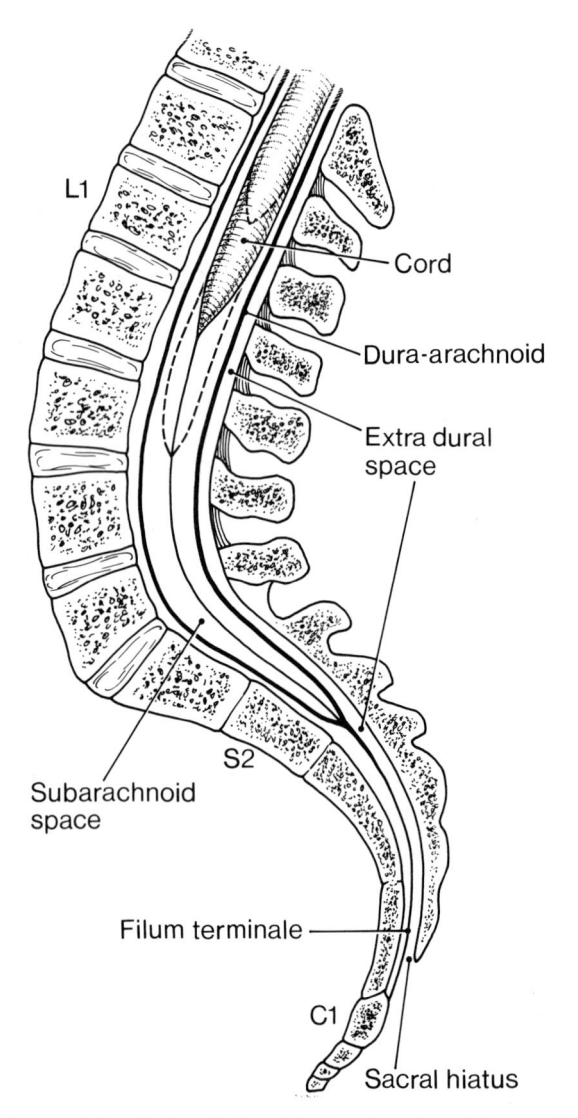

Fig. 2.14 In the adult male the spinal cord is 42 to 45 cm long. It is generally stated to end at the lower border of the 1st lumbar vertebra, but Reimann and Anson (1944) found this to be so in only 50 per cent of 129 adults examined by them. In 121 of these cases (94 per cent) the cord ended opposite either the 1st or the 2nd lumbar vertebra: of the remainder, five finished opposite the 12th thoracic, and three as low as the 3rd lumbar vertebra. Compare with Fig. 2.13.

The subdural space

This is a potential space between the dura and the pia-arachnoid, and local analgesic solutions, contrast medium (Schultz and Brogdon, 1962) and even a catheter (Boys and Norman, 1975) have been proved to enter it. Its presence may lead to inadequate block (Cohen and Kallos, 1972) or even to total central neural blockade (Sechzer, 1963).

The dura and arachnoid are in such close contact that in the process of lumbar puncture it is most unusual to pierce the dura without piercing its companion membrane. In the cervical region, however, the subdural space is easier of access and is also wider laterally adjacent to the nerve roots, a fact which has been made use of for the injection of analgesic and neurolytic solutions in the treatment of pain due to malignant disease (Mehta and Maher, 1977). In describing the technique of lumbar puncture, it is common to omit any reference to the arachnoid; and in fact the subarachnoid space is sometimes loosely, though incorrectly, referred to as the subdural space.

Pia mater

The pia mater is a delicate, highly vascular membrane closely investing the cord and brain, clinging to the surface of the latter throughout its irregular contours. It gives a covering to each nerve root which becomes continuous with the epineurium of the nerve, and consists of two layers.

Nerve supply of the meninges

The posterior (unlike the anterior) aspect of the dura and arachnoid is not supplied with afferent nerve fibres, so that pain is not felt when the dura is pierced by a lumbar puncture needle. The anterior aspect is supplied by twigs from the spinal nerves, each of which enters an intervertebral foramen, divides and passes upwards for one segment and downwards for two segments (Edgar and Nundy, 1966).

Extradural space

The extradural (peridural, epidural) space is that part of the vertebral canal not occupied by the dura mater and its contents. It

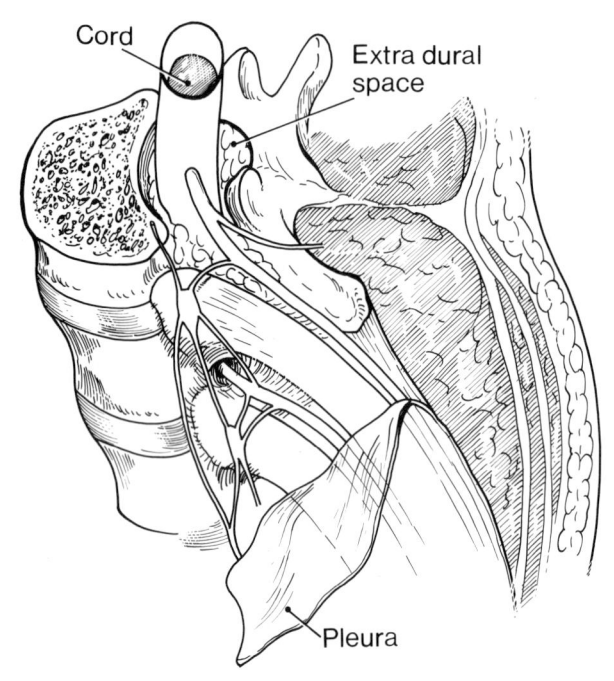

Fig. 2.15 The extradural space. The fat has been removed from the 8th intervertebral foramen. (After Macintosh and Mushin, 1947.)

lies between the dura and the periosteum lining the canal, and corresponds to the very restricted space within the skull between the two layers of the cranial dura mater enclosing the venous sinuses (Figs 2.13, 2.15 and 2.40).

The extradural space extends from the sacral hiatus to the base of the skull. Except in the lower sacral region it is annular in shape, and narrow. The anterior and posterior nerve roots in their dural coverings pass across the very narrow space to unite in the intervertebral foramen to form the segmental nerves. The rest of the extradural space is occupied by numerous small veins and by fatty areolar tissue which is continuous around the nerves through the intervertebral foramina with the fat in the paravertebral spaces. The extradural space and its communications can be outlined easily by the instructive exercise of injecting a liberal quantity of methylene blue through the sacral hiatus of a cadaver. A varying amount runs out around the nerves through the various sacral foramina, and through the lumbar, thoracic and cervical intervertebral foramina, but the upward spread is limited by the attachment of the dura to the circumference of the foramen magnum. The sciatic nerves will be found to be stained for a considerable distance into the thighs, and if the thorax is opened a blob of blue is found in practically every intercostal (Nunn and Slavin, 1980) and thoracic paravertebral space between the heads of adjoining ribs. Here the dye has seeped out from the extradural space, through the foramina, and extended along the intercostal spaces for varying distances; but this staining is not uniform, since occasionally some of the intervertebral foramina are partially occluded by fibrous tissue.

The experiment demonstrates the unpredictability of the spread of a limited quantity of analgesic solution in the extradural space, on account of the numerous openings through which the fluid can escape. The aim of extradural injection is to block, by spread of local analgesic solution, the nerve roots in their very short course across the extradural space to their intervertebral foramina.

As in other parts of the body, the amount of fat in the areolar tissue of the space depends on the obesity of the subject: but in any case it is greatest in the median plane posteriorly where the summit of the vertebral arch is commonly separated from the rounded posterior aspect of the dura by approximately 5 to 6 mm, and antero-laterally where it is continuous with the pads of fat surrounding the spinal nerves in the intervertebral foramina. Between the postero-lateral walls of the lumbar vertebral canal and the dura, the space is narrower, and the fat less evident. Anteriorly, in a thin subject, the space is only potential, since here the dura lies close to the posterior longitudinal ligament on the posterior aspects of the vertebral bodies.

The extradural space extends from the foramen magnum to the sacral hiatus, the dural sac from the foramen magnum to the lower border of S.2. The anaesthetist takes advantage of this discrepancy in caudal analgesia, when he introduces a needle through the sacral hiatus into the caudal part of the sacral canal — the lowermost part of the extradural space — without piercing the dura. The spread of the local analgesic solution injected into the extradural space is not accurately predictable, because of the resistance offered by the fatty areolar tissue and because of the numerous foramina through which the fluid can leak; but it is reliable enough to make extradural analgesia a practical method of providing pain relief.

Investigations into the topography of the extradural space have been carried out after injecting polyester resin into cadavers (Husemeyer and White, 1980). The shape was found to be triangular with the apex dorso-medial. In some cadavers, a dorso-medial fold of dura mater was demonstrated which sometimes divided the extradural space into a ventral and two dorso-lateral compartments, not necessarily freely communicating with each other. It was shown that the median thickness of the space might be only 2 mm. These observations could explain occasional patchy analgesia and inadvertent dural puncture when the mid-line approach is used (Luyendijk and van Voorthuisen, 1966; Husemeyer and White, 1980). Local analgesic drugs injected into the extradural space can affect both the brain and the cord (Bromage et al, 1963). The solution can pass from the extra- to the intradural space in the region of the root sleeves in the intervertebral foramina (Rexed and Wennstrom, 1959).

The space occupied by the venous plexus varies with the amount that the veins are distended and is related to the intrathoracic pressure.

Subarachnoid or intradural space

The subarachnoid space is lined externally by the arachnoid, internally by the pia mater, and innumerable cobweb-like trabeculae run between the two membranes, though sparsely in the cisterns. It is traversed by the cranial and spinal nerves. It houses the main blood vessels of the central nervous system, and extends along the smaller arteries and capillaries into the nervous tissue of the brain and spinal cord (Fig. 2.16): here the cerebrospinal fluid takes the place of the tissue fluid (lymph) found in other regions of the body — see p. 93. In the cervical and thoracic regions the space is annular and the distance between the arachnoid and the pia covering the cord, even in an adult, is only about 3 mm (Fig. 2.18), so that a spinal tap here is fraught with the danger of injuring the cord with the needle. The cord commonly finishes at the lower border of the 1st lumbar vertebra so that below this level the subarachnoid space is no longer annular but is practically circular in section (Fig. 2.18) and has a diameter of about 15 mm. Lumbar puncture should be carried out in the lower lumbar region. As will be seen later, the approach of the needle to the subarachnoid space here is easy. The fact that the cord terminates above this level renders it immune from injury, the constituent nerve roots of the cauda equina escape damage on account of their relative mobility, and the absence of the cord greatly increases the cross-sectional area of the subarachnoid space, the ultimate target at which the needle is aiming.

ANATOMY 61

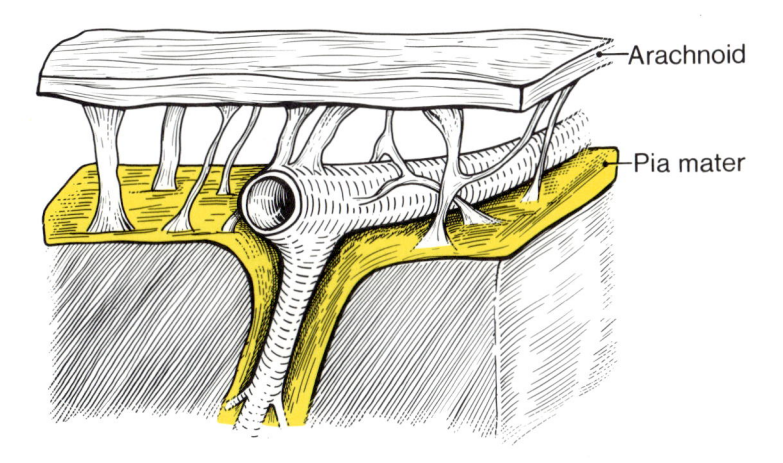

Fig. 2.16 From Kuntz (Kuntz, 1950). Delicate strands of arachnoid tissue cross the narrow subarachnoid space to be attached to the pia.

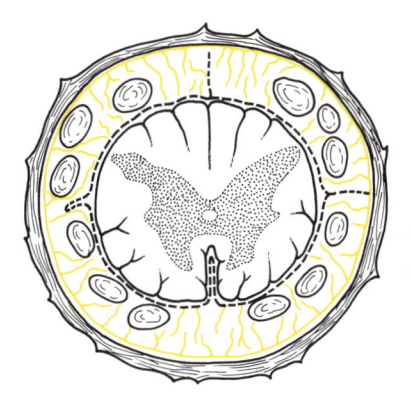

Fig.2.17 Section through the 12th thoracic segment of the cord at the level of the 9th thoracic vertebra. The anterior and posterior roots of the 10th, 11th and 12th thoracic nerves are seen. (After Ranson, 1953.)

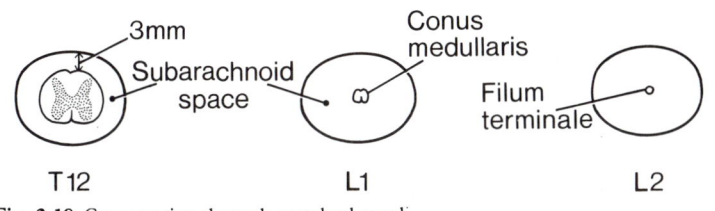

Fig. 2.18 Cross section through vertebral canal

In the skull the pia and arachnoid membranes are, for the most part, in fairly close apposition, especially at the summit of the cerebral convolutions, but since the pia closely follows the irregularities of the brain surface and dips into sulci which are bridged by the arachnoid a large number of gaps occur between the two membranes which are filled with cerebrospinal fluid. In certain situations, such as the base of the brain, these spaces are of considerable size, and are referred to as *cisterns*. Examples of these are the cisterna magna formed where the arachnoid does not follow the pia closely into the angle between the medulla and undersurface of the cerebellum (Fig. 2.19), and the cisterna pontis which is a wide space on the ventral aspect of the pons.

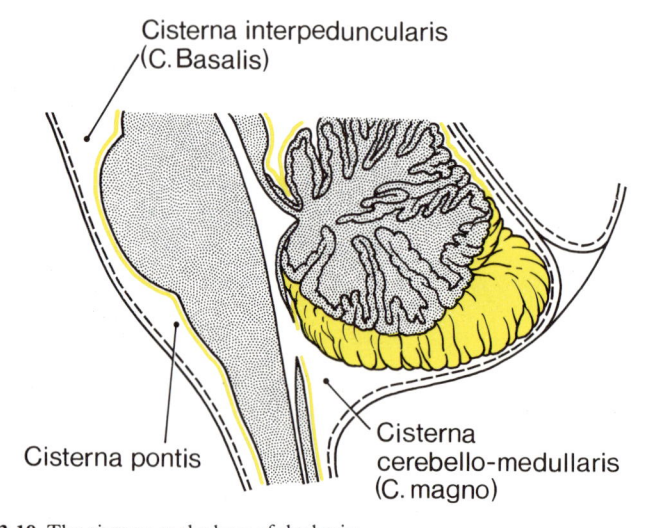

Fig. 2.19 The cisterns at the base of the brain.

There is evidence that the entire central nervous system is surrounded by a membrane similar to and continuous with the pia-arachnoid, and that cerebrospinal fluid passes along spinal nerves in both centrifugal and centripetal directions (Steer and Horney, 1968).

Ligamenta denticulata

The two ligamenta denticulata are so named because of their resemblance to the teeth of a saw. They consist of two serrated folds of the pia which surrounds the cord, and they project at right angles

ANATOMY 63

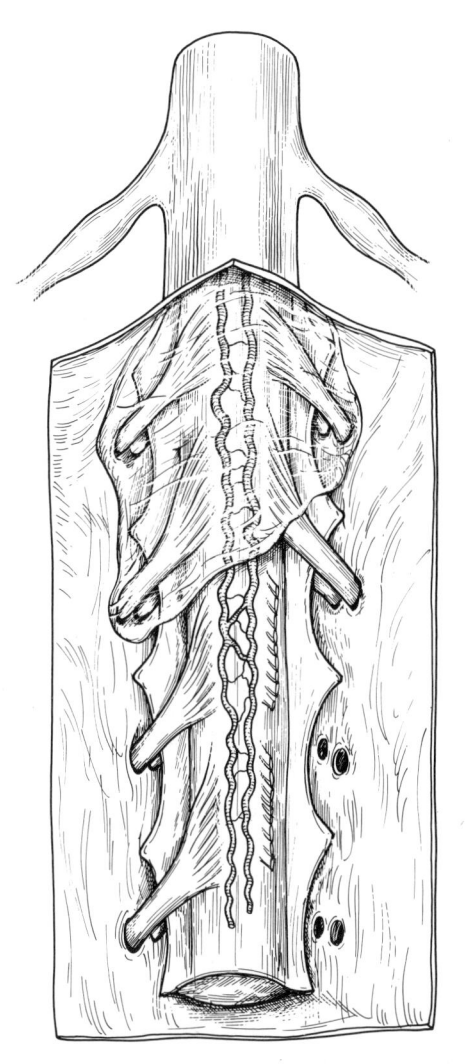

Fig. 2.20 The dura has been opened to show the denticulate ligaments and the posterior aspect of the cord in the upper thoracic region. In the middle of the picture the flimsy arachnoid can be seen. On the lower right-hand side the anterior and posterior nerve roots have been removed showing the points where they pierce the dura separately, but closely associated.

in the mid-lateral line from the cord to the dura. The bases of the ligaments extend continuously from the bulb almost to the conus medullaris, that is along practically the whole length of the cord, separating the anterior from the posterior nerve roots (Fig. 2.20).

From the bases, 21 pairs of teeth, corresponding in number to the cervical, thoracic and 1st lumbar nerves, project on either side, and the apices of the teeth are attached to the inner surface of the dural sac at points midway between the exits of successive spinal nerves. The lowest tooth of the ligament curves downwards and is crossed in front and behind by the roots of the 1st lumbar nerve (Figs 2.20 and 2.25). The ligaments support the cord, and anchor it fairly firmly in the centre of the dural sac.

Posterior subarachnoid septum

The cord is further steadied and the intradural space again subdivided by the posterior subarachnoid septum. The fine strands of this incomplete and inconstant partition pass from the mid-line of the dorsal surface of the cord directly backwards to be attached to the arachnoid.

Neither the denticulate ligament nor the subarachnoid septum exercise any detectable influence on the spread of local analgesic injected into the subarachnoid space.

Cauda equina

In early fetal life the cord is as long as the vertebral canal. During development, however, increase in length of the cord does not keep pace with the growth of the vertebrae, so that soon a great disproportion results between the length of the bony column and the spinal cord it protects. At birth the tip of the cord has risen from the level of the 2nd coccygeal vertebra to the lower border of the 3rd lumbar vertebra, a distance of nine segments. After birth the growth in length of the cord still lags behind that of its bony enclosure, but the difference is less marked so that by the time growth ceases, the end of the cord has risen generally by another two segments to the lower border of the 1st lumbar vertebra (Figs 2.14 and 2.21).

If growth of the cord had kept pace with that of the vertebrae the nerve roots would run transversely from the cord to their corresponding intervertebral foramina. This happens in the cervical region, but because of the relative inequality in the rate of growth of bony column and cord, the thoracic nerve roots run an increasingly oblique course; and the direction of the lower lumbar and sacral roots is practically vertical. Since the latter roots are necessarily given off before the spinal cord ends at the level of say the 1st lumbar vertebra, most of them must perforce run almost vertically downwards for several centimetres behind the bodies of the

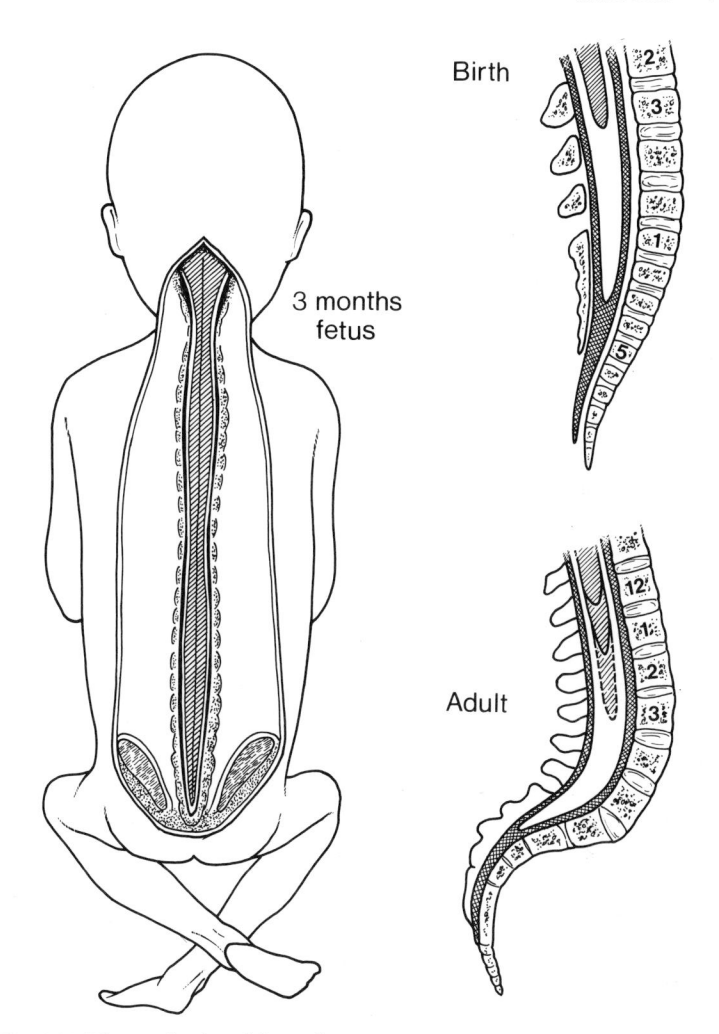

Fig. 2.21 The termination of the cord.

remaining four lumbar vertebrae before passing through the dura to reach their corresponding lumbar and sacral foramina. The 1st lumbar nerve has the highest and most lateral point of origin from the conus medullaris. The 2nd lumbar nerve arises immediately below this: and the sequence continues until the lowest sacral and the coccygeal nerve roots leave the tip of the conus and so occupy the central part of the intradural space (Fig. 2.25). The general appearance of the nerve roots in this region readily suggests the description of cauda equina or horse's tail.

The nerve roots here are completely immersed in cerebrospinal fluid, and since they enjoy a considerable range of mobility, they are immune from injury during straightforward lumbar puncture. No doubt they are frequently touched by the invading needle, but they float easily to one side and escape damage in the same way as the elusive apple does when being 'bobbed' for in a bucket of water.

The sacrum

This bone is formed by the fusion of five vertebrae, is triangular in outline and becomes progressively smaller from above downwards. It is convex posteriorly. Above, it articulates with the 5th lumbar vertebra and below with the coccyx. Ligaments above and below the lumbo-sacral joint support the weight of the body. The pelvic surface is smooth and has four transverse ridges which take the place of the intervertebral discs; the fifth is between the sacrum and the coccyx. On each side the sympathetic trunk lies medial to the sacral foramina, four in number, while lateral to these foramina the pyriformis muscle separates the trunk from the sacral plexus. Local analgesic solution may pass freely through these foramina. The posterior surface is indented and closed in the middle line by the fusion of adjacent laminae and spinous processes.

The sacral hiatus, very variable in shape and size, is caused by the failure of fusion of the 5th and often of the 4th laminae. It is covered by the sacro-coccygeal membrane. The sacral canal follows the curve of the sacrum and in cross-section is triangular. Both the anterior and the posterior foramina open into it. In the average adult patient the dural sac extends to the lower border of the 2nd sacral vertebra which is on the level of the posterior superior iliac spines. The filum terminale extends from the cord, through the dura to the coccygeal periosteum. The canal contains, in addition to the dural sac and its contents, the sacral nerves, loose fat, veins and the filum terminale. The upper opening of the canal is oblique owing to the inclination of the sacrum. It points upwards and forwards, and may retard upward spread of injected solution (see Fig. 2.14).

Figure 2.22. The 2nd lumbar vertebra has been cut through vertically, close to the median plane. The left pedicle and lamina of the 3rd vertebra have been cut through and the intervening piece, which includes the superior articular and transverse processes, has been removed. See inset.

Figure 2.23. Articulated vertebral column. Interlaminar foramina are seen between T.12 and L.1, all the lumbar vertebrae, and L.5 and

ANATOMY 67

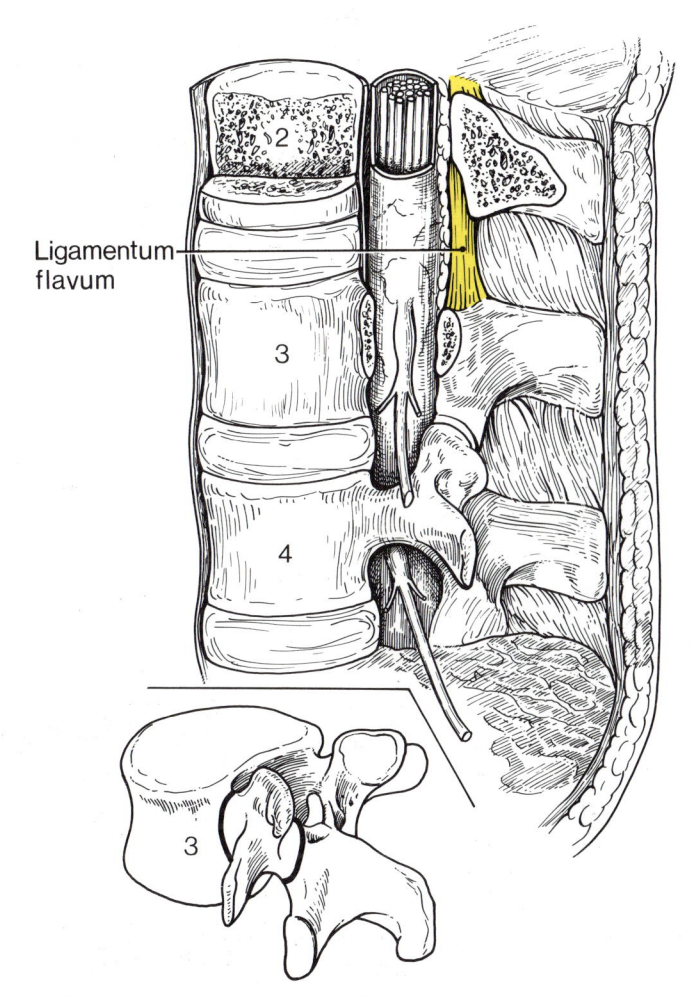

Ligamentum flavum

Fig. 2.22 Suggested by a drawing by Mr L. Schlossberg, by courtesy of Dr R. A. Hingson.

S.1, offering approaches to the extradural space and dura mater.

The triangular sacral hiatus is formed by failure of the laminae of the 5th sacral vertebra to fuse. A needle inserted through the tough, taut, fibrous membrane covering the hiatus at once enters the extradural space. Owing to the curvature of the sacrum and to the fact that the dural sac terminates some distance above — opposite the lower border of the 2nd sacral vertebra (Figs 2.14, 2.24) — this approach is never made deliberately to the subarachnoid space.

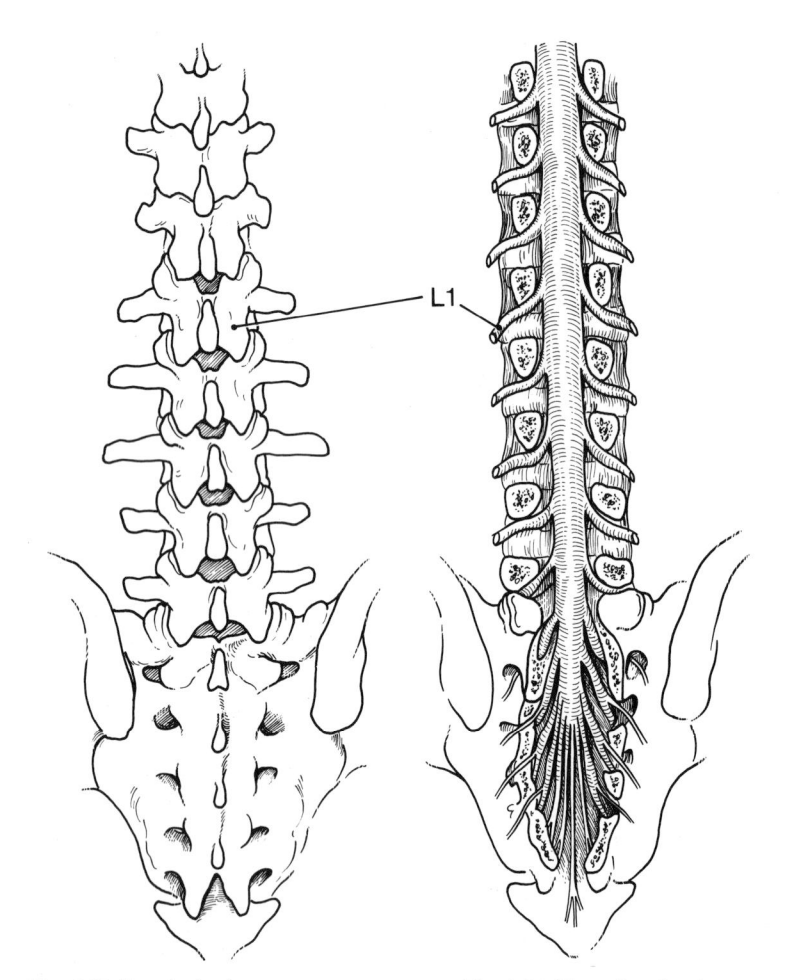

Fig. 2.23 Vertebral column

Fig. 2.24 Dissection showing extradural space

Nevertheless, inadvertent puncture of the dura occurs from time to time when caudal extradural analgesia is intended, and if this accident is not detected early it may well provide alarming complications, for the large volume of solution necessary for caudal extradural analgesia would then be injected intradurally. However, intradural injection of an appropriate dose of local analgesic solution will result in block of the lower nerves.

Figure 2.24. The extradural space has been exposed by removing the laminae of the sacral vertebrae, and by cutting through the pedicles and taking away the vertebral arches of the lumbar and thoracic vertebrae. The extradural fat has been cleared away.

The extradural space is continuous from the sacral hiatus to the foramen magnum and communicates with the paravertebral spaces through the intervertebral foramina. Spread of any given quantity of fluid injected into the extradural space is not accurately predictable because of the resistance offered by the loose areolar tissue which occupies it, and because of escape through the numerous intervertebral foramina.

The lower limit of the theca is seen opposite the lower border of S.2, and the 3rd, 4th and 5th sacral nerves, the coccygeal nerve and the filum terminale are shown emerging from it and descending in the caudal part of the sacral canal.

Figure 2.25. The dura mater and arachnoid have been opened, showing the cord ending at the lower border of L.1. The filum terminale, pulled aside in its upper course, continues, leaving the intradural space at its extremity; from here it passes through the sacral canal, and out of the sacral hiatus, to be anchored to the posterior surface of the body of the 1st segment of the coccyx.

On the right the nerve roots, except for L.1, have been removed in their subarachnoid course; the holes for their escape through the arachnoid-dura are seen.

The ligamenta denticulata (p. 62) end just above the lower end of the spinal cord, and the bases of the lower serrations separate the anterior and posterior roots of several lumbar nerves as they pass vertically downwards to their exits. The lowest denticulation, recognised by its obliquity, serves as a guide for the neurosurgeon to the roots of L.1, which pierce the dura just below it.

In this specimen the dural sac ends very slightly higher than usual. When attempting caudal extradural analgesia, the anaesthetist must bear in mind the possibility that the sac may terminate abnormally low and be penetrated by the needle inserted through the sacral hiatus.

Figure 2.26. *Top*. Section through T.12. (See corresponding arrow, Fig. 2.25.) A lumbar puncture at this level might injure the cord. The bases of the denticulate ligaments are seen separating the fibres of the anterior and posterior roots of four lumbar nerves on either side.

Middle. Section through L.1. The conus medullaris can be injured by lumbar puncture at this level. The denticulate ligament has ended. The nerve roots within the dura are L.2–5, which have taken origin higher up, and S.1–2 which have just left the conus.

Bottom. Section through L.2. (See corresponding arrow,

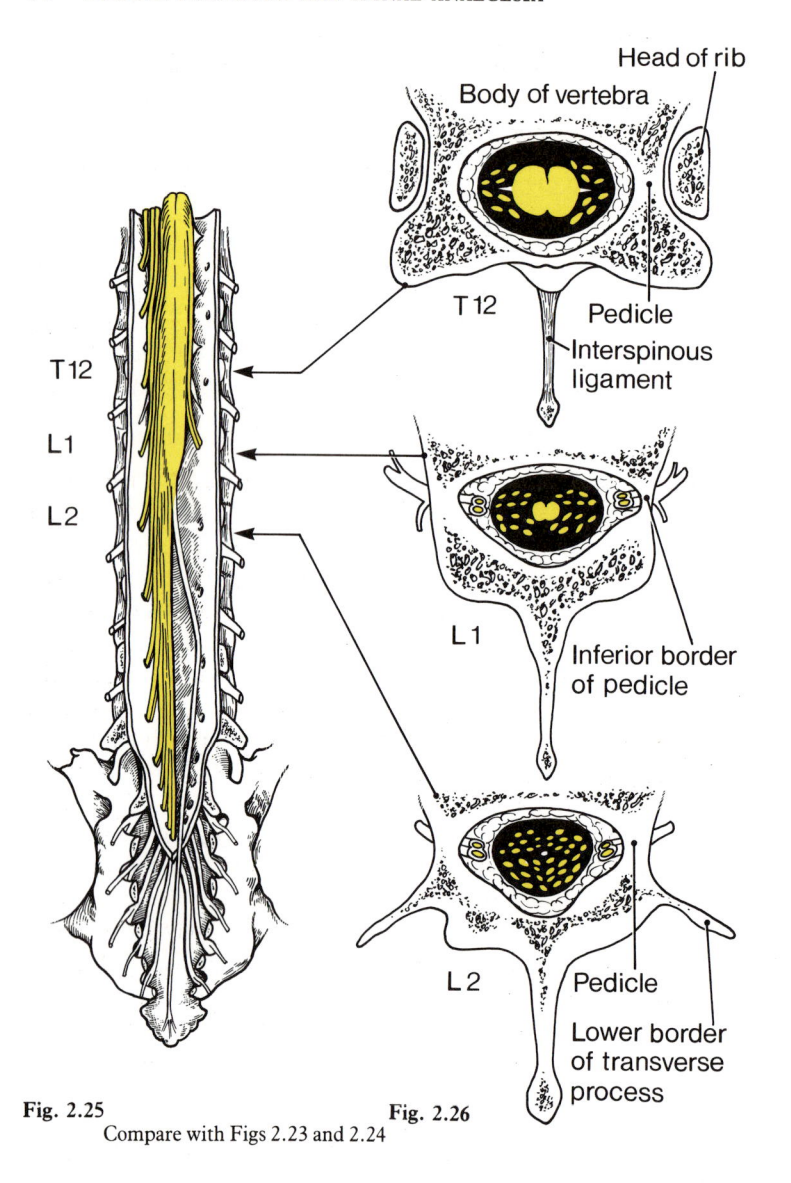

Fig. 2.25.) Lumbar puncture carried out below this level is reasonably free from the danger of injuring the cord which usually terminates at L.1. The theca contains at this level the individual lumbar and sacral nerve roots, each of which, cushioned by cerebrospinal fluid, enjoys considerable mobility as it runs downwards from the cord to its exit from the dura. The descending

nerve roots do not pierce the dura and unite to form the nerve trunk until they reach the level of their particular intervertebral foramen.

The 2nd lumbar nerve has left the dura immediately below this section, and is seen passing through the extradural space to reach the intervertebral foramen just below the border of the pedicle. Outside the dura the nerve is relatively fixed and therefore much more likely to give rise to pain if encountered by the lumbar puncture needle well out of its course. Pain down the thigh is a sure sign that the needle has penetrated the ligamentum flavum and is deep enough for dural puncture, although it has passed too much to one side. All the anaesthetist has to do is to withdraw the needle slightly and reinsert it to the same depth directing the point a little away from the side on which the pain was felt (see Fig. 7.18).

Figure 2.27. The bodies of L.1, 2, 3 and most of 4 have been removed by sawing through the pedicles, and across the lower border of the body of L.4. The roots of the 4th lumbar nerve in their dural coverings run across the extradural space, and the nerve is seen leaving the inter-vertebral foramen. In the 3rd lumbar interspace, the extradural fat and vessels have been left intact. The left 3rd lumbar nerve, cut from its dural attachment, is seen leaving the intervertebral foramen immediately in front of the lateral margin of the ligamentum flavum, which can be discerned through the fat.

In the space above, the fat and vessels have been cleared away to show the posterior boundaries of the extradural space — the ventral aspect of the upper halves of the laminae and the ligamenta flava.

In the uppermost space, the ligamenta flava and the capsules surrounding the articular facets have been removed. Even allowing for the fact that the specimen is in the extended cadaveric position, the interlaminar foramen is much smaller than visualised before the ligamenta flava are removed. When the spine is flexed the inferior articular facets of one vertebra ride up on the superior facets of the vertebra below, considerably increasing the size of the interlaminar space.

Figure 2.28. *Top*. The approach to the vertebral canal is barred by the lower borders of the laminae of L.2. The ligamentum flavum is seen attached to the anterior surface of the lamina of the upper vertebra.

Bottom. The section has passed through the apex of the interlaminar foramen.

Figure 2.29 *Top*. The section here, in fact, passes through the lowermost part of the interlaminar foramen, and a gap in the bone filled by ligamentum flavum just allows access to the vertebral canal.

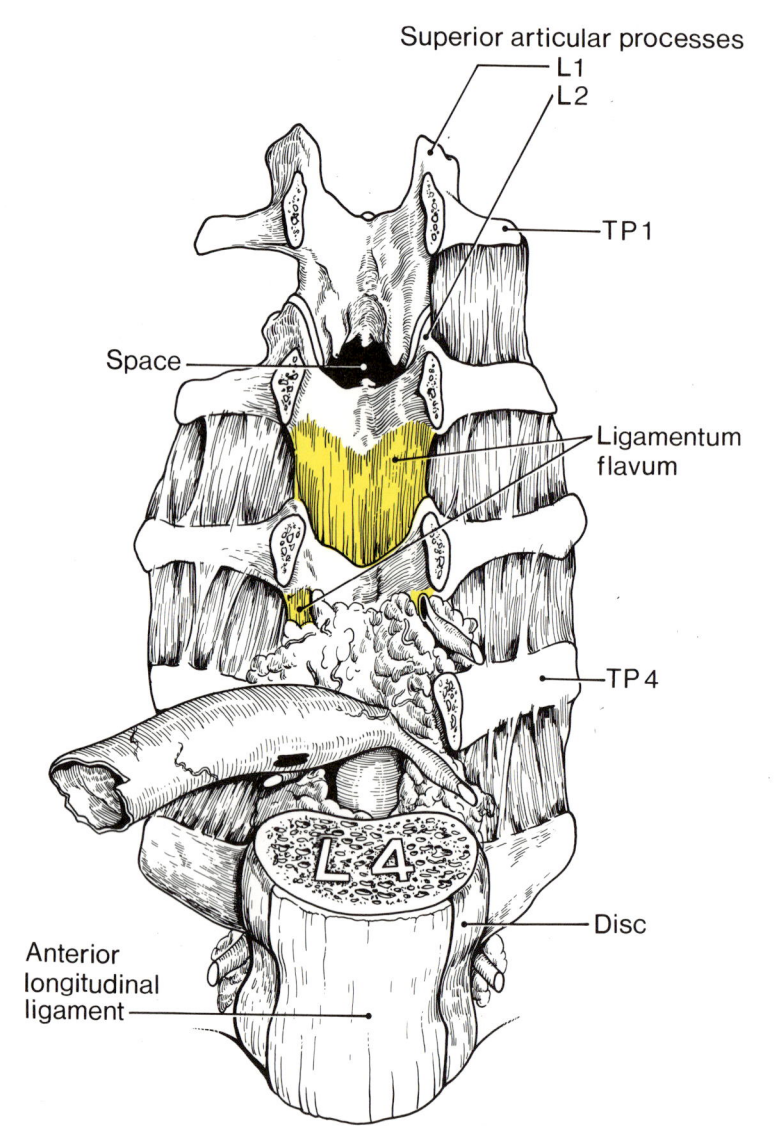

Fig. 2.27 Dissection showing lumbar vertebral canal

The ligament is seen attached to the posterior surface of the lamina of the lower vertebra.

Bottom. Immediately below the level of the interlaminar foramen. The approach to the vertebral canal is barred by the upper borders of the laminae.

ANATOMY 73

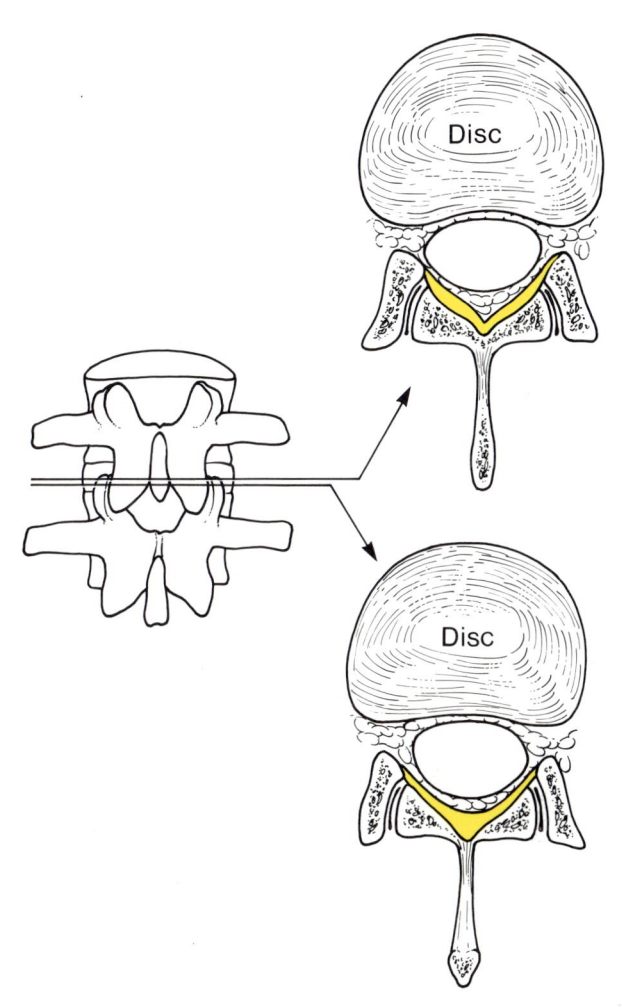

Fig. 2.28 Section through the disc between L.2, 3.

Figure 2.30. An intervertebral disc on top of a lumbar vertebra has been cut through to show the annular fibrous outer cover surrounding the gelatinous nucleus pulposus.

The supraspinous and interspinous ligaments and the ligamenta flava are continuous. The ligamentum flavum is closely connected with the anterior aspect of the capsule surrounding the articular processes. It lies immediately posterior to the lumbar nerve roots (not shown) running from the dural sac across the extradural space to reach the intervertebral foramen. The facets of the superior

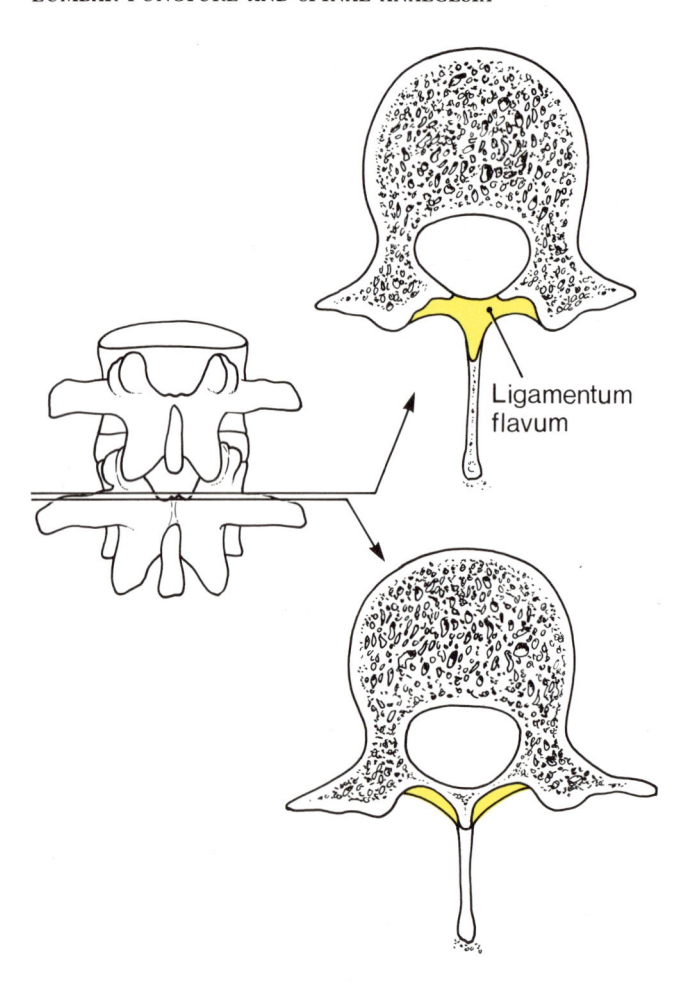

Fig. 2.29 Section through the uppermost part of the lamina of L.3.

articular processes of the lumbar vertebra are seen within their capsules. When the inferior articular processes of the upper vertebra are *in situ*, the breadth of the ligamentum flavum through which a lumbar puncture needle can be passed is much narrowed. The fat in the extradural space is most extensive posteriorly in the median plane, diminishing considerably on the two sides where ligamentum flavum and dura almost touch, and then increasing in volume laterally to become continuous with the fat in the intervertebral foramen.

The anterior part of the extradural space between the dura and the

ANATOMY 75

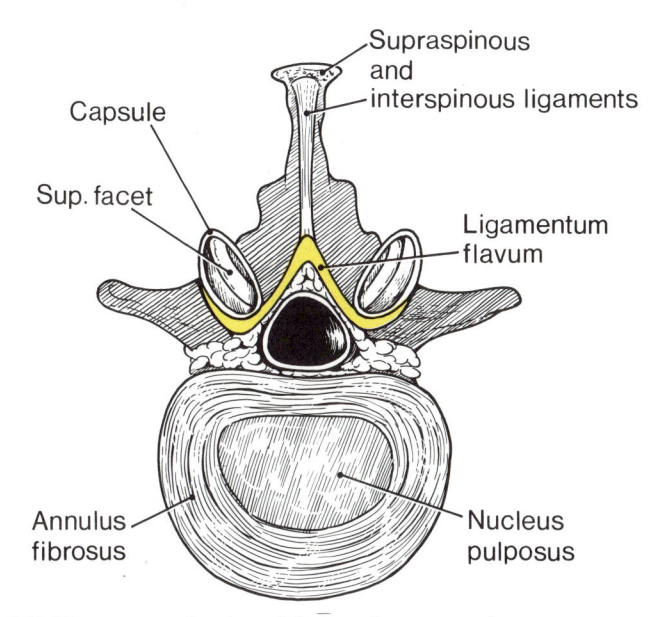

Fig. 2.30 Transverse section through lumbar disc

posterior aspects of the vertebral bodies and discs is very narrow but contains vessels and sometimes a thin strip of fat.

From the picture it will be realised that if it is intended to identify the extradural space, it is better for the needle to penetrate the ligamentum flavum as near the median plane as possible, where the space is deepest. If the needle is pushed through the ligament to one side of the median plane, it is very easy for it to go through the very narrow extradural space and dura with the same movement.

Figure 2.31. The laminae have been cut into as indicated by the

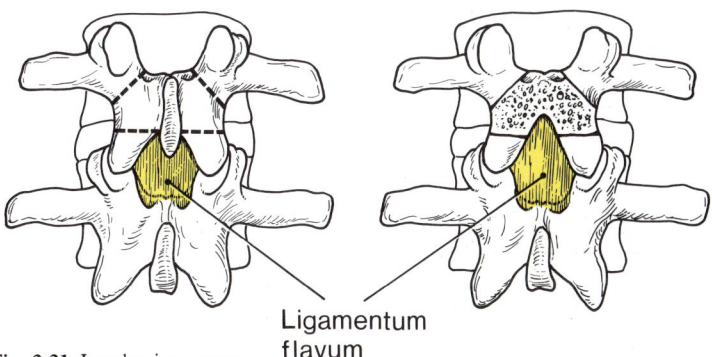

Fig. 2.31 Interlaminar space

interrupted lines and the spine has been removed. If the point of the needle is directed slightly cephalwards during lumbar puncture, it has a better chance of entering the ligamentum flavum than if it is inserted at right angles to the skin.

Figure 2.32. Almost the whole of the cerebellum has been removed and the pia-ependymal roof of the fourth ventricle is shown semi-diagrammatically. The fourth ventricle, the aqueduct of the midbrain and the third ventricle are enclosed by the interrupted lines. The median aperture (foramen of Magendie) is shown and the two lateral openings (ff. Luschka) are indicated. Above the tentorium the cerebrum has been cut coronally and the optic tracts are seen lying on the sides of the midbrain. Below the tentorium the 5th, the 7th and 8th, the 9th, 10th and 11th, and the 12th nerves run across the cranial subarachnoid space to enter their foramina. Below the foramen magnum the cervical nerve roots are seen running across the spinal subarachnoid space to enter their corresponding intervertebral foramina.

This picture explains why a patient loses consciousness if the spinal analgesic solution spreads much higher than was intended.

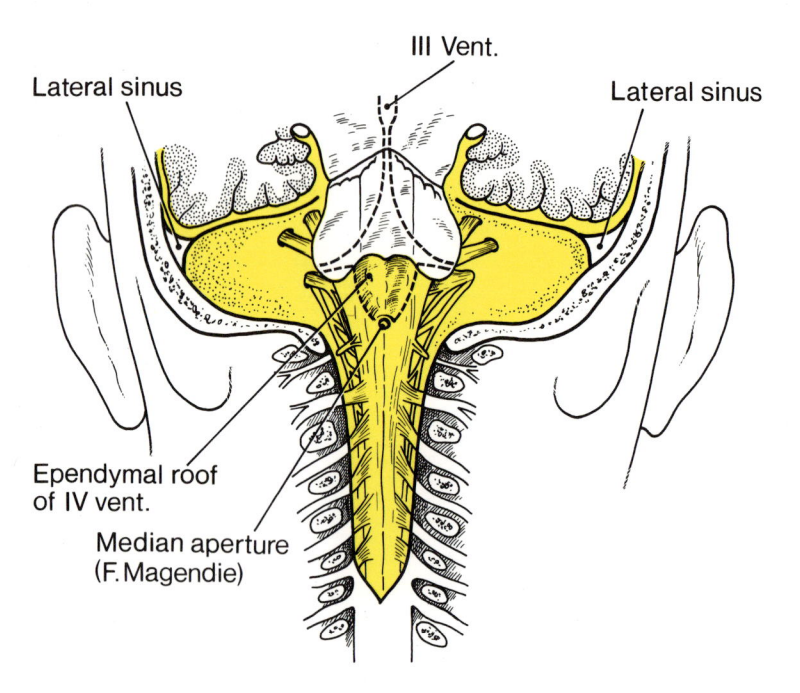

Fig. 2.32 The cerebrospinal fluid pathways.

It is commonly observed that if analgesia extends to the upper thoracic region the patient tends to become drowsy. Moreover, if now a general anaesthetic (e.g. thiopentone) is superimposed only a very small amount is necessary to produce unconsciousness; and respiratory arrest follows the administration of doses which would not have this effect if the patient were not under spinal block.

Consciousness is maintained by 'an awareness of the body' and of the environment. Consciousness lapses in the absence of sensory impulses to the cortex. It is clear, and the authors can testify from personal experience, that the higher a spinal analgesic spreads the more the awareness of the body is diminished. The area from which the cortex receives stimuli is lessened. If the solution spreads to the foramen magnum, sensory stimuli from the body are eliminated and the patient remains awake by virtue of stimuli reaching the cortex from the cranial sensory nerves.

When a person courts sleep, he does what he can to eliminate outside stimuli. A conscious patient is certainly in possession of some at least of his five senses. If a patient is deprived of all five senses can he remain conscious? The subject is one suitable for discussion by the philosopher, but the practical answer is probably contained in the observation that the higher a spinal analgesic solution spreads, the greater the tendency for the patient to become drowsy and lose consciousness in a way no more unpleasant than going to sleep. Tactile sensibility of the trunk is eliminated early, and if spinal analgesia extends high enough to spread through the cranial subarachnoid space, taste, hearing, sight and smell are also soon lost. Contact with the outside world is now lost and the patient becomes unconscious.

It is well known that in local analgesia and central neural blockade, sensory nerve fibres are affected before motor. If the concentration of analgesic is low enough there can be sensory loss without motor paralysis. In really high spinal analgesia the skin over the neck (C.2, 3, 4) can be insensitive when the diaphragm, supplied by the motor roots of the phrenic (C.3, 4, 5), still functions. When the spinal analgesia is more extensive still, the patient loses consciousness. Even now diaphragmatic activity may be enough to sustain life. On the other hand respiration may cease and there is no means then of knowing whether the motor roots of the phrenic are affected, or whether some of the analgesic solution has entered the fourth ventricle and reached the respiratory centre located there. In either case the treatment is the same. Give artificial ventilation preferably with added oxygen, until the local analgesic is eliminated and normal respiration begins again. The duration of the respiratory paralysis depends on the drug used: in the case of lignocaine the time is about an hour, and with cinchocaine or bupivacaine the period may be up to two or even three hours. Provided the patient is kept well ventilated and well oxygenated during this time, he will be little the worse for the misadventure.

Figure 2.33. The visceral motor nerve supply to the abdominal and pelvic organs are derived from both sympathetic and parasympathetic components of the autonomic nervous system. Sympathetic preganglionic axons arise from cells in the intermedio-lateral horn of the cord from T.5 to L.1 (or 2) inclusive. Leaving the cord, they travel with the anterior roots across both the intra- and the extradural spaces and they are of course myelinated. Leaving the extradural space, these fibres separate from the anterior roots and pass in the white rami communicantes through the paravertebral ganglia and fuse to form the three splanchnic nerves on each side. These enter the abdomen by piercing the crura of the diaphragm and end in the coeliac (splanchnic) and the other pre-aortic plexuses from which they reach the viscera with the arterial supply, after synapsing, as postganglionic fibres.

Visceral afferent impulses from the abdomen travel along fibres which accompany the efferent sympathetic fibres, pass through the paravertebral sympathetic ganglia and proceed up the splanchnic

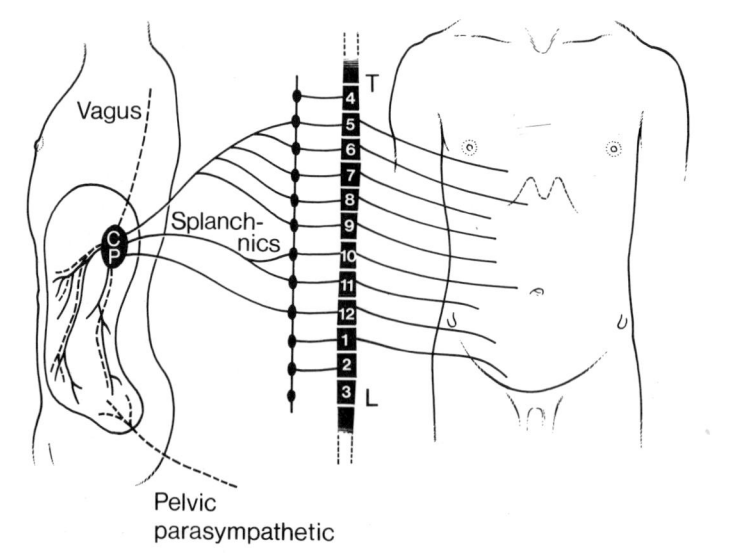

Fig. 2.33 Diagram of afferent nerve supply

nerves to enter the spinal nerves via the white rami. They then make for the posterior root ganglia up to T.5 where they have their cell stations.

The visceral parasympathetic nerves leave the central nervous system in two distinct parts. That section of the cranial parasympathetic outflow which supplies the viscera consists of fibres in the vagus nerves which run their course outside the vertebral canal to enter the abdomen, passing through the hole in the diaphragm with the oesophagus at the level of the 10th thoracic vertebra, innervate the stomach, and communicate freely with the coeliac plexus through which they are distributed to the rest of the alimentary canal up to the distal part of the transverse colon. The sacral parasympathetic or sacral outflow consists of fibres which leave the 2nd, 3rd and 4th sacral nerves to supply the splenic flexure, descending colon, and pelvic organs.

The abdominal wall is supplied by nerve fibres which enter and leave the cord between the 5th or 6th thoracic and 1st or 2nd lumbar segments of the cord. It is seen therefore, that if spinal analgesia reaches as high as T.5, the abdominal wall will be rendered insensitive and paralysed. Also the sympathetic nerve supply of the abdominal viscera will be interrupted, but the fibres of the vagi, because of their extravertebral course, remain unaffected.

When the abdomen is opened, the facts that the vagi contain sensory fibres and that they remain active can be demonstrated by traction on the mesentery: nausea and a poorly localised but distressing abdominal discomfort result, the blood-pressure falls and sweating of the head and neck is sometimes observed. Provided the mesentery is not pulled on, an abdominal operation under reasonably high central neural blockade can be carried out painlessly. In upper abdominal surgery a certain amount of traction appears to be almost inevitable, and in these cases the surgeon is well advised to infiltrate with local analgesic the vagus nerves on both the anterior and posterior surfaces of the lower end of the gullet to abolish the transmission of unpleasant stimuli via these fibres.

Motor paralysis of the splanchnic nerves is revealed by the contracted tape-like condition of the gut, and this effect is accentuated by the unopposed and unimpaired tonic action of the vagi on the muscle of the intestinal wall. This condition is the exact opposite of the contraction of the sphincters and the distension of the gut which frequently follows the operation of vagotomy in the treatment of peptic ulcer, for here the action of the splanchnic nerves on the gut is unopposed.

In high central neural blockade the heart rate is affected. The rate at which the heart beats is an indication of the preponderance of the influence of the sympathetic or the parasympathetic nervous system on that organ. The rate is increased by the action of the sympathetic cardiac accelerator fibres which leave the 2nd, 3rd and 4th thoracic segments, and the rate is decreased by stimulation of the vagus. If a spinal analgesic reaches as high as the upper thoracic nerve roots some of the sympathetic fibres to the heart are put out of action. The action of the vagus now predominates and the heart rate slows, commonly to 45 to 60 per minute.

Figure 2.33 can be used too to emphasise the point that both the good and the bad effects of central neural blockade depend not on the mass of local analgesic drug injected, but on the height which the drug reaches. Let us assume that bupivacaine solution is injected and reaches the 5th or 6th thoracic segment of the spinal cord. All the desirable results of this — the freedom from pain below this level, the relaxation, and the lack of response to surgical stimuli are due to the fact that the drug has reached just this level. Similarly any ill effects — for example, low blood-pressure and impaired respiratory exchange due to paralysis of intercostal muscles — are attributable to the same cause. The good and the bad effects depend not in the least on whether the patient is given a certain amount of bupivacaine; they depend on the level within the dural canal reached by the drug. If in each case the drug reaches the same cord level the results are indistinguishable.

Figure 2.34. Lumbar vertebrae 1, 2, 3. The last thoracic and first

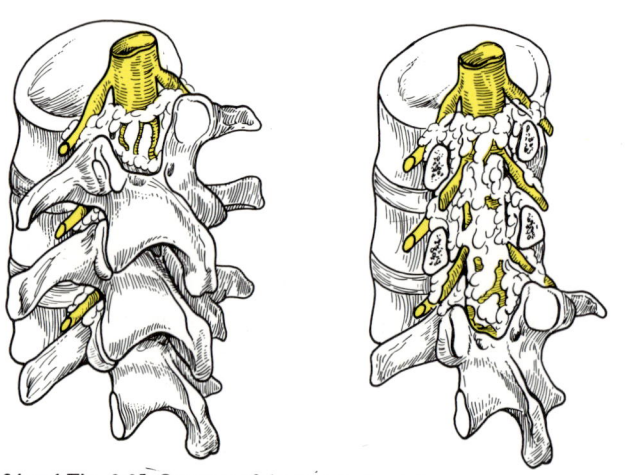

Fig. 2.34 and **Fig. 2.35** Contents of the vertebral canal

two lumbar nerves on the left side are seen leaving the intervertebral foramina surrounded by fat, which is continuous with the fat in the extradural space.

Figure 2.35. The pedicles have been sawn through, and the vertebral arches of L.1 and 2 have been removed, showing the contents of the vertebral canal.

Figure 2.36. The fat and vessels of the extradural space have been cleared leaving the main structures in the vertebral canal, the cord and membranes running vertically, and the spinal nerve roots in their dural sheaths running almost horizontally, to reach their intervertebral foramina.

Figure 2.37. The cord and membranes have been removed to show the posterior longitudinal ligament forming the continuous anterior boundary of the vertebral canal.

Fig. 2.36 Dural sac in vertebral canal

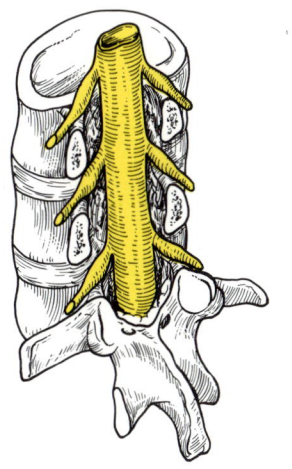

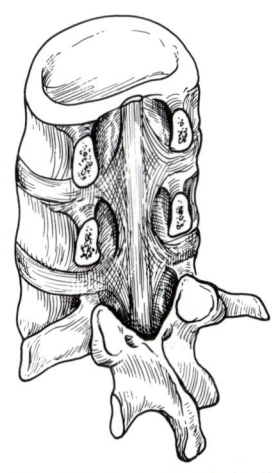

Fig. 2.37 Posterior longitudinal ligament

Figure 2.38 and 2.39. The skin over the back is commonly connected by fibrous strands with the supraspinous ligament, a local condensation of the lumbar aponeurosis. When a fat patient is sitting, the resultant furrow between the layers of fat over the lumbar muscles is central (Fig. 2.38). If she lies down on one side the furrow may remain almost in the mid-line; but usually it sags considerably below the line joining the spinous processes (Fig. 2.39). The spines are not readily palpable, but the anaesthetist must not be tempted to be guided by sight when deciding where to insert his needle: for if he accepts the furrow as a landmark he will start

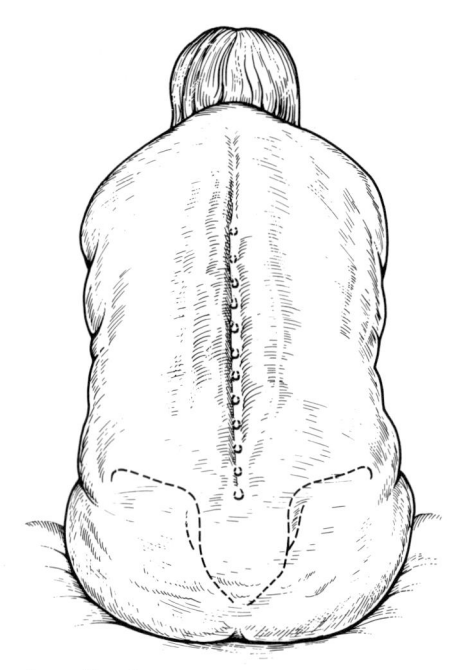

Fig. 2.38 Furrow in median plane

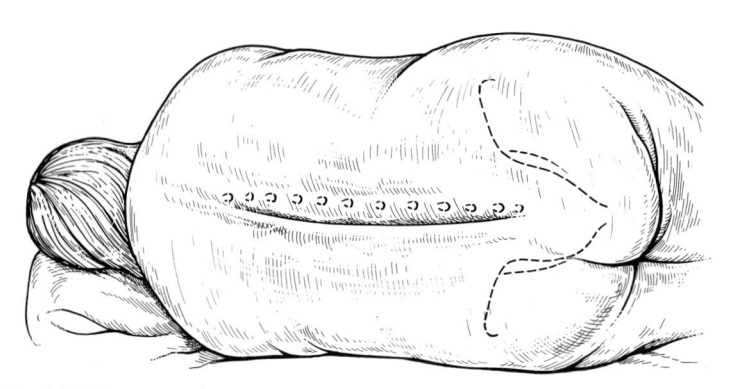

Fig. 2.39 Furrow sagging

frequently well lateral to where he imagines himself to be. He should dig his fingers deeply into the back to find the mid-line. Individual spinous processes will not be recognised, but the general direction taken by them will.

With the really fat patient the difficulties of lumbar puncture may be increased for two reasons. The first is the uncertainty in defining the outline of any one spinous process from which the course of the needle is set; and the second is that the depth at which the cerebrospinal fluid will be encountered cannot be predicted accurately. It is in these cases, where the course of the needle may have to be changed once or twice before success is achieved, that the anaesthetist is advised to avail himself of a director (p. 179), and to keep to the mid-line throughout.

The distance the needle must be inserted before the extradural space is reached is remarkably constant in the average individual, but it is much more difficult to estimate in the fat subject. Gutiérrez (Gutiérrez, 1939) in a personal series of 3200 cases, found the distance varied from 2.5 to 8 cm, but in 80 per cent of this large series the range narrowed down to 4 to 5 cm. The increased depth in fat people is due primarily to the fat in the subcutaneous tissue, but depends also on the angulation of the needle. If the needle happens to go in almost at right angles (Fig. 2.40A), the depth will be much less than if it has to be angulated steeply (B1) to avoid the lamina.

The distance between the ligamentum flavum and the dura varies from an average of 5 to 6 mm in the lumbar region to 1.5 or 2 mm in the lower cervical region; at the upper thoracic level it may be 3 to 4 mm. In some patients in the median plane it may be as little as 2 mm (Husemeyer et al, 1978).

Figure 2.40. The posterior surface of the lamina of a lumbar vertebra slopes downwards and backwards. The upper border lies at the same depth as the ligamentum flavum which is attached to it; the

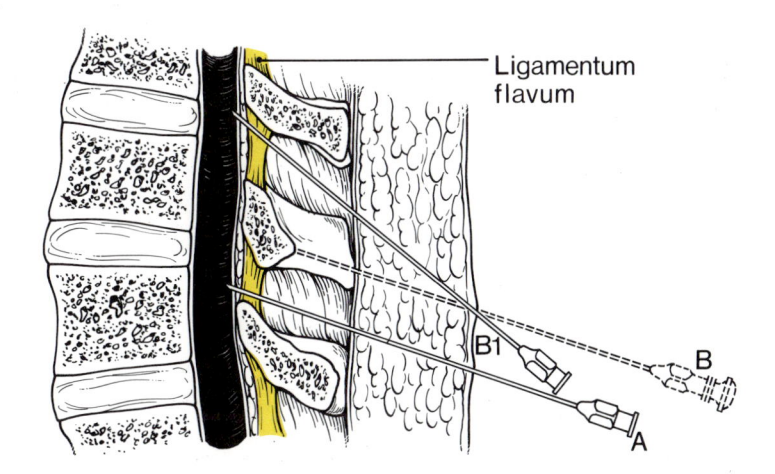

Fig. 2.40 Differences in direction of needle

lower border is considerably more superficial. In patients of average build the distance from the skin to ligamentum flavum varies a little from 4 to 5 cm. A lumbar puncture needle with distance markings (Lee, 1960) is often helpful in these and other patients. If, therefore, the needle, slightly out of the median plane, encounters bone at a shallow depth, it is the lower border of the lamina on which it impinges; if the obstruction is deep it is the upper border. This information is of great help when deciding what alteration should be made in the angle at which the needle is reinserted.

Figure 2.41. Although the distribution of the intercostal nerves overlaps slightly, the skin over the abdominal wall and the lower part of the thorax is generally regarded as being innervated in serial bands from the corresponding segments of the cord. The skin over the lowest part of the abdominal wall is supplied by L.1. If the analgesic spreads to the 10th thoracic nerve roots, analgesia of the skin extends up to the umbilicus. The 6th or 7th intercostal nerve supplies the skin at the level of the xiphisternum.

When central neural blockade is induced for an upper abdominal operation, it can be predicted with considerable assurance that analgesia of the parietes will reach, and stop at, the nipple line. If a heavy solution is injected the reason can be found in Figures 8.2 and 8.15. But even if a totally different technique is followed, skin analgesia is practically sure to stop at the same landmark. The explanation lies in the fact that the skin over the upper part of the thorax has a double innervation: it is supplied not only by the corresponding intercostal nerves but by the descending branches of the cervical plexus which join the 3rd and 4th cervical segments of the cord. Even if the spinal analgesic solution were to spread as high as C.5 — high enough to anaesthetise the skin of the upper extremities — the skin over the thorax above the nipple line, and over the shoulders, would still be sensitive.

In assessing the level that the block has reached, a knowledge of myotomes and their nerve supply is sometimes useful. For example, hip flexion is controlled by L.2 and 3; hip extension by L.4 and 5; knee-joint flexion by L.3 and 4, and extension by L.5 and S.1; dorsiflexion of the ankle joint by L.4 and 5; plantar flexion by S.1 and 2 (Last, 1978).

Cutaneous sensibility is as follows: middle finger, C.7; apex of axilla, T.3; tip of xiphisternum, T.7; umbilicus, T.10; inguinal ligament, T.12; front of knee, L.3; medial side of calf, L.4; lateral side of calf, L.5; outer border of foot, S.1; back of knee, S.2.

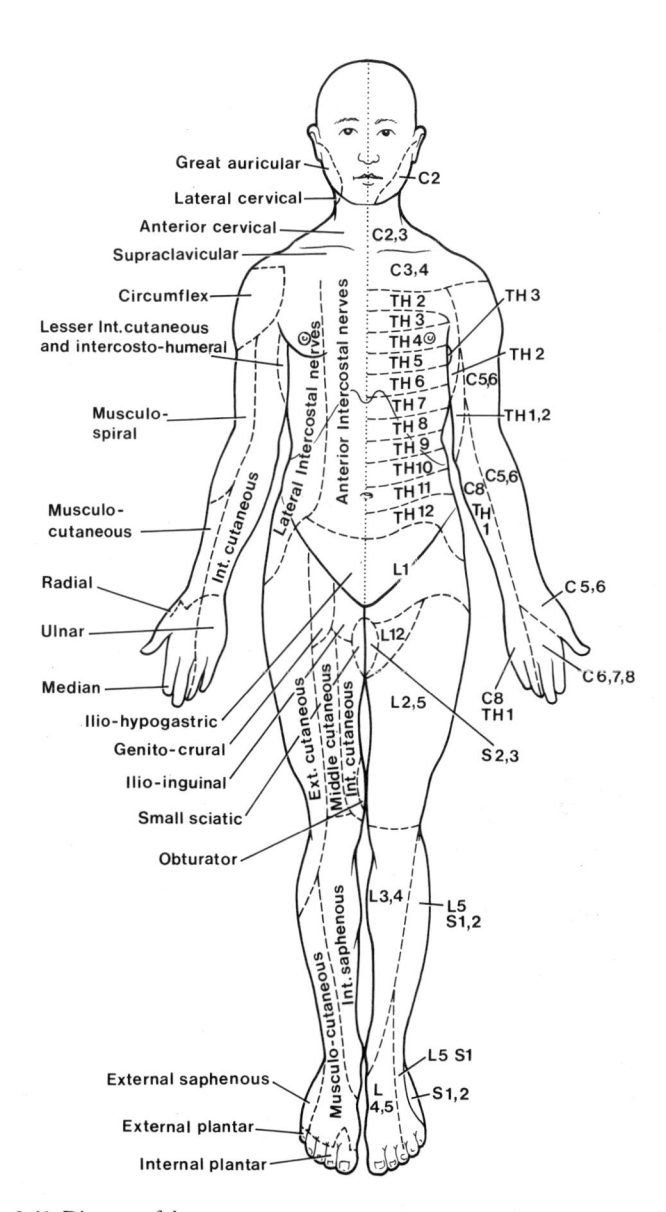

Fig. 2.41 Diagram of dermatomes

REFERENCES

Ballin, N. C. (1981) Paraplegia following epidural analgesia. *Anaesthesia*, **36**, 952.
Batson, O. V. (1940) The function of the vertebral veins and their role in the spread of metastases. *Annals of Surgery*, **112**, 138.
Boys, J. E. & Norman, P. F. (1975) Accidental subdural injection. *British Journal of Anaesthesia*, **47**, 1111.
Bozeman, P. M. & Chandra, P. (1980) Epidural and subarachnoid block; unilateral analgesia following. *Anesthesiology*, **52**, 356.
Bromage, P. R., Joval, A. C. & Binney, J. C. (1963) Local anesthetic drugs: penetration from spinal epidural space into neuraxis. *Science*, **140**, 292.
Chaudhari, L. S., Kop, B. R. & Dhruva, A. J. (1978) Paraplegia and epidural analgesia. *Anaesthesia*, **33**, 722.
Cohen, C. A. & Kallos, T. (1972) Failure of spinal anesthesia due to subdural catheter placement. *Anesthesiology*, **37**, 352.
Corning, J. L. (1900) *Medical Record* (NY), **58**, 601–604; cf. p. 602.
Costello, T. G. & Fisher, A. (1983) Neurological complications following aortic surgery. *Anaesthesia*, **38**, 230.
Crisp, E. J. (1955) *Guy's Hospital Gazette*, **69**, 475–482.
Critchley, E. M. R. (1982) Lumbar spinal stenosis. *British Medical Journal*, **284**, 1588.
Djindjian, R. (1970) Angiography of the spinal cord and canal. *Proceedings of the Royal Society of Medicine*, **63**, 181.
Domisse, G. F. (1976) *Arteries and Veins of the Human Spinal Cord from Birth*. Edinburgh: Churchill Livingstone.
Edgar, M. A. & Nundy, S. J. (1966) Innervation of the spinal dura mater. *Journal of Neurology and Psychiatry*, **29**, 530.
Gilliatt, L. A. (1958) *Journal of Comparative Neurology*, **110**, 75.
Grant, J. C. B. (1952) *A Method of Anatomy*, p. 625, 5th edn. London.
Gutiérrez, A. (1939) *Anestesia Extradural*, p. 40. Buenos Aires.
Heile, B. (1913) Der epidurale Raum. *Archiv für Klinische Chirurgie*, **101**, 845.
Husemeyer, R. P. & White, D. C. (1980) Topography of the epidural space. *Anaesthesia*, **35**, 7.
Husemeyer, R. P., White, D. C. & Smolenski, T. (1978) The shape of the lumbar extradural space with reference to accidental puncture. *British Journal of Anaesthesia*, **50**, 631P.
Kuntz, A. (1950) *A Text-book of Neuro-anatomy*, p. 148, 5th edn. London.
Last, R. J. (1978) *Anatomy: Regional and Applied*, 6th edn. Edinburgh: Churchill Livingstone.
Lee, J. Alfred (1960) A specially marked needle to facilitate extradural block. *Anaesthesia*, **15**, 156.
Luyendijk, W. & van Voorthuisen, A. E. (1966) *Acta Radiologica (Diagnosis)*, **5**, 1051.
Macintosh, R. R. & Mushin, W. W. (1947) Observations on the epidural space. *Anaesthesia*, **2**, 100.
Mehta, M. & Maher, R. (1977) Injection into the extra-arachnoid subdural space. *Anaesthesia*, **32**, 760.
Mixter, W. J. & Barr, J. S. (1934) Rupture of the intervertebral disc with involvement of the spinal canal. *New England Journal of Medicine*, **211**, 210.
Naffziger, H. G. & Boldrey, E. S. (1946) Surgery of the spinal cord. In Bancroft, F. W. & Pilcher, C. (eds) *Surgical Treatment of the Nervous System*, p. 377. Philadelphia.
Nunn, J. F. & Slavin G. (1980) Posterior intercostal nerve block for pain relief after cholecystectomy. *British Journal of Anaesthesia*, **52**, 253.
Ranson, S. W. (1953) *The Anatomy of the Nervous System*, p. 20, 9th edn. Revised by S. L. Clark, Philadelphia.

Reimann, A. F. & Anson, B. J. (1944) Vertebral level of termination of the spinal cord, with report of a case of sacral cord. *Anatomical Record*, **88**, 127.

Rexed, B. A. & Wennstrom, K. G. (1959) Arachnoidal proliferation and cystic formation in the spinal nerve root pouches in man. *Journal of Neurology*, **16**, 73.

Schultz, E. H. & Brogdon, B. G. (1962) The problem of subdural placement in myelography. *Radiology*, **79**, 91.

Sechzer, P. H. (1963) The subdural space in spinal anesthesia. *Anesthesiology*, **24**, 869.

Sharrock, N. E. (1979) Recordings of and anatomical explanations for false positive loss of resistance during extradural analgesia. *British Journal of Anaesthesia*, **51**, 253.

Steer, J. L. & Horney, F. D. (1968) Evidence for the passage of cerebrospinal fluid along spinal nerves. *Canadian Medical Association Journal*, **98**, 71.

Taylor, J. A. (1940) Lumbo-sacral subarachnoid tap. *Journal of Urology*, **43**, 561.

Wells, C. E. C. (1966) Clinical aspects of spinovascular disease. *Proceedings of the Royal Society of Medicine*, **59**, 790; and (1967) Annotation. *Lancet*, **2**, 143.

3

Cerebrospinal fluid

The term cerebrospinal fluid was first used by Magendie the French physiologist (1783–1855) in 1825 (Magendie, 1825) who also brought to light the earlier work of Dominicus Cotunnius (1736–1822) of 1764.

Source

The cerebrospinal fluid is mostly derived from the choroid plexuses which are formed in all four ventricles of the brain by the invagination of vessels into the intradural space. These vascular protrusions, supported in a matrix of pia, are thrown into many folds which carry on their surfaces a great number of minute lobulated tufts into each of which afferent and efferent vessels may be traced; the capillaries are in intimate contact with the ependyma, the single layered epithelium lining the ventricle (see Figs 3.1 and 3.2).

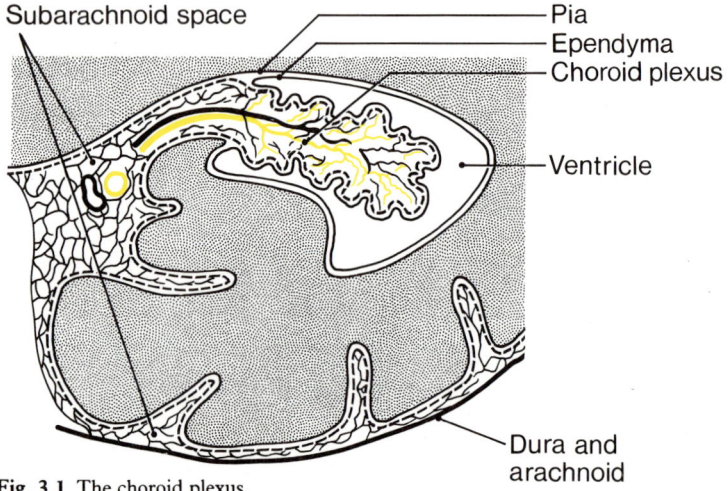

Fig. 3.1 The choroid plexus.

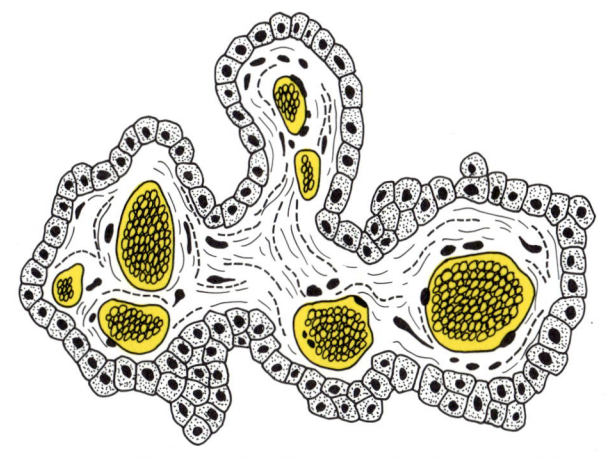

Fig. 3.2 Section of a villus of the choroid plexus. (After Maximov and Bloom, 1952.)

Method of formation

It is now held that, besides permitting selective filtration, the cells of the ependyma have a secretory function (Voetmann, 1949). This theory is strengthened by the vacuolation which is seen when the cells are examined microscopically.

The present uncertainty which prevails about the method of its formation is made evident in some quarters by referring to cerebrospinal fluid somewhat vaguely as a 'selective transudate'.

It is estimated that an amount equal to the total volume is secreted every four hours but an increased rate of production is not seen under physiological conditions. Decreased production occurs in hypothermia, respiratory and metabolic acidosis, and after the administration of such drugs as acetazolamide, frusemide, ouabain, spirolactone and vasopressin.

Absorption is probably due to the hydrostatic pressure differences between sinus blood and the CSF and not to osmotic pressure differences (Plum and Siesjo, 1975).

Circulation

As much as 500 ml may be secreted in 24 hours (Cutler, 1968). The bulk is formed in the lateral ventricles and passes through the interventricular foramina (of Monro) to mix with the fluid produced in the third ventricle in the diencephalon (Fig. 3.3 & 3.4). From here it passes along the aqueduct of Sylvius in the mesencephalon to

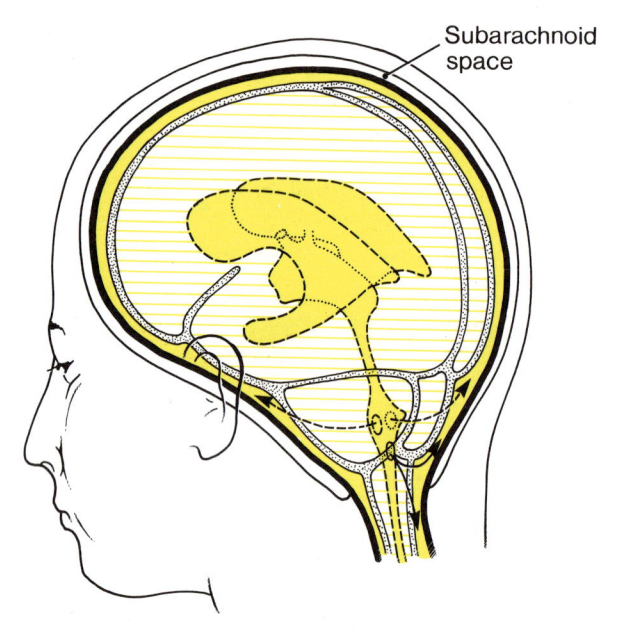

Fig. 3.3 The cerebral ventricles.

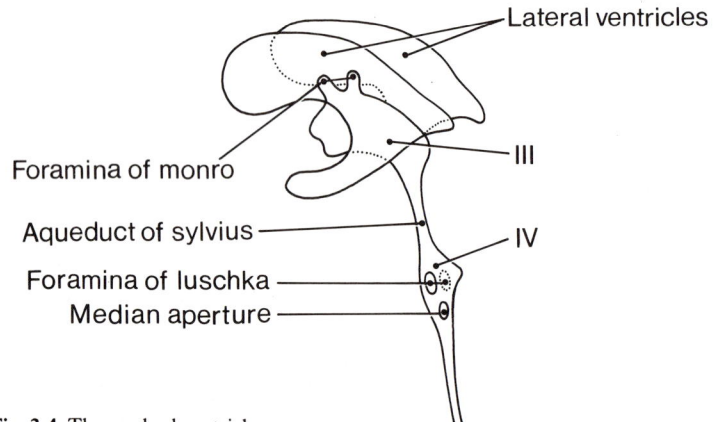

Fig. 3.4 The cerebral ventricles.

the fourth ventricle, which is superior to the brainstem between the pons, medulla and cerebellum, and reaches the subarachnoid space by flowing through the three openings in the roof of this ventricle; the two foramina of the lateral recesses (Luschka) lead forward from either side to the region of the cisterna pontis, and the median aperture (of Magendie) drains backwards into the cerebellomedullary cistern. The flow is mainly but not entirely from within the ventricular system, outwards. These cisterns at the base of the brain communicate freely with the spinal subarachnoid space, but the main circulation of fluid continues in the cerebral subarachnoid space upwards through the opening in the tentorium cerebelli, and then over the cerebral hemispheres. The cerebrospinal fluid passes back into the bloodstream by filtration and osmosis. Transference takes place chiefly in the supratentorial region, through arachnoid villi and granulations, Pacchionian bodies (Fig. 3.5), formed where the arachnoid bulges into and penetrates the meningeal dura to come into direct contact with the endothelium of the great venous sinuses.

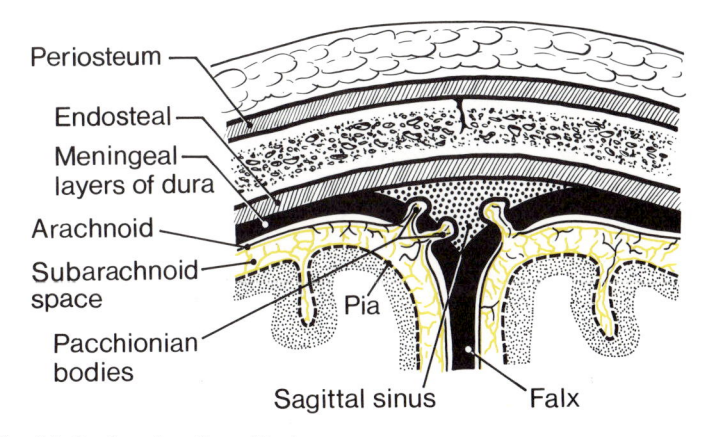

Fig. 3.5 Section of surface of brain

Some authorities (Davies, 1962) hold that there is no active circulation of cerebrospinal fluid in the spinal subarachnoid space but that osmosis, alterations in posture, and arterial pulsations tend to keep the composition of the fluid constant. Others believe that there is a slow circulation downwards and that fluid passes directly into venous plexuses in the spinal subarachnoid space (Nash, 1942; Howarth and Copper, 1949), and that some leaves the dural sac along the course of the segmental nerves to be absorbed by the lymphatics (Field and Brierly, 1948) (Fig. 3.6).

There is no suggestion that any circulation of cerebrospinal fluid there may be in the spinal subarachnoid space influences the distribution of analgesic solutions injected there. Moreover, in the rare event of an analgesic solution reaching as high as the foramen magnum, it is easier for it to spread in the cerebral subarachnoid

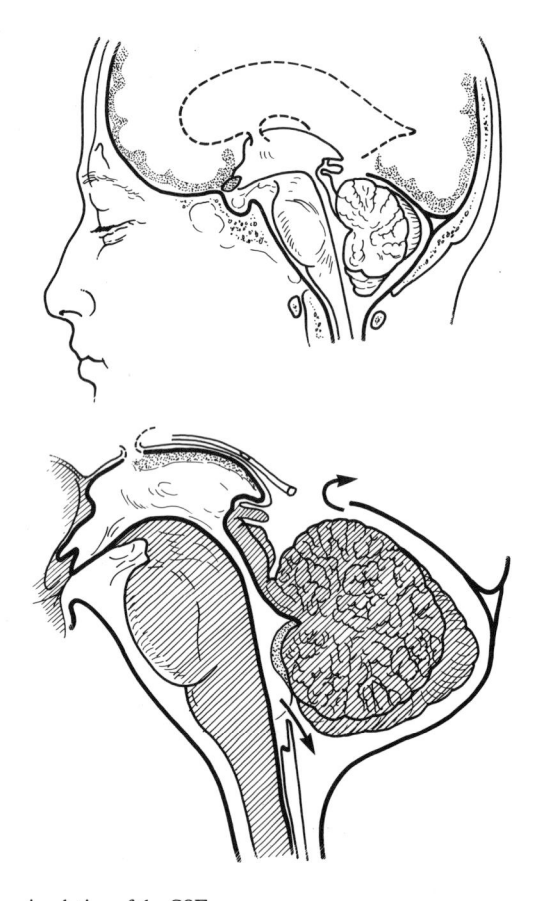

Fig. 3.6 The circulation of the CSF.

space anaesthetising the cranial nerves as they pass across it, than it is for the solution to enter the foramina of Luschka and Magendie 'against the stream' and gain access to the respiratory and cardiac centres situated in the floor of the fourth ventricle. The cerebrospinal fluid comes into contact with the nerve cells of the cortex and the basal ganglia (Davies, 1962).

Composition

The cerebrospinal fluid is clear, colourless, and does not clot on standing. It has the same pH as serum, 7.4, so that it is just alkaline. The P_{CO_2} is 50 mmHg and the sodium bicarbonate concentration is about 22 mmol/l (Thompson and Johnson, 1982). The specific gravity of the fluid at body temperature, referred to water at 4°C, is 1.003. The protein content, up to 0.3 g per 1, is very low, and the antibody value is correspondingly poor. The glucose content of 1.5 to 4.0 mmol/l is also low, and the chloride content is the main factor in keeping the cerebrospinal fluid in osmotic equilibrium with the plasma. In normal health the cells present in the cerebrospinal fluid are almost entirely lymphocytes and their number does not exceed 5 per ml.

Functions

The cerebrospinal fluid does not contain any substances not found in the blood: this lends colour to the idea that its purpose is mainly a physical one. By acting as a mechanical buffer the fluid absorbs and distributes the force of a blow on the head, thus affording considerable protection to the brain and cord. It acts as a hydraulic shock absorber. The deep collections of fluid in the cisternae around the base of the brain serve admirably as a water cushion. The fluid here floats the brain. As Livingstone points out (Livingstone, 1950), 'The comparative densities of cerebrospinal fluid and nervous tissue are such that a brain and spinal cord weighing about 1500 grams when removed from the craniospinal chambers would have a net weight *in situ* of less than 50 grams.' The cerebrospinal fluid is also a compensatory mechanism whereby the pressures in the cranial and spinal cavities are equalised and kept within physiological limits.

There is no evidence of the presence of lymphatics anywhere throughout the central nervous system; the removal of waste products arising from the activity of the nerve cells, therefore, must be effected by some other means. As an artery penetrates the brain substance, it carries with it a thin layer of pia (Fig. 2.16), and the potential perivascular space is thus continuous with the subarachnoid space (Fig. 3.5). Cerebrospinal fluid is in free communication with the interstitial fluid of the brain, the two making up the cerebral extracellular fluid. This transports humoral messages from one part of the brain to another and removes the waste products of cerebral cellular metabolism. The pH of extracellular fluid regulates pulmonary ventilation and cerebral blood flow. The acid base balance appears to be regulated differently from that of blood (Plum and Siesjo, 1975).

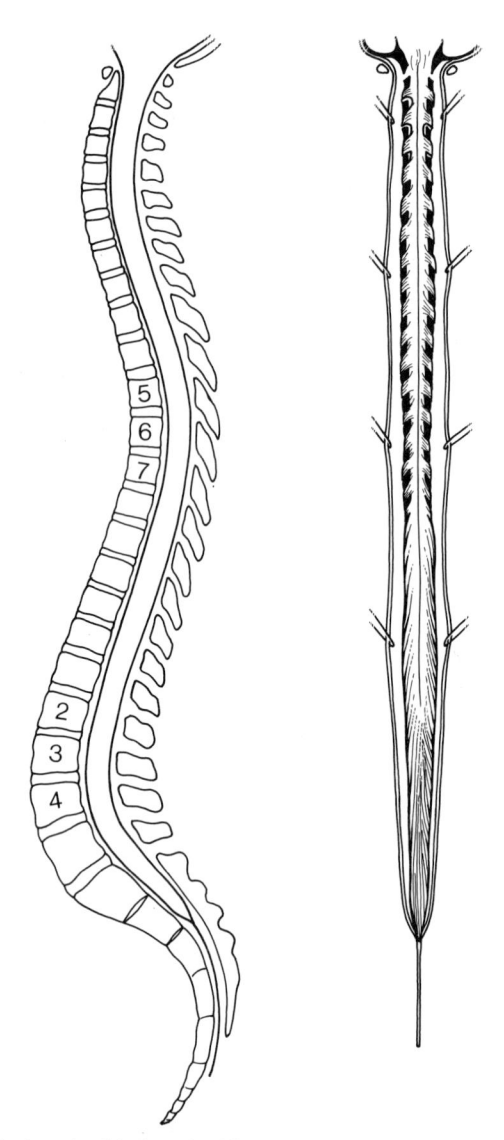

Fig. 3.7 The intradural (subarachnoid) space.

Volume

In an adult the volume is about 135 ml. Of this, 35 ml is contained in the ventricles, 25 ml in the intracranial subarachnoid space, and 75 ml within the spinal theca (O'Connell, 1970).

Pressure

There are small rhythmic fluctuations in the pressure of the cerebrospinal fluid. These fluctuations, readily seen on a manometer attached to a lumbar puncture needle, are related to cardiac impulse and respiration and may play their part in circulation and absorption of the fluid.

When the patient sits up, the column of cerebrospinal fluid bulges the spinal theca into the loosely filled extradural space. The pressures in the ventricles, and even in the basal cisterns, are now slightly below atmospheric so that a ventricular or cisternal puncture will not yield fluid except on suction. The pressure within the theca depends almost entirely on the hydrostatic pressure of the fluid above the level at which the needle is inserted. For this reason readings taken with the patient in the sitting position give no indication of the real cerebrospinal fluid pressure. This can be measured only when the patient is horizontal (Fig. 3.8). Then the pressures in the ventricles, cisternae and lumbar sac are equal. Normally the figures lies within the range of 70 to 170 mm water.

One of the functions of cerebrospinal fluid is to stabilise the pressure within the skull. Since the walls are rigid, any change in volume of one of the contents, brain, blood or cerebrospinal fluid must be compensated for by a change in the opposite direction in the others. The blood volume of the brain fluctuates according to physiological requirements and any increase must be accompanied by a decrease in the volume of cerebrospinal fluid: otherwise the

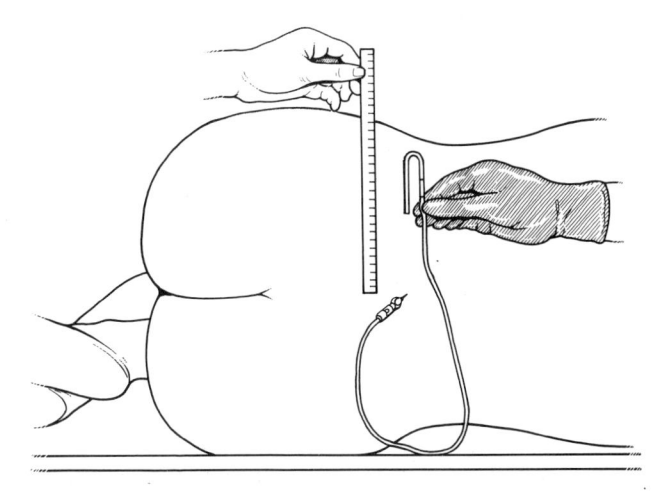

Fig. 3.8 Measurement of the CSF pressure.

brain will be compressed. The pressure of the fluid rises and this in turn accelerates the rate of its absorption.

The principal factors which influence the pressure of cerebrospinal fluid are:

1. *Forces responsible for production and absorption.* The rate of secretion is independent of the intraventricular pressure, but the rate of absorption is directly proportional to this pressure, ceasing when the pressure falls below that in the intracranial venous sinuses, 66 mm water. Thus a positive cerebrospinal pressure is always assured (Cutler, 1968).

2. *Hydrostatic pressure.* The pressure in the lumbar region is highest when the patient is erect.

3. *Pressure in the veins in the cranium and spinal canal.* Changes in intrathoracic pressure are transmitted to the venous system and hence to the cerebrospinal fluid. This is well marked in coughing, straining and respiratory obstruction. If lumbar puncture is performed and respiratory obstruction is allowed to occur, as can easily happen in the lateral, fully-flexed position in the anaesthetised patient, cerebrospinal fluid spurts from the needle. If the patient is moved from the lateral to the prone position, the pressure falls by about 80 mm water, though the fall may not be marked if there is much pressure on the abdomen.

An immediate transient rise in the cerebrospinal fluid pressure is caused, too, by deliberately obstructing the internal jugular vein — Queckenstedt's test (Queckenstedt, 1916). Cerebral venous engorgement due to congestive heart failure may also give a very high cerebrospinal fluid pressure. (O'Connell, 1970).

4. *The tension of CO_2 in the blood* (Woolf and Lennox, 1930). Any increase, whether derived from adding this gas to the inspired mixture, or from deficient elimination due to respiratory depression, central or peripheral, enlarges the cerebral vascular volume, causing a marked rise in cerebrospinal fluid pressure. So does a low oxygen tension, and volatile anaesthetic agents.

5. *Leakage of cerebrospinal fluid*, e.g. following a previous lumbar puncture.

6. *Infection or irritation of the meninges.* Quite apart from overt infection, an appreciable rise in cerebrospinal fluid pressure is on occasions seen after simple lumbar puncture or after a spinal analgesic. The cause is sometimes ascribed to 'aseptic chemical meningitis'.

7. *Changes in the osmotic pressure of the blood.* These affect both the formation and absorption of cerebrospinal fluid. Anything which

decreases water elimination increases the pressure of CSF whilst a low pressure is to be expected in a dehydrated patient.

When the anaesthetist embarks on an extradural block and uses a liquid for the loss of resistance test he occasionally sees liquid dripping from the needle after disconnecting his syringe. He must then decide what is the nature of the liquid. Is it test fluid (local analgesic or saline) or is it CSF? Three easy tests are available to help him. He may pull back the glove from his wrist and estimate the temperature of the drops on his skin; CSF is usually warmer than his injected liquid. He may allow a few drops to fall into a syringe after its plunger has been removed, which contains 2.5 per cent solution of thiopentone which has a pH of about 10; local analgesic solution will precipitate forming a cloud (Catterberg, 1977). Thirdly, the glucose in CSF will turn a test strip containing glucose oxidase, blue, providing the strip is fresh from its container (Berry, 1958). This occasional difficulty in diagnosing the nature of the liquid drops is one reason why the authors prefer to use the loss of resistance to air.

REFERENCES

Berry, A. (1958) A test for spinal fluid. *Anaesthesia*, **13**, 100.
Catterberg, J. (1977) Local anesthetic versus spinal fluid. *Anesthesiology*, **46**, 309.
Cutler, R. W. P. (1968) Formation and absorption of cerebro-spinal fluid in man. *Brain*. **91**, 707.
Davies, D. V. (ed.) (1962) *Gray's Anatomy*, p. 1129, 34th edn. London: Longman.
Field, E. J. & Brierly, J. B. (1948) Lymphatic connexions of the subarachnoid space. *British Medical Journal*, **1**, 1167.
Howarth, F. & Copper, E. R. A. (1949) Departure of substances from the spinal theca. *Lancet*, **2**, 937.
Livingstone, R. B. (1950) Cerebrospinal fluid. In Fulton, J. F (ed.) *A Textbook of Physiology*, p. 908, 16th edn. Philadelphia.
Magendie, F. (1825) Memoire sur un liquide qui se trouve dans la cràne et le canal vertébrale. *Journal of Physiology and Experimental Pathology*, **5**, 27; and (1827), **7**, 1.
Maximov, A. A. & Bloom, W. (1952) *A Textbook of Histology*, p. 201, 6th edn. Philadelphia.
Nash, J. (1942) *Surgical Physiology*, p. 358. Springfield: Thomas.
O'Connell, J. E. A. (1970) Cerebrospinal fluid mechanics. *Proceedings of the Royal Society of Medicine*, **63**, 507.
Plum, F. & Siesjo, B. (1975) Recent advances in cerebrospinal fluid physiology. *Anesthesiology*. **47**, 788.
Queckenstedt, H. (1916) Zur Diagnose der Rückenmarkskompression. *Deutsche Zeitschrift für Nervenheilkunde*, **55**, 352.
Thompson, E. J. & Johnson, M. H. (1982) Electrophoresis of CSF proteins. *British Journal of Hospital Medicine*, **28**, 600.
Voetmann, E. (1949) On the structure and surface area of the human choroid plexuses. *Acta Anatomica*, **8**, Suppl. 10, 1.
Wolff, H. G. & Lennox, W. G. (1930) Cerebral circulation; effect on pial vessels in variation in oxygen and carbon dioxide content of blood. *A. M. A. Archives of Neurology and Psychiatry*. **73**, 1097.

4

Physiology of central neural blockade

The physiological responses to intra- and extradural blockade result from autonomic blockade with its effects on both the vascular beds and cardiac action; from abolition of somatic pain and the reflex responses associated with it, and from the effects of the blockade of motor fibres.

Autonomic nervous system

Sympathetic preganglionic axons arise from cells in the intermedio-lateral horn of the spinal cord from T.1 to L.2 inclusive. They travel with the anterior roots as myelinated fibres and pass in white rami to the paravertebral sympathetic ganglia where the pilomotor, sudomotor and vasomotor fibres synapse with a number of postganglionic fibres and then pass in the grey rami communicantes to join the spinal nerves. These fibres which also convey motor impulses to the gut above the middle of the transverse colon, pass through the paravertebral ganglia of the sympathetic chain to unite into the three splanchnic nerves. These, after entering the abdomen through the crura of the diaphragm, synapse with postganglionic fibres in the coeliac and other retroperitoneal preaortic plexuses. Somatic afferent fibres from the viscera travel with the efferent sympathetic nerves and go through the paravertebral ganglia without synapsing, and proceed in the white rami to the posterior spinal nerves, where in the posterior root ganglia, they have their cell stations.

The actions of local analgesic solutions on nerve fibres

In the years following 1924, Erlanger and Gasser (Erlanger et al, 1924; Erlanger and Gasser, 1929; Erlanger and Gasser, 1930; Erlanger and Gasser, 1937) investigated 'the differential action of cocaine on the fibres of the nerve trunk' and proposed a classification of nerve fibres into 'A', 'B', and 'C'. This classification was widely accepted, and it aids the understanding of differential effects of local analgesic drugs on nerve fibres.

'A' fibres are medullated and can be further subdivided into alpha, beta, gamma and delta, according to size, varying from 20μ to 1μ in diameter. The larger the fibre, the faster the conduction rate of nerve impulses: this ranges from 120 to 2 metres per second, between large and small fibres. In recent years, the classification of 'A' fibres has been complicated by the discovery of two types of gamma efferent fibres (Boyd and Davey, 1968); a relatively rapidly conducting, well myelinated group, and a relatively slowly conducting, thinly myelinated group. At the same time, afferent fibres have been studied and separated into three groups according to diameter size (Lloyd, 1943); group 1 (12 to 20μ,) group 2 (6 to 12μ) and group 3, (1 to 6μ). It is now suggested that 'A' efferents be classified as alpha, beta, gamma and delta, and 'A' afferents be subdivided into 1, 2 and 3 (Granit, 1966; Whitwam, 1976).

'B' fibres are medullated autonomic fibres and form the familiar white rami of the preganglionic sympathetic nervous sytem. They have a diameter of between 1 and 3μ.

'C' fibres are non-medullated and may be found in both somatic and autonomic systems. They form the postganglionic sympathetic grey rami and the fibres have a diameter of less than 1μ with a slow conduction rate of about 2 metres per second.

Local analgesic drugs prevent the passage of the action potential along the fibre. Blockade takes place exclusively at the nodes of Ranvier of myelinated nerves. Three adjacent nodes where the myelin is absent must be blocked before nerve conduction is completely interrupted. The minimal concentration to cause block in a given nerve fibre can be expressed as the C_m. C_m is related to the diameter of the nerve fibre. 'A' delta fibres which carry sensations of pain and temperature have a C_m of about half that of 'A' gamma fibres which are concerned with motor function and proprioception. It is thus possible to use a strength of local analgesic solution which will abolish the sensations of pain and temperature but will allow motor function and position sense to be retained. The C_m of 'B' fibres (sympathetic) and 'A' delta fibres (pain) are similar, but because the highest preganglionic fibres leave the cord at the level of T.1, and because sympathetic blockade is, on average two segments higher than the sensory level in intradural block (Greene, 1958), sensory denervation to T.3 or above will result in total interruption of the sympathetic output. Recent work, however, suggests that the differential sensitivity of nerve fibres to local analgesic drugs varies according to circumstances and the drugs used (Rosenberg and Heinonen, 1983) though the results of different workers do not agree (Gissen et al, 1980), perhaps because of experimental temperature differences which have been shown to be important (Rosenberg and Hearner, 1980). Sensory block occurs principally by action on the dorsal root ganglia (Galindo and Witcher, 1979), on the sensory afferent dorsal spinal nerve roots and also on the spinal cord after traversing the dura mater (Bromage, 1975). Some afferent fibres may travel in the anterior roots (Sherrington, 1894; Sykes and Coggeshall, 1973).

Muscle tone is abolished during spinal analgesia even if the 'A' alpha fibres are unaffected. This is because normal muscle tone is maintained by the stretch reflex. Stimuli from stretch receptors in the muscle pass up the afferent nerve to the spinal cord with resultant discharge of action potential along the efferent pathway. If the afferent fibres fail to conduct due to local analgesia, the stretch reflex is blocked and resting muscle tone abolished. Muscle contraction may still however occur if the impulses reach the dorsal horn cells from higher up in the central nervous system, whether by conscious action or reflexly in association with straining respiration or coughing.

It is a common observation that smaller doses of local analgesic drug are required in intradural than in extradural spinal analgesia. Intradural spinal analgesia is associated with blockage of all nerve fibres; muscles are paralysed because 'A' alpha fibres are blocked and conscious movement is not possible. In extradural block, however, motor blockade is unlikely to be complete and good analgesia often coexists with the ability to move the limbs on command. This is the basis of the 'test dose' in extradural block which may result in inability to move the toes if inadvertent subarachnoid injection has occurred. The authors have frequently observed the patient's ability to move the legs during successful extradural blockade, but they have also noticed that the patient is unable to cough forcefully during high levels of block, an indication that there is some degree of motor block. The quality of motor paresis during extradural analgesia is influenced by the concentration of solution used and also by the nature of the agent chosen. Etidocaine is associated with a greater degree of motor paralysis than bupivacaine, for example.

Analgesic drug injected into the intradural space causes sympathetic block before sensory block, while motor fibres, being the largest in diameter, are affected somewhat later. Recovery takes place in the order of sympathetic function, sensation to pinprick, somatic motor activity and proprioception, at least following intradural block with amethocaine (Pflug et al, 1978), and it has been suggested that a patient should be allowed to walk, postoperatively, in the absence of hypotension, provided there is sensation round the anus, plantar extension of the foot is as strong as originally, and there is return of proprioception of the big toe. Cardiovascular depression may persist (Daos and Virtue, 1963) even when motor and sensory function have returned. Sympathetic function can however appear to return first (Roe and Cohn, 1973; Kim et al, 1977), perhaps because the segmental innervation of sensory function is lower than the sympathetic outflow, which is not below L.2. On the other hand, even with saddle block of the sacral roots, slight sympathetic block can occur due to upward spread of a dilute concentration, which may be significant in the shocked or hypovolaemic patient. When hyperbaric solutions are used, sensory block is likely to extend about two segments above the level of motor block (Walts et al, 1964; Freund et al, 1967). The sacral parasympathetic fibres are almost always blocked in intradural analgesia. Local analgesic drug molecules move in both directions across the dura. When the drug is injected intradurally it can be demonstrated in the extradural space and vice versa. This may be an important route by which the local analgesic agent is eliminated from the cerebrospinal fluid (Bromage, 1975).

The spread of solution in the extradural space (Ch. 9) differs greatly from that following intradural injection. Larger concentrations of analgesic drug are needed to provide satisfactory sensory and motor block, and motor fibres may be relatively unaffected. This may be because the nerve roots are covered by dural sheaths and molecules of solution of the analgesic drug have to penetrate this membrane to reach the nerve trunk. It has been shown that Indian ink suspensions which have a particle size of 0.4 to 1.5μ can cross the dura in the region of the dural sheath (Brierley and Field, 1948; Woolam and Millen, 1953) and it seems reasonable to suppose that the analgesic agent may take a similar pathway. Whether this is so or not, it is clear that the analgesic drug can act also on the nerve trunk distal to the sheath as well as on the white and grey rami communicantes and visceral afferents. Spread to the spinal cord itself certainly occurs (Bromage et al, 1963) possibly associated with the presence of arachnoid villi (Shantha and Evans, 1972). It is interesting that blockade of the cord has been shown sometimes to be present even after the effect on peripheral nerves has gone (Urban, 1973) and that some features characteristic of an upper motor neurone lesion have been demonstrated (Bromage, 1974). However, the presence of local analgesic drug in the spinal cord is not necessarily associated with extensive block of nerve fibres within the cord, since the pattern of regression of spinal analgesia follows nerve root dermatome sequence, rather than what would be expected if cord blockade had occurred (Forbes and Roizen, 1978). The presence of local analgesic drug within the cord is determined by accessibility, lipid solubility and tissue blood-flow. Accessibility depends on the number of Virchow-Robin spaces, the extensions of the subarachnoid space accompanying vessels as they penetrate neural substance (Fig. 2.16) per unit surface area of cord. Lipid solubility is an important factor since myelin contains lipid and the posterior and lateral spinal tracts are heavily myelinated; hence more local analgesic drug can be found in these tracts than in the anterior nerve roots which contain less myelin. Regional blood flow variations within nervous tissue determine the rate of removal of local analgesic drug.

Such considerations are of enormous interest in the study of the mode of action of extradural block and in the pathophysiology of neurological sequelae, but they have little practical importance to the clinical anaesthetist. There are however differences in the level of autonomic, sensory and motor block as compared with intradural analgesia. In extradural block, sympathetic and sensory paralysis occur to the same segmental levels, while motor fibres may be spared in varying degree, according to the nature and concentration of the local analgesic agent, and the level of sensory and motor block may differ by a greater distance than in intradural analgesia (Walts et al, 1964; Freund et al, 1967). The difference in dose requirements between intra- and extradural analgesia also means that extensive and profound block is likely to occur if a solution prepared for extradural use is inadvertently injected into cerebrospinal fluid.

For further information regarding the action of local analgesic drugs on nervous tissue the reader is referred to the comprehensive monograph of de Jong (de Jong, 1977).

Respiration

Spinal analgesia results in noticeably quiet respiration with little obvious movement in the field of operation during abdominal surgery. This contrasts with the conspicuous movements sometimes seen during intermittent positive pressure ventilation. It has long been suspected that this tranquillity is paid for in terms of underventilation and consequent changes in blood gas tensions. Careful measurements, however, have not upheld these suspicions (Moir, 1963; Moir and Mone, 1964; de Jong, 1965) and the consensus of opinion is that changes both up and down, are negligible. With the help of a Wright's anemometer the anaesthetist can verify that even high spinal analgesia has little effect on respiratory minute volume. Only the diaphragm and the fifth to ninth ribs take part in quiet respiration, and in spinal analgesia the completely reflexed anterior abdominal wall allows easier descent of the diaphragm and abdominal contents, thus compensating for intercostal paralysis. It must be borne in mind, too, that there will be more intercostal muscles in action than the level of skin analgesia would suggest (Walts et al, 1964; Freund et al, 1967). Expiration is unaffected since it is passive in the absence of obstruction. Although resting respiratory parameters show little changes of clinical significance following high levels of block, ventilatory reserve and vital capacity are reduced (Takasaki and Takahashi, 1980). Forced expiratory volume is reduced, especially in cigarette smokers (Aldrete et al, 1973). Intercostal paralysis does impair the ability to cough forcibly and to expel secretions. (Egbert et al, 1961).

In high spinal analgesia there is reduced venous return to the heart (preload) with consequent reduction in pulmonary arterial pressure and in pulmonary blood volume. Alveolar dead-space increases after spinal block (Askrog et al, 1964), nevertheless the $PaCO_2$ rises very little. Thus spinal analgesia *per se* does not interfere significantly with pulmonary gas exchange (de Jong, 1965), but related factors such as respiratory depression from premedicant drugs or from any other cause, interference with the movement of the diaphragm by packs, tumours, retractors or a steep tilt, can easily upset the balance. Obesity is associated with a reduced inspiratory capacity in high spinal analgesia (Catenacci and Sampathacher, 1969). Inability of the patient to talk above a whisper suggests involvement of the phrenic roots, and oxygen should be given, if necessary with IPPV. During the first 24 hours after operation the $Paco_2$ may be lower after spinal analgesia than after general anaesthesia (Linderholm and Norlander, 1958). Spinal analgesia in patients with chronic obstructive airways disease has remarkably little effect on resting pulmonary ventilation (Paskin et al, 1969). Such changes as are found in ventilatory mechanics do not affect arterial oxygen and carbon dioxide tensions *per se*.

The use of an extradural catheter so that repeated injections of local analgesic drug can be made to maintain pain relief allows good respiratory movement, so that FRC does not fall postoperatively and airways closure does not cause hypoxia. Extradural block is more effective than systemic opiates in preventing arterial hypoxaemia following upper abdominal surgery (Simpson et al, 1961; Spence and Smith, 1971) but it confers no marked advantages following lower abdominal surgery (Drummond and Littlewood, 1977).

Apnoea may sometimes be seen after high block. The most serious cause is inadequate medullary blood flow consequent on reduced cardiac output; indeed spontaneous respiration is a valuable monitor of the adequacy of cerebral blood flow during hypotension. Total spinal analgesia, causing apnoea, may follow inadvertent intradural injection of an extradural dose of local analgesic solution. Another possible explanation of the development of unexpectedly high block is accidental injection into the extra-arachnoid subdural space during attempted extradural block (Boys and Norman, 1975; Mehta and Maher, 1977). Other causes of apnoea include the toxic effect of the local analgesic drug in the systemic circulation (Scott, 1981), the lack of arousal stimuli, posture, and depressant drugs used in premedication or paramedication. Because of the resistance shown by large motor roots to weak analgesic solutions, true paralysis of the phrenic nerve (C.3, 4 and 5) is rare. The anaesthetist must be watchful for respiratory depression, so that, if necessary, ventilation can be aided.

The incidence of postoperative pulmonary complications is unaffected by whether the patient receives a spinal or a general anaesthetic (King, 1933; Dripps and Deming, 1946; Urbach et al, 1946). Bromage reported that emphysematous patients breathe more easily after extradural block (Bromage, 1954) and this is seen too after intradural analgesia. The relief may stem from reflex bronchodilatation resulting from the effect of hypotension on baroceptors in the carotid sinus and aortic arch (Daly and Schweitzer, 1951). Reduction of output from the right side of the heart resulting in reduced pulmonary blood volume may also play a part in this phenomenon.

The authors are of the opinion that block up to the level of T.8 is itself, during or after operation, unlikely to handicap the respiratory function.

The cardiovascular system

The preganglionic sympathetic fibres leave the cord between T.1 and L.2 and run in the anterior roots of the corresponding somatic nerves across the subarachnoid and extradural spaces. Spinal analgesia affects the cardiovascular system insofar as a number of these sympathetic fibres are paralysed (Tuffier and Hallion, 1900; Smith and Porter, 1915). The more extensively the solution spreads, the more the area of analgesia and the greater the sympathetic involvement.

High spinal block, whether intra- or extradural is likely to be accompanied by a fall in arterial pressure, stroke volume, cardiac output and peripheral resistance (Ward et al, 1966a). There is dilatation of peripheral vessels on both the arterial and the venous sides of the circulation, but the importance of the latter is not always appreciated. In normal man, the total peripheral resistance decreases only about 18 per cent following complete sympathetic block (Sancetta et al, 1952) and this is not sufficient to account for the degree of hypotension often seen in the clinical environment. Changes in venous return or preload, associated with pooling of blood on the venous side, are more important than often realised, leading to diminished venous return and reduced cardiac output. The increase in peripheral blood flow, noticed clinically, as veins dilate and skin temperature increases, is largely due to increases in skin blood flow and does not necessarily mean that the deeper tissues are better perfused (Wright and Cousins, 1972). Sympathetic blockade of the segments T.1 to T.4 is likely to result in bradycardia due to unopposed vagal action and consequent reduction in cardiac output and hypotension, especially in the aged (Dohi et al, 1979). Changes in heart rate may also reflect changes in right atrial pressure, a decrease in pressure being associated with cardiac slowing, and an increase with tachycardia, this being one mechanism whereby cardiac output adjusts to changes in venous return.

Spinal analgesia results in a decrease in both myocardial oxygen requirements and myocardial oxygen supply. It is likely that, within limits, the overall effect of spinal block on the myocardium will be beneficial. It should be noted that overzealous treatment with inotropic and chronotropic drugs may in fact be harmful, if it causes an increase in myocardial oxygen requirement without concomitant rise of oxygen delivery.

Absorption of analgesic drug following extradural injection may be significant enough to produce generalised pharmacological effects, including those on the heart although the central nervous system is the primary target for local analgesic toxicity. The convulsive dose is many times lower than the lethal cardiovascular dose (Liu et al, 1983). It has been shown that under certain circumstances, and in the presence of an intact sympathetic nervous system, lignocaine may cause a rise in cardiac output (Kao and Jalar, 1959; Jorfeldt et al, 1968), but in the context of high spinal (and autonomic) block, the effect is likely to be depressant.

Adrenaline absorption may result in beta-stimulation with a rise in cardiac output but a reduction in overall peripheral resistance, so that the total effect in extradural block is likely to be a greater fall in mean arterial pressure than if plain analgesic agent had been used (Bonica et al, 1966).

There are significant differences between the physiological effects of intradural and extradural analgesia on the cardiovascular system. These are due principally to the pharmacological actions of the local analgesic drugs and adrenaline, which are much greater because of the larger doses necessary in extradural block, but also to the fact that no zone of differential sympathetic block between autonomic and sensory blockade occurs, as in the case of intradural block.

Age is an important factor whenever hypotension is considered in association with spinal analgesia. The young patient with a healthy cardiovascular system is able to compensate well and at the age of 20 years, serious falls in arterial pressure are unlikely (Bonica et al, 1970). On the other hand, the older patient with arteriosclerosis may suffer untoward hypotension in the presence of high block, while the ill, debilitated hypovolaemic subject or those with a fixed cardiac output may exhibit profound falls and even cardiac arrest. Care is necessary in the presence of heart block or beta blockade. It is a mistake to consider that spinal techniques are safer than general anaesthesia in these ill and handicapped patients.

Occasionally, even in a high central neural blockade, the blood-pressure does not drop at all unless the position of the patient is altered. But the pressure here is unstable and any movement may trigger a sudden fall, particularly if it involves the patient in effort. Any change of position should be carried out slowly, and as little as necessary, with a knowledge of the likely effect. The manouevre must be performed gently, utilising as many strong arms as are available.

A central neural block should not be given unless the anaesthetist is prepared to face up to a fall in blood-pressure. How the fall should be dealt with is a matter on which opinions differ considerably, but certainly immediate resort should not be made to vasopressors. A good head of pressure is essential for a person sitting erect or playing football, but a surprisingly low one will drive blood round the patient lying horizontal during spinal analgesia. With a low pressure the work load on the heart is greatly reduced and experience suggests that the decreased coronary circulation is adequate. This view is supported by experimental work in dogs which received extradural analgesia without adrenaline (Klassen et al, 1980). The rate pressure product (product of heart rate and peak systolic pressure), is unlikely to exceed the threshold of 11 000 at which myocardial ischaemia may be considered to occur. Such considerations may not, however, be universally applicable (Baragh and Kiprian, 1980).

With a spinal block, a fall in blood-pressure is to be expected. If this is at all severe, we advise that oxygen should be added to the inspired mixture even though this may result in a diminution of cardiac output and a theoretical diminution in the oxygen availability to the tissues (Ward et al, 1966a). Routinely the legs should be raised and any pillow removed to facilitate the cerebral circulation, including that to the vasomotor and respiratory centres. Though the Trendelenburg position increases cardiac output by facilitating venous return from the legs, there is no evidence that cerebral vascular perfusion is increased (Gunteroth et al, 1964; Taylor and Weil, 1967). The authors have, however, on many hundreds of occasions adopted this position when the patient's blood-pressure has been low, but are not aware that they have ever caused any harm by so doing. If venous return is interfered with by any large abdominal tumour (such as the full term pregnant uterus) compressing the inferior vena cava against the spinal column, the patient should be rolled to the left side to relieve possible obstruction.

Spinal analgesia, whether intradural or extradural, causes enlargement of the vascular bed, and it is logical to be ready to fill it again. Blood loss is tolerated badly as the homeostatic vasoconstrictive responses to haemorrhage are in abeyance. Early and adequate fluid replacement is necessary. Before the operation is started it is prudent, certainly with high levels of block, to have an intravenous drip set up so that preloading with intravenous fluids up to as much as 2000 ml can be undertaken and blood loss replaced quickly by blood or other fluids. Prompt and adequate replacement may be as important as the choice of a particular fluid. Tissue oxygenation may be improved by infusing fluids which decrease the haematocrit reading, thus lowering viscosity and improving blood flow (Messmer et al, 1972; Sunder-Plassman et al, 1973; Messmer and Sunder-Plassman, 1974). In the absence of biochemical guidance we incline, for this purpose, more to compound sodium lactate solution (Hartmann) or Dextran than to dextrose or saline solutions. The infusion of 500 to 1000 ml will, in most patients, raise the pressure some 20 mmHg and maintain it for half an hour or longer because of the delayed renal secretion associated with the hypotension. The use of large volumes of intravenous fluids is, however, likely to lead ultimately to increased urinary output with an increased need for bladder catheterisation, with a further risk of urinary tract infection.

Low blood-pressure allied to bradycardia can often be raised by the intravenous injection of a small dose of atropine (0.2 mg) repeated as indicated. As the slow pulse yields to the vagal blocking effect of the atropine, so is the hypotension reversed. Small doses of atropine are especially useful in the treatment of hypotension associated with bradycardia which may be seen in the immediate postoperative period.

It is difficult for the anaesthetist to remain inactive when faced with a progressive fall in blood-pressure. We advise that he should remain so, but only as long as the patient looks well and the skin is pink, dry and has a good capillary circulation. There is seldom cause for worry if a peripheral pulse, such as the superficial temporal or facial is palpable. It has been suggested that a fall of arterial pressure of more than one-third below preoperative levels might be an indication for the use of corrective measures (Greene, 1982). The pressure can be raised by vasopressors but the rise does not necessarily benefit the patient. When the patient is supervised by a careful anaesthetist, consideration should be given as to whether vasopressors are likely to do more harm than good. The surgical advantages of hypotension are lost, and the increased pressure may merely reflect vasoconstriction and the bypassing of blood around tissues badly in need of perfusion. Alpha adrenergic agonists such as methoxamine and phenylephrine may cause an increase in peripheral resistance and left ventricular work, with the result that the cardiac output may actually fall. Instead of being improved tissue hypoxia and metabolic acidosis may be made worse. Ephedrine and mephentermine are rational choices once the decision to administer a pressor drug has been made (see Ch. 5). A drug which causes constriction on the venous side but allows arteries to remain dilated would be useful as preload would increase while afterload remained low. Unfortunately such a drug does not at present exist.

Lumbar extradural block may enhance fibrinolysis if the block ascends above T.8, and so there is a possible contraindication to the use of the technique in patients where a risk of fibrinolysis exists such as prostatectomy (Simpson et al, 1982).

Pulmonary hypertension

There are case reports where extradural block has been used successfully in the presence of pulmonary hypertension (Spinnato et al, 1981; Mallampati, 1983). Pulmonary sympathetic innervation is from segments T.2 to T.4, but denervation may not affect pulmonary arterial pressures even when there is a fall in systemic arterial pressure. There is little information regarding the effect of extradural block on pulmonary haemodynamics in normal subjects.

The liver

A reduction in hepatic blood flow of about 28 per cent has been reported when mean arterial pressure falls 27 per cent (Mueller et al, 1952) but this is without clinical significance.

There is no evidence that the effects of spinal analgesia on the liver are any more harmful than are those of general anaesthesia. Nor does spinal analgesia affect patients with liver dysfunction any differently from general anaesthesia.

Extradural block to the level of T.5 with plain lignocaine is associated with a decrease of hepatic blood flow and a decrease in splanchnic vascular resistance, although when adrenaline is added to the injected solution hepatic blood flow is maintained initially within normal limits as a result of increased cardiac output and decreased splanchnic vascular resistance (Kennedy et al, 1971).

The lowest blood-pressure level at which the liver ceases to function adequately is not known.

Genito-urinary system

The preganglionic nerve supply to the kidneys leaves the intermediolateral horn cells of the spinal cord between the eleventh thoracic and the first lumbar segments. Renal vascular resistance is little influenced by nervous control (Green and Kepchar, 1959). Renal blood flow is maintained by autoregulation as long as mean arterial pressure remains above 55 mmHg, but the renal vessels are constricted by alpha adrenergic agonist drugs. Dopamine is without this effect and may therefore be indicated if renal failure is feared. Studies have shown that during spinal analgesia in healthy volunteers glomerular filtration rate and effective renal plasma flow are reduced (Kennedy et al, 1969), but recovery of function follows provided the cells are kept oxygenated in the meantime. The relative excretion of the different electrolytes in the urine due to acute denervation by spinal analgesia differs from that seen when the denervation is longer lasting (Pearce and Sonnenberg, 1965).

The bladder wall, supplied by the parasympathetic system, is paralysed during spinal analgesia but the sphincter is not relaxed. Urinary retention may outlast skin analgesia as the slender parasympathetic fibres from S.2–4 are very susceptible to the analgesic solution; moreover because of their anatomical position, they may be bathed in the solution for a relatively long time. In prolonged blockade, urinary catheterisation may be necessary.

Engorgement of the flaccid penis due to paralysis of the nervi erigentes (S.2–3) is often the first sign of the onset of a successful block. Spermatorrhoea is sometimes seen.

The tone of the ureters, supplied from L.1 and 2, is not materially altered.

Gastrointestinal tract

The gut is supplied by parasympathetic and sympathetic fibres. The former contract the muscle and narrow the lumen, while stimulation of the sympathetic results in the opposite effects. The parasympathetic fibres reach the alimentary tract from two widely separated sources, (1) the medulla, via the vagus, and (2) the distal end of the cord (S.2–4) via the hypogastric nerves. The vagal distribution is to the oesophagus and onwards as far as the splenic flexure, at which point the sacral parasympathetic fibres take over. The sympathetic fibres to the whole of the alimentary tract (excluding the oesophagus) are given off from segments of the cord between T.5 and L.2. It will be seen that a lumbar injection will inactivate the sacral parasympathetic nerve supply, and that the extent to which the sympathetic is paralysed depends on the height to which analgesia extends. The vagus nerve is virtually out of reach so that its action remains unaffected. Spinal analgesia up to the level of T.5 results in a narrowing of the gut, increase in peristalsis and of secretion, and a relaxation of the sphincters. Peristalsis may be increased, not in frequency, but in force and the pressure within the bowel lumen increases too (Eckenhoff and Cannard, 1960).

Peristalsis is, however, decreased by morphine, and by any atropine in the premedication. The contracted state of the bowel allows more room for the surgeon to do his work and is one of the practical benefits of spinal analgesia. Nevertheless, some surgeons find that intra (and extra) dural block interferes with bowel anastomosis because of the contracted state of the intestine (Fig. 2.33) Spinal block in animals has been shown to increase colonic blood supply and oxygen availability (Aitkenhead et al, 1980) so that the use of spinal techniques during and after operation on the large bowel may reduce the incidence of anastomotic breakdown.

There is some evidence that intestinal tone and bowel sounds are regained more rapidly after spinal than after general anaesthesia. Gastric emptying time is delayed much less when extradural analgesia is used for relief of postoperative pain, than when narcotic analgesics are employed (Nimmo et al, 1978) and so nausea and vomiting are likely to be less troublesome. Spinal analgesia has been employed for the relief of paralytic ileus (Tuohy, 1952), but perforation of the gut wall has been reported in areas which are ischaemic. Some consider spinal analgesia to be an unwise choice in cases of strangulated herniae since diminution in the size of the gut may result in preoperative spontaneous reduction — with intra-abdominal perforation should the gut include a gangrenous area.

Nausea and vomiting may cause much misery to the conscious patient under spinal analgesia, and this is necessarily accompanied by poor operative conditions. Possible causes are afferent impulses along the unblocked vagus, increased peristalsis, backward flow of bile into the stomach through the relaxed sphincter of Oddi and pylorus, acute hypotension, cerebral hypoxia, drugs used for premedication and psychological factors. If intravenous atropine does not relieve the patient (Ward et al, 1966b), light general anaesthesia will be required.

Sympathetic paralysis will be followed by enlargement of the spleen and this may cause recurrent bleeding if the viscus is ruptured.

Endocrine system

The adrenals are supplied by sympathetic nerves coming from cord segments T.11 to L.2. They pass in the inferior splanchnic nerves to the glands without synapsing.

The adrenal cortex. Blood cortisol levels increase during surgery under general anaesthesia as a response to stress (Moore and Ball, 1952; Hammond et al, 1958). This rise may be less during central neural blockade but in the case of major abdominal or thoracic surgery, the rise in blood cortisol is little different whether general or extradural block is employed (Bromage, 1971; Lines, 1971).

In any case the effect is only postponed until the block has worn off, so that postoperative cortisol levels are not related to the anaesthetic method employed.

During the operation general anaesthesia causes a reduction in the number of circulating eosinophils; spinal analgesia is not associated with lymphopaenia or granulocytosis after operation, while the endocrine metabolic response to surgery and postoperative immunosupression are prevented (Roche et al, 1950; Rem et al, 1980). Whatever method of pain relief is employed there is a marked decrease in eosinophil count four hours postoperatively (Jarvinen et al, 1959).

The adrenal medulla. Denervation of the medulla has little effect on circulating catecholamines which is not surprising since these are secreted for the most part from effector organ sites throughout the body. Low block may be beneficial in patients with cardiovascular disease as adrenergic responses are inhibited (Pflug and Halter, 1981). Central neural blockade has been recommended as a good method of pain relief in suitable patients for the removal of phaeochromocytoma (Greene, 1969). There is theoretical support for the use of spinal analgesia for abdominal and other surgery in those hyperthyroid patients who have not been made euthyroid before operation (Brewster et al, 1956).

Central neural blockade prevents the hyperglycaemic response of surgical stress (Moore and Ball, 1952; Hammond et al, 1958; Oyama and Matsuki, 1970; Möller et al, 1982; Traynor et al, 1982) but has no effect on glucose tolerance and insulin release due to stress in the postoperative period (Buckley et al, 1982). The block may have a beneficial effect in diabetic patients as glucose utilisation may be facilitated (Houghton et al, 1978), though there is evidence that the response to insulin may be augmented by splanchnic blockade (Griffiths, 1953) and the anaesthetist should bear in mind the possibility of hypoglycaemia developing in patients receiving insulin (Bromage, 1978).

REFERENCES

Aitkenhead, A. R., Gilmore, D. E., Hothersall, A. P. & Ledingham, I. M. (1980) Effects of subarachnoid nerve block on arterial PO_2 and colonic blood-flow in dogs. *British Journal of Anaesthesia*, 52, 1071.

Aldrete, J. A., Woodward, S. T. & Turk, L. H. (1973) Influence of cigarette smoking on the changes produced by spinal anesthesia on expiratory forced volumes and flow rates. *Anesthesia and Analgesia*, 52, 809.

Askrog, V. F., Smith, T. C. & Eckenhoff, J. E. (1964) Changes in pulmonary ventilation during spinal anesthesia. *Surgery, Gynecology and Obstetrics*, 119, 653.

Baragh, P. G. & Kiprian, C. (1980) The rate-pressure product in clinical anesthesia; boon or bane? *Anesthesia and Analgesia*, 59, 229.

Bonica, J. J., Berges, P. V. & Morikawa, K. (1970) Circulatory effects of peridural block: 1. Effects of level of analgesia and dose of lidocaine. *Anesthesiology*, 33, 619.

Bonica, J. J., Kennedy, W. F. (Jun.), Ward, R. J. & Tolas, A. G. (1966) A comparison of the effects of high subarachnoid and epidural anaesthesia. *Acta Anaesthesiologica Scandinavica* Suppl., 23, 429.

Boyd, I. A. & Davey, M. R. (1968) *Composition of Peripheral Nerves*. Livingstone: Edinburgh.

Boys, J. E. & Norman, P. F. (1975) Accidental subdural analgesia: a case report, possible implications and relevance to massive extradurals. *British Journal of Anaesthesia*, 47, 1111.

Brewster, W. R. (Jun.), Isaacs, J. P., Osgood, P. F. & King, T. L. (1956) The hemodynamic and metabolic interrelationships in the activity of epinephrine, norepinephrine and the thyroid hormones. *Circulation*, 13, 1.

Brierley, J. P. & Field, E. J. (1948) The connexions of the spinal subarachnoid space with the lymphatic system. *Journal of Anatomy* (London), 82, 153.

Bromage, P. R. (1954) *Spinal Epidural Analgesia*. Edinburgh: Livingstone.

Bromage, P. R. (1971) Influence of prolonged epidural blockade on blood sugar and corticol responses to operations upon the upper part of the abdomen and the thorax. *Surgery, Gynecology and Obstetrics*, 132, 1051.

Bromage, P. R. (1974) Lower limb reflex changes in segmental epidural analgesia. *British Journal of Anaesthesia*, 46, 504.

Bromage, P. R. (1975) Mechanism of action of extradural analgesia. *British Journal of Anaesthesia*, 47, 199.

Bromage, P. R. (1978) *Epidural Anesthesia*. Philadelphia: Saunders. p. 394.

Bromage, P. R. Joyal, A. C. & Binnie, J. C. (1963) Local anesthetic drugs: penetration from the spinal extradural space into the neuraxis. *Science*, 140, 392.

Buckley, F. P., Kehlet, H., Brown, N. S. & Scott, D. B. (1982) Postoperative glucose tolerance during extradural anaesthesia. *British Journal of Anaesthesia*, 54, 325.

Catenacci, A. J. & Sampathacher, K. R. (1969) Ventilatory studies in the obese patient during spinal anesthesia. *Anesthesia and Analgesia*, 48, 48.

Daos, F. G. & Virtue, R. W. (1963) Sympathetic block persistence after spinal and epidural anesthesia. *Journal of the American Medical Association*, 183, 285.

Daly, M. De B. & Schweitzer, A. (1951) Reflex bronchomotor responses to stimulation of receptors in the region of the carotid sinus and arch of the aorta in the dog and cat. *Journal of Physiology* (London), 113, 442.

de Jong, R. H. (1965) Arterial carbon dioxide and oxygen tensions during spinal block. *Journal of the American Medical Association*, 191, 698.

de Jong, R. H. (1977) *Local Anesthetics*, 2nd edn. Springfield: Thomas.

Dohi, S., Naito, H. & Takahashi, T. (1979) Age related changes in blood pressure and duration of motor block in spinal anesthesia. *Anesthesiology*, 50, 319.

Dripps, R. D. and Deming, M. V. (1946) Postoperative atelectasis and pneumonia. *Annals of Surgery*, 124, 94.

Drummond, G. B. & Littlewood, D. G. (1977) Respiratory effects of extradural analgesia after lower abdominal surgery. *British Journal of Anaesthesia*, **49**, 999.

Eckenhoff, J. E. & Cannard, T. H. (1960) Influence of anesthetic agents and adjuvants upon intestinal tone. *Anesthesiology*, **21**, 96.

Egbert, L. D., Tamersoy, K. & Deas, T. C. (1961) Pulmonary function during spinal anesthesia: the mechanism of cough depression. *Anesthesiology*, **22**, 882.

Erlanger, J. & Gasser, H. S. (1929) The role of fibre size in the establishment of a nerve block by pressure or cocaine. *American Journal of Physiology*, **88**, 581.

Erlanger, J. & Gasser, H. S. (1930) The actual potential in fibres of slow conduction in spinal roots and somatic nerves. *American Journal of Physiology*, **92**, 43.

Erlanger, J. & Gasser, H. S. (1937) *Electrical signs of nervous activity*. Philadelphia: Pennsylvania University Press.

Erlanger, J., Gasser, H. S. & Bishop, G. H. (1924) The compound nature of the action current as disclosed by the cathode ray oscillograph. *American Journal of Physiology*, **70**, 624.

Forbes, A. R. & Roizen, M. F. (1978) Does spinal anesthesia anesthetise the spinal cord? *Anesthesiology*, **48**, 440.

Freund, F. G., Bonica, J. J., Ward, R. J., Takamatsu, T. J. & Kennedy, W. F. (1967) Ventilatory reserve and level of motor block during high spinal and epidural anesthesia. *Anesthesiology*, **28**, 834.

Galindo, A. & Witcher, T. (1979) Vulnerability of sensory pathways to local anesthetics. *Anesthesiology*, **51**, S.212.

Gissen, A. J., Covino, B. G. & Gregus, J. (1980) Differential sensitivity of mammalian nerve fibres to local anesthetic agents. *Anesthesiology*, **53**, 467.

Granit, R. (ed.) (1966) Muscle afferents and motor control. *Proceedings of the First Nobel Symposium*. Stockholm: Almquist and Wiksell.

Green, H. D. & Kepchar, J. H. (1959) Control of peripheral resistance in major systemic vascular beds. *Physiological Reviews*, **39**, 617.

Greene, N. M. (1958) The area of differential block during spinal analgesia with hyperbaric tetracaine. *Anesthesiology*, **19**, 357.

Greene, N. M. (1969) *Physiology of Spinal Anesthesia*, p. 68 2nd edn. Baltimore: Williams and Wilkins.

Greene, N. M. (1982) Perspective in spinal anesthesia. *Regional Anesthesia*, **7**, 55.

Griffiths, J. A. (1953) The effects of general anaesthesia and hexamethonium on the blood sugar in the non-diabetic and the diabetic surgical patient. *Quarterly Journal of Medicine*, **22**, 405.

Gunteroth, W. G., Abel, F. L. and Mullins, G. L. (1964) The effects of the Trendelenburg position on blood pressure and carotid flow. *Surgery, Gynecology and Obstetrics*, **119**, 245.

Hammond, W. G., Vandam, L. D., Davis, J. M., Carter, R. D., Ball, M. R. & Moore, F. D. (1958) Studies on surgical endocrinology, IV. Anesthetic agents as stimuli to changes in corticosteroids and metabolism. *Annals of Surgery*, **148**, 199.

Houghton, A., Hickey, J. B., Ross, S. A. & Dupre, J. (1978) Glucose tolerance during anaesthesia and surgery: a comparison of extradural and general anaesthesia. *British Journal of Anaesthesia*, **50**, 495.

Jarvinen, P. A., Kivalo, I. & Vara, P. (1959) Effects of different anaesthesia methods of eosinopenic response to surgical stress. *Acta Anaesthesiologica Scandinavica*, **3**, 75.

Jorfeldt, L., Löfstrom, B., Pernow, B., Persson, B., Wahren, J. & Widman, B. (1968) The effects of local anaesthetics on the central circulation and respiration in man and dog. *Acta Anaesthesiologica Scandinavica*, **12**, 153.

Kao, F. F. & Jalar, U. H. (1959) The central action of lignocaine and its effects on cardiac output. *British Journal of Pharmacology and Chemotherapy*, **14**, 522.

Kennedy, W. F., Everett, G. B., Cobb, L. A., & Allen, G. D. (1971) Simultaneous systemic and hepatic hemodynamic measurements during high peridural anesthesia in normal man. *Anesthesia and Analgesia*, **50**, 1069.

Kennedy, W. F., Sawyer, T. K., Gerbershagen, H. V., Cutler, R. E. Allen, G. D. & Bonica, J. J. (1969) Systemic cardiovascular and renal hemodyanamic alterations during peridural anesthesia in normal man. *Anesthesiology*, 31, 414.

Kim, J. M., La Salle, A. D. & Parmley, R. T. (1977) Sympathetic recovery following lumbar epidural and spinal analgesia. *Anesthesia and Analgesia*, 56, 352.

King, D. S. (1933) Postoperative pulmonary complications. *Anesthesia and Analgesia*, 12, 243.

Klassen, G. A., Bramwell, R. S., Bromage, P. R. & Zbrowska-Sluis, D. T. (1980) Effect of acute sympathectomy by epidural anesthesia on the canine circulation. *Anesthesiology*, 52, 8.

Linderholm, H. & Norlander, O. (1958) Carbon dioxide tension and bicarbonate content of arterial blood in relation to anaesthesia and surgery. *Acta Anaesthesiologica Scandinavica*, 2, 1.

Lines, J. G. (1971) Plasma cortisol responses during neurosurgical and abdominal operations. *British Journal of Anaesthesia*, 43, 1136.

Liu, P. L., Feldman, H. S., Giasi, R. et al (1983) Comparative central nervous system toxicity of lidocaine, etidocaine, bupivacaine and tetracaine in awake dogs, following rapid intravenous administration. *Anesthesia and Analgesia*, 62, 375.

Lloyd, D. P. C. (1943) Neuron patterns controlling transmission of ipsilateral hind limb reflexes in the cat. *Journal of Neurophysiology*, 6, 293.

Mallampati, S. R. (1983) Low thoracic epidural anesthesia for elective cholecystectomy in a patient with congenital heart disease and pulmonary hypertension. *Canadian Anaesthetists' Society Journal*, 30, 72.

Mehta, M. & Maher, R. (1977) Injection into the extra-arachnoid subdural space. *Anaesthesia*, 32, 760.

Messmer, K., & Sunder-Plassman, L. (1974) Haemodilution. *Progress in Surgery*, 13, 216.

Messmer, K., Lewis, D. H., Sunder-Plassman, L., Klovekorn, W. P., Mendler, P. & Holper, K. (1972) Acute normovolaemic haemodilution. *European Surgical Research*, 4, 55.

Moir, D. D. (1963) Ventilatory function during epidural analgesia. *British Journal of Anaesthesia*, 35, 3.

Moir, D. D. Mone, J. G. (1964) Acid-base balance during epidural analgesia. *British Journal of Anaesthesia*, 36, 480.

Möller, I. W., Rem, J., Brandt, M. R. & Kehlet, H. (1982) Effects of post-traumatic epidural analgesia on the cortisol and hyperglycaemic response to surgery. *Acta Anaesthesiologica Scandinavica*, 26, 58.

Moore, F. D. & Ball, M. R. (1952) *The Metabolic Response to Surgery*. Oxford: Blackwell.

Mueller, R. P., Lynn, R. B. & Sancetta, S. M. (1952) Studies of hemodynamic changes in humans following induction of low and high spinal anesthesia. 2. The changes in splanchnic vascular resistance in humans not undergoing surgery. *Circulation*, 6, 894.

Nimmo, W. S., Littlewood, D. G., Scott, D. B. & Prescott, L. F. (1978) Gastric emptying following hysterectomy with extradural analgesia. *British Journal of Anaesthesia*, 50, 559.

Oyama, T. & Matsuki, A. (1970) The effects of spinal anaesthesia and surgery on carbohydrate and fat metabolism in man. *British Journal of Anaesthesia*, 42, 723.

Paskin, S., Rodman, T. & Smith T. C. (1969) Effects of spinal anesthesia on the pulmonary function in patients with chronic obstructive pulmonary disease. *Annals of Surgery*, 169, 35.

Pearce, J. W. & Sonnenberg, H. (1965) Effects of spinal section and renal denervation on the renal response to blood volume expansion. *Canadian Journal of Physiology and Pharmacology*, 43, 211.

Pflug, A. E., Aasheim, G. M. & Forbes, C. (1978) Sequence of return of neurological function and criteria for safe ambulation following subarachnoid block (spinal anaesthesia). *Canadian Anaesthetists' Society Journal*, 25, 133.

Pflug, A. E. & Halter, J. B. (1981) The effect of spinal anesthesia on adrenergic tone and neurobehavioural responses to surgical stress in humans. *Anesthesiology*, 55, 120.

Rem, J., Brandt, M. R. & Kehlet, H. (1980) Prevention of postoperative lymphopaenia and granulocytosis by epidural analgesia. *Lancet*, 1, 283.

Roche, M., Thorne, G. W. & Hills, A. G. (1950) The levels of circulating eosinophils and their response to ACTH in surgery. *New England Journal of Medicine*, 242, 307.

Roe, C. F. & Cohn, F. L. (1973) Sympathetic blockade during spinal anesthesia. *Surgery, Gynecology and Obstetrics*, 136, 265.

Rosenberg, P. H. & Hearyner, J. E. (1980) Temperature dependent nerve blocking action of lidocaine and halothane. *Acta Anaesthesiologica Scandinavica*, 24, 314.

Rosenberg, P. H. & Heinonen, E. (1983) Differential sensitivity of A and C nerve fibres to long-acting amide local anaesthetics. *British Journal of Anaesthesia*, 55, 163.

Sancetta, S. M., Lynn, R. B., Simeone, F. A. & Scott, R. W. (1952) Studies in hemodynamic changes in humans following induction of high and low spinal anesthesia. I. General considerations of the problem. The changes in cardiac output, brachial arterial pressure, peripheral and pulmonary oxygen contents and peripheral blood flow induced by spinal anesthesia in humans not undergoing surgery. *Circulation*, 6, 559.

Scott, D. B. (1981) Editorial. Toxicity caused by local anaesthetic drugs. *British Journal of Anaesthesia*, 53, 553.

Shantha, T. J. & Evans, J. A. (1972) The relationship of epidural anesthesia to neural membranes and arachnoid villi. *Anesthesiology*, 37, 543.

Sherrington, C. S. (1894) On the anatomical constitution of nerves of skeletal muscles; with remarks on recurrent fibres in the ventral spinal nerve roots. *Journal of Physiology* (London), 17, 211.

Simpson, B. R., Parkhouse, J., Marshall, R. & Lambrechts, W. (1961) Extradural analgesia and the prevention of postoperative respiratory complication. *British Journal of Anaesthesia*, 33, 628.

Simpson, P. J., Radford, S. K., Foster, S. J., Cooper, G. M. & Hughes, A. O. (1982) The fibrinolytic effects of anaesthesia. *Anaesthesia*, 37, 3.

Smith, G. C. and Porter, W. T. (1915) Spinal analgesia in the cat. *American Journal of Physiology*, 38, 108.

Spence, A. A. & Smith, G. (1971) Post operative analgesia and lung function: a comparison of morphine with extradural block. *British Journal of Anaesthesia*, 43, 144.

Spinnato, J. A., Kraynack, B. J. & Cooper, M. N. (1981) Eisenmenger's syndrome in pregnancy: epidural anesthesia for elective Cesarean section. *New England Journal of Medicine*, 304, 1215.

Sunder-Plassman, L., Lesch, F., Klovekron, W. P. & Messmer, K. (1973) Limited hemodilution in hemorrhagic shock in dogs. *Researches in Experimental Medicine*, 159, 167.

Sykes, M. T. & Coggeshall, R. F. (1973) Unmyelinated fibres in human L. 4 and L.5 ventral roots. *Brain Research*, 63, 490.

Takasaki, M. & Takahashi, T. (1980) Respiratory function during cervical and thoracic extradural analgesia in patients with normal lungs. *British Journal of Anaesthesia*, 52, 1271.

Taylor, J. & Weil, M. H. (1967) Cerebral circulation in the head-down position. *Researches in Experimental Medicine*, 124, 1005.

Traynor, C., Paterson, C., Paterson, J. L., Ward, D., Morgan, M. & Hall, G. M. (1982) Effects of extradural analgesia and vagal blockade on metabolic and endocrine response to upper abdominal surgery. *British Journal of Anaesthesia*, **54**, 319.

Tuffier, T. & Hallion, L. (1900) *Comptes Rendus Hebdomadaires des Séances et Mémoires de la Société de la Biologie*, **52**, 897.

Tuohy, E. B. (1952) The adaptation of continuous spinal anesthesia. *Anesthesia and Analgesia, Current Researches*, **31**, 372.

Urbach, K. F., Lee, W. R. Sheely, L. L. Lang, F. L. & Sharp, R. P. (1946) Spinal or general anesthesia for inguinal hernia repair. *Journal of the American Medical Association*, **190**, 25.

Urban, B. J. (1973) Clinical observations suggesting a changing site of action during induction and recession of spinal and epidural anesthesia. *Anesthesiology*, **39**, 496.

Walts, L. F., Koepke, G. & Margules, R. (1964) Determination of sensory and motor levels after spinal anesthesia with tetracaine. *Anesthesiology*, **25**, 634.

Ward, R. J., Danziger, F., Akamatsu, T., Freund, F. & Bonica, J. J. (1966a) Cardiovascular response to oxygen therapy for hypotension of regional anesthesia. *Anesthesia and Analgesia*, **45**, 140.

Ward, R. J., Kennedy, W. F., Bonica, J. J., Martin, W. E., Tolas, A. G. & Akamatsu, T. (1966b) Atropine and vasopressors for the treatment of hypotension in high subarachnoid anesthesia. *Anesthesia and Analgesia*, **45**, 621.

Whitwam, J. G. (1976) Classification of peripheral nerves fibres. *Anaesthesia*, **31**, 494.

Woolam, D. H. M. & Millen, J. N. (1953) An anatomical approach to poliomyelitis. *Lancet*, **1**, 364.

Wright, C. J. & Cousins, M. J. (1972) Blood-flow distribution in the human leg following epidural sympathetic block. *Archives of Surgery*, **105**, 334.

5

Pharmacology

LOCAL ANALGESIC AGENTS

Local analgesic agents are drugs which, in clinical dosage, produce reversible block by impeding impulse transmission in peripheral nerves, spinal roots, or nerve endings. Applied to an accessible neural structure, these drugs obtund sensation and reduce motor tone and sympathetic effects in the innervated part distal to the site of application, without depressing consciousness or sensation in other parts of the body. Extremely good local analgesic agents are in world-wide use today but controllable duration of action is one property still lacking. The first drug to be used was, of course, cocaine. It was isolated by Gaedicke in 1855 but was not employed clinically until 1884 (Koller, 1884b).

Because of the toxicity of cocaine, substitutes were sought. The first to be used was tropococaine, obtained from the coca plant of Java by Giesel in 1891, and was used by one of the authors as late as the middle 1930s. With the advance of organic chemistry the Frenchman, Fourneau, introduced a further improvement in 1904, amylocaine (Fourneau, 1904), naming the new drug Stovaine, a play on the English translation of his name. Stovaine achieved immediate popularity but was itself soon superseded by the even less toxic procaine (Novocaine) synthesised by the German biochemist Einhorn (Einhorn 1905) and given widespread publicity by the great German master of local analgesia Heinrich Braun (Braun, 1905).

For the next 20 years, analgesia still had to be restricted to operations which would finish within the hour, but in 1928 Eisleb synthesised a new ester-bonded local analgesic agent, amethocaine hydrochloride, superior to procaine because of its longer duration of action and greater potency (Eisleb, 1931). Another long-acting drug appeared in 1929 under the name of Percaine (Uhlmann, 1929), which is now known as cinchocaine, dibucaine or Nupercaine.

In more recent times, several very good local analgesic drugs manufactured in Sweden have been introduced clinically, making the practice of spinal analgesia the popular and practical procedure that it is today. Lignocaine was synthesised by Löfgren and Lundqvist in 1943 and introduced clinically by Gordh in 1948 (Gordh, 1949). Mepivacaine was synthesised by Ekenstam and Egner in 1956 and introduced clinically by Dhuner in 1957. Prilocaine was synthesised by Löfgren and Tegner in 1959, tested pharmacologically by Wiedling and used clinically by Eriksson and Gordh in 1959 (Eriksson and Gordh, 1959). Bupivacaine was synthesised by Ekenstam in 1957 and used clinically by Telivuo in 1963. Etidocaine was synthesised by Takman in 1971 and used clinically by Lund in 1972.

The preparations available for intradural and extradural injection are summarised in Table 5.1.

Concurrent with the use of spinal agents, physiological and pharmacological observations and experience have been assessed and published.

The primary pharmacological action of local analgesic agents is by interference with the excitation-conduction process in peripheral nerve fibres and nerve endings. Local analgesic agents are water soluble salts of lipid soluble alkaloids and contain either an ester (COO-) or amide (NH.CO-) link in the molecule. Each molecule is composed of an aromatic portion, an intermediate chain and an amide portion. The ester-linked group (procaine-like) has an ester link between the aromatic end of the molecule and the intermediate chain, and the amide-linked group (lignocaine-like) has an amide link between the aromatic portion and the intermediate chain. The ester-linked drugs (cocaine, procaine, amethocaine) are hydrolysed by plasma esterases. The amide-linked drugs (cinchocaine, lignocaine, prilocaine, mepivacaine, bupivacaine and etidocaine) are inactivated by hepatic amidases, have good tissue penetration and some have a relatively prolonged duration. They are weak bases and the rate of excretion depends on the urine pH. All the amide-linked drugs cross the placenta and the fetus is less able to metabolise the amide group than the ester-linked group.

Para-aminobenzoic acid is a metabolite formed by hydrolysis of ester-linked compounds. This substance is capable of inducing allergic type reactions in a small percentage of the general population. The amide-linked agents (e.g. lignocaine) are not metabolised to para-aminobenzoic acid and reports of allergic phenomena are extremely rare (Covino, 1982). However, Brown et al (1981) reported an allergic reaction to bupivacaine (preservative

Table 5.1 Local analgesic drugs for intradural and extradural injection

Group	Name	Synonyms	Preparations for intradural use	Preparations for extradural use	Duration
Ester-linked	Procaine	Novocaine Planocaine Ethocaine Neocaine Nesacaine	5 per cent with glucose or crystals dissolved in CSF	2 to 5 per cent	Short
	Chloroprocaine		Not recommended	1.5 to 3 per cent	Short
	Amethocaine	{ Tetracaine Pantocaine Pontocaine }	0.5 to 1 per cent with glucose 5 to 10 per cent (hyperbaric)	0.25 per cent	Long
Amide-linked	Lignocaine	{ Xylocaine Duncaine Lidocaine }	5 per cent with 5 to 8 per cent glucose	1.5 to 2 per cent	Medium
	Mepivacaine	Carbocaine	4 per cent with glucose 0.5 per cent plain	1.5 to 2 per cent	Medium
	Bupivacaine	Marcain(e)	0.5 per cent with 8 per cent glucose	0.25 to 0.75 per cent	Long
	Etidocaine	Duranest		0.25 to 1.5 per cent	Long
	Prilocaine	{ Citanest Xylonest Distanest }	5 per cent with 5 per cent glucose (hyperbaric)	2 per cent to 3 per cent	Medium
Quinoline derivative	Cinchocaine	{ Nupercaine Dibucaine }	0.5 per cent with 6 per cent glucose (hyperbaric); 1 in 1500 in 0.5 per cent NaCl (hypobaric)		Long

free), documented by concurrent immunological changes, in a patient who had given a history of allergy to lignocaine. McLeskey (1981) noted that methylparaben, the most frequently used commercial preservative for local analgesic drugs, is very similar in chemical structure to that of para-aminobenzoic acid. Therefore, any investigations for allergy suspected to be caused by an amide type local analgesic agent must be done on the preservative free drug.

The analgesic profile of a chemical compound is dependent on its lipid solubility, protein binding, dissociation constant, non-nervous tissue diffusibility, and intrinsic vasodilator activity (Covino, 1982). Lipid solubility appears to be a primary determinant of intrinsic analgesic potency. Those local analgesic agents which are highly lipid soluble penetrate the nerve membrane more easily and this is reflected biologically in increased potency. The protein binding characteristics of local analgesic agents primarily influence the duration of action. Procaine is poorly bound to proteins and possesses a relatively short duration of action. Conversely, amethocaine, bupivacaine and etidocaine are highly bound to proteins and display long duration of anaesthesia. The relationship between protein binding of local analgesic agents and their duration of action is again consistent with the basic structure of the nerve membrane. Proteins account for approximately 10 per cent of the nerve membrane, therefore agents which penetrate the axolemma and attach more firmly to the membrane proteins will tend to possess a prolonged duration of activity. On the basis of differences in duration of action, it is possible to classify the clinically useful injectable local analgesic compounds (Covino, 1982):

Group I   Agents of short duration of action — e.g. procaine, chloroprocaine.
Group II   Agents of intermediate duration of action — e.g. lignocaine, mepivacaine, prilocaine.
Group III   Agents of long duration of action — e.g. amethocaine, bupivacaine, etidocaine, cinchocaine.

It appears that with the older amide-linked drugs, such as lignocaine, there is a relatively wide margin between central nervous system toxicity and cardiovascular depression (Scott, 1981). Because lignocaine occasionally causes apnoea, cardiovascular depression is often secondary to hypoxia rather than the primary effect of the drug. Recently this separation of central nervous system and cardiovascular toxicity has been questioned in regard to the longer acting drugs bupivacaine and etidocaine (Albright, 1979; Tucker, 1982). Case reports have appeared suggesting that severe cardiac depression, often leading to cardiac arrest, may occur soon after the appearance of convulsions. Scott reminds us (Scott, 1981) that hypoxia develops very quickly in a convulsing patient. The rapidity with which hypoxia and respiratory acidosis may occur has been illustrated recently (Moore et al, 1980) and central nervous system toxicity from local analgesics is greatly enhanced by acidosis and hypercapnia (Engelsson and Matousek, 1975).

Covino (1982) noted that under conditions of normal acid base status, bupivacaine and etidocaine are four times more toxic than lignocaine, but as bupivacaine is four times as potent as lignocaine, there is little difference in the therapeutic ratio of these agents with regard to the cardiovascular system. The possibility exists that under clinical conditions in which hypoxia and acidosis may be present, the more potent local analgesics such as bupivacaine may prove to be relatively more harmful with regard to the cardiovascular system than agents such as lignocaine.

Liu et al (1983) investigated the comparative central nervous system toxicity of serially administered intravenous doses of lignocaine, bupivacaine, etidocaine and amethocaine on awake dogs. The mean cumulative dose required for convulsive activity was 4 mg/kg amethocaine, 5 mg/kg bupivacaine, 8 mg/kg etidocaine, and 22 mg/kg lignocaine. The cumulative convulsive dose of lignocaine was significantly greater than that of the other three agents. They suggest that a comparison of the in vivo potency and the acute central nervous system toxicity of these agents show little difference in the therapeutic ratio between the less potent analgesics such as lignocaine and the more potent drugs amethocaine, bupivacaine and etidocaine. The relative central nervous system toxicity of the different agents, as determined in awake dogs, was compared with the relative cardiovascular toxicity previously evaluated in ventilated dogs anaesthetised with pentobarbitone. The dose of lignocaine, etidocaine, amethocaine and bupivacaine required to produce irreversible cardiovascular depression was 3.5 to 6.7 times greater than that which produced convulsions. These results suggest that the central nervous system is the primary target organ for the toxic effects of both highly lipid soluble and highly protein bound local analgesic agents (i.e. bupivacaine, etidocaine and amethocaine) and less lipid soluble and less protein bound drugs (i.e. lignocaine) following rapid intravenous administration.

Tachyphylaxis, the phenomenon of acute tolerance to drugs, is exhibited by local analgesic agents. Repeated injections produce a successively diminishing effect in duration and quality of blockade (Bromage et al, 1964). Bromage et al (1969) studied extradural tachyphylaxis in man using lignocaine, mepivacaine and prilocaine and noted results which have important clinical implications in the management of continuous extradural analgesia. There was an augmentation of analgesia associated with a relatively short interval between injections. The most significant interval was the period between the disappearance of analgesia from the previous dose and the time of the next injection, i.e. the 'interanalgesic interval'. Analgesic potency tended to be augmented if the interanalgesic interval was short but augmentation declined and gave way to decay of effect and tachyphylaxis if the interval exceeded 10 minutes. Tachyphylaxis increased with the length of interanalgesic interval up to 60 minutes and was fairly constant thereafter. They noted that if analgesia was allowed to wear off completely, each delayed dose required an increase of 25 to 30 per cent above that of its immediate predecessor. Therefore, clinical conditions that reduce the need for frequent re-injections reduce the number of occasions for tachyphylaxis to develop, and the use of long-acting agents and the addition of adrenaline to prolong their action further will both tend to postpone the effects of acute tolerance. It is also advisable to start with as small a dose as is practicable.

Working with bupivacaine, Bromage noted augmentation of response when re-injections were made at frequent intervals before analgesia had receded. There was a greater spread and more intense sensory and motor block even when very dilute solutions of bupivacaine were used. Repeated injections of 0.125 per cent bupivacaine gradually intensified the quality of analgesia and sometimes produced an appreciable degree of motor block too.

Wüst et al (1979) noted tachyphylaxis during continuous extradural anaesthesia with bupivacaine 0.125 per cent and 0.25 per cent given for postoperative pain relief. These authors noted increasing tolerance to the agent and both concentration and volume necessary to block the required number of segments had to be increased. Following interruption of the injection for four hours the initial dose response returned. There was a tendency to a decreased effectiveness of a given dose in relation to metabolic acidosis.

ESTER-LINKED LOCAL ANALGESIC AGENTS

Cocaine hydrochloride BP and USP

Cocaine, a naturally occurring local analgesic agent, is of great historical importance but has no place in present-day central neural blockade.

Procaine hydrochloride BP (Novocaine, Planocaine, Ethocaine, Neocaine, Allocaine, Syncaine, Kerocain, Servocaine, Scurocaine)

The remarkable lack of toxicity of procaine is chiefly due to its rapid hydrolysis by serum cholinesterase, but the use of procaine in central neural blockade is very limited since the advent of superior agents. The crystalline form of procaine may be used intradurally by dissolving 50 to 300 mg in aspirated CSF and re-injecting the solution slowly. The 2 per cent solution has been used extradurally, but the onset of action is slow and duration is only 30 to 45 minutes. The powers of penetration are inferior to those of lignocaine. Ansbro et al (1953) found that 5 per cent concentration was necessary for satisfactory clinical results in the extradural space, and in a series of 700 cases they used an induction dose of 20 ml of 5 per cent procaine (i.e. one gram). Sung and Truant (1954) suggested procaine had advantages over lignocaine for nerve blocks in patients with connective tissue disease, as it is less fat soluble and is broken down more rapidly. Eisele and Reitan (1971) reported prolonged effects with lignocaine in scleroderma and Raynaud's phenomenon. Procaine has also been suggested as the agent of choice where is a history of malignant hyperpyrexia (Cousins and Mather, 1980).

Chloroprocaine hydrochloride (Nesacaine)

2-chloroprocaine is an ester-linked local analgesic agent which has been in frequent use in the United States since 1952. It has been popular because of its rapid onset of action, and very low toxicity due to rapid hydrolysis of the molecule by plasma cholinesterase. It does not easily cross the placental barrier. Duration of analgesia is relatively short, approximately 45 minutes, and the level of analgesia may wane suddenly. The 3 per cent solution is necessary to provide adequate extradural analgesia for surgical operations but 1.5 to 2 per cent concentrations are adequate for obstetric analgesia. Because of its rapidity of action, chloroprocaine has been used for short surgical procedures and in vaginal deliveries where its low toxicity is an advantage for the fetus. Chloroprocaine is the most acid of local analgesic agents commonly used. The 3 per cent solution has a pH of 3.3. Intradural injection is not recommended. The possibility of neurotoxicity caused by inadvertent intradural injection of chloroprocaine has been the subject of much recent controversy in the United States (Flowerdew, 1982; Marx and Finster, 1982; Moore et al, 1982). Intradural injection may cause prolonged blockade, and if it is inadvertently injected it is advisable to irrigate it out (Covino et al, 1980; Ravindran et al, 1980; Reisner et al, 1980). A considerable number of animal experiments have been undertaken and official reviews of human and animal data made. The available data tend to support the conclusion that local analgesic agents used with clinical judgement do not injure nervous tissue directly (Schnider, 1982). However, the controversy continues.

Amethocaine hydrochloride BP

Amethocaine (Pantocaine, Pontocaine, Decicain, Butethanol, Anethaine, Tetracaine (USP) Pantokain, Dikain) was first synthesised in 1928. Like procaine, it is an ester of para-aminobenzoic acid, and is hydrolysed into the latter drug by plasma cholinesterase. Hydrolysis of amethocaine in the body takes about four times longer than that of procaine, and is more easily exceeded by the rate of absorption. Amethocaine is about 10 times as toxic as procaine when injected intravenously.

A concentration of 0.25 to 0.5 per cent with adrenaline 1:200 000 achieves satisfactory extradural blockade for operative surgery (Bromage, 1969; Watt et al, 1970). Its duration of action is longer than that produced by lignocaine with adrenaline, but usually shorter than that of bupivacaine with adrenaline. The onset of action is slower than that produced by lignocaine but amethocaine has been frequently mixed with procaine or lignocaine to combine the short latency of these agents with the prolonged action of amethocaine. Bromage (1978a) notes that 0.5 per cent amethocaine solution in the extradural space produces profound motor block but only marginally satisfactory sensory block, and is therefore not a suitable agent for either obstetric or postoperative analgesia.

There have been several recent trials comparing intradural amethocaine with other agents. McClure (1982) investigated the effects of baricity and posture using amethocaine 0.5 per cent hyperbaric and 0.5 per cent isobaric, and hyperbaric and plain 0.5 per cent bupivacaine. He concluded that a hyperbaric solution is preferable for abdominal surgery, but when a block is required for surgery to the legs or perineum and minimal circulatory effects are desired, an isobaric solution is recommended. Löfström et al (1982) found that hyperbaric amethocaine 1 per cent produced analgesia and motor blockade of longer duration than hyperbaric mepivacaine 4 per cent but shorter than that produced by hyperbaric bupivacaine 0.5 per cent and 0.75 per cent. Tattersall (1983) compared the effects of 1 per cent hyperbaric amethocaine solution with those produced by 15 mg plain bupivacaine 0.5 per cent intradurally. He found that bupivacaine had a more limited spread of analgesia which lasted longer and was accompanied by less hypotension and fewer complications than amethocaine.

Amethocaine can be obtained in either a 1 per cent solution to which an equal volume of 10 per cent glucose can be added, giving an 0.5 per cent concentration, or in ampoules containing 20 mg of micro-crystals to which 5 to 10 per cent dextrose solution can be added to ensure that the solution is hyperbaric. Solutions of amethocaine may be sterilised by boiling or autoclaving, but repeated or prolonged autoclaving is undesirable. They are rapidly inactivated by alkalis. Solutions prepared under sterile conditions remain sterile and bactericidal (Zaidi and Healey, 1977). Amethocaine may be a useful alternative where amide-linked agents are contraindicated, such as a history of malignant hyperpyrexia (Cousins and Mather, 1980).

AMIDE-LINKED LOCAL ANALGESIC AGENTS

Cinchocaine hydrochloride BP

Cinchocaine (Nupercaine, Dibucaine USP, Percaine, Sovcaine) is a complex amine derived from quinoline and first synthesised in 1925. It is very highly lipid soluble, and a most potent local analgesic agent. It is detoxicated in the liver but elimination is relatively slow.

Cinchocaine is an excellent intradural agent and hyperbaric cinchocaine ('heavy Nupercaine') 1:200 solution in 6 per cent glucose with a dosage of 0.5 to 2.0 ml has been popular and successful for nearly 50 years. It has a specific gravity of 1.025. Hypobaric cinchocaine 1:1500 solution is still used in some countries and has a specific gravity of 1.0035. Cinchocaine has a very slow onset of action in the extradural space, and because of its toxicity and the availability of superior agents, there is little justification for extradural use. Because of the low pKa, care must be taken to avoid the addition of any alkali which causes precipitation of base and inactivation of the drug. This is a real possibility when glass syringes and needles have to be sterilised for re-use. Flushing through of resterilised syringes and needles, with rejection of the flushing liquid, would avoid this problem. Rubin (1982) compared 0.5 per cent bupivacaine, hyperbaric and plain, with hyperbaric cinchocaine 0.5 per cent in 6 per cent glucose, and found hyperbaric bupivacaine a useful alternative to cinchocaine. Both sensory loss and motor blockade were produced earlier by the hyperbaric solutions than by the glucose free bupivacaine.

Lignocaine hydrochloride BP

Lignocaine (Xylocaine, Duncaine, lidocaine USP) is a basic anilide synthesised by Löfgren and Lundqvist in 1943 and first used by Gordh in 1948. It has a pKa of 7.86 and is only moderately lipid soluble. It is very stable, not decomposed by boiling, acids or alkalis. Lignocaine has a long shelf life and can be resterilised by heat without loss of potency or fear of toxic changes (Whittet, 1954). It should not be left in contact with copper or nickel in syringes or gallipots, as ions are liberated which are irritating to the tissues; it is inactivated by iodine. Lignocaine appears to diffuse over a wider field and has greater penetrating powers than equal volumes of other local analgesic drugs; it is very reliable in its action. It is the most thoroughly studied and widely used of all local analgesic agents and has become the standard against which the performance and toxicity of other drugs are measured. Potency and toxicity are approximately twice those of procaine.

Lignocaine 1.5 per cent with adrenaline 1:200 000 is an excellent agent for extradural analgesia for operative surgery. Analgesia develops within 6 to 8 minutes and lasts 2 to 3 hours. Amethocaine crystals, dissolved to make a concentration of 1:1000 may be added to the lignocaine-adrenaline solution to extend the duration of analgesia if required. 2 per cent lignocaine with adrenaline may prove useful where superior relaxation of muscles is desirable. The 1 per cent concentration is useful where sensory blockade only is required, e.g. postoperative or obstetric analgesia. Following injection, absorption of lignocaine causes drowsiness and amnesia which is useful for sedation in patients undergoing surgery. The addition of adrenaline ensures that less drug is absorbed into the bloodstream at any one time, maintaining minimal blood levels, and concurrently therefore, more lignocaine is left in the spinal canal to enhance the quality and duration of the central neural blockade (Bromage, 1978b). Phenylephrine may be added as vasoconstrictor instead of adrenaline. Metabolism of lignocaine is by microsomes in the liver, and metabolites are excreted by the kidney. Like prilocaine, its metabolism can give rise to the formation of methaemoglobin, although in practice this is not a problem, Tachyphylaxis may be exhibited when subsequent doses of lignocaine are given within hours of the first injection.

Hyperbaric lignocaine has not gained favour for intradural block in Britain because of the variable and often too rapid nature of its spread within the theca. Fisher and Bryce-Smith (1971) used lignocaine 5.0 per cent with 7.5 per cent glucose in a study with comparable solutions of cinchocaine and prilocaine, and found that lignocaine produced inferior results. One of the main difficulties was that the amount of glucose added gave a specific gravity of 1.035 to 1.040, and such a heavy solution tended to flow rapidly, making control of level difficult to the point of danger. Nevertheless, hyperbaric lignocaine is used in the USA, India, Scandinavia, the United Kingdom and elsewhere.

In 1963, the carbonation of lignocaine was investigated with encouraging results. Bromage (1965; Bromage et al, 1967; Bromage and Gertel, 1970) and Cousins and Bromage (1971) undertook several studies comparing the hydrochloride and carbonated salts of local analgesic agents. They found that the speed and intensity of sensory and motor block were enhanced when the carbonated solutions of lignocaine and prilocaine were used, in comparison with the hydrochloride salts. The normally resistant segments L.5 and S.1 were very adequately anaesthetised with carbonated lignocaine. Benefits were confirmed by Schulte-Steinberg et al (1970) and Catchlove (1973). Hemmings et al (1983) suggest that carbonated lignocaine may be useful for sacral extradural use when rapid perineal analgesia is required for vaginal delivery.

In order to retain maximum efficacy of a carbonated local analgesic agent, the containing vial should be freshly opened, and the agent drawn into a syringe by slow aspiration through a wide bore cannula in order to avoid loss of carbon dioxide from the solution. In vivo, carbon dioxide diffuses out of the drug, raising the environmental pH and increasing the percentage of the un-ionised base that is available for diffusion intracellularly (Soderman and Duke, 1983).

The principle of carbonation of local analgesic agents is of considerable practical importance, but unfortunately the manufacturing process is relatively difficult and expensive and the products are not easily available in the United Kingdom.

Prilocaine hydrochloride

Prilocaine (Citanest, Xyonest, Distanest, Propitocaine) is an amide of orthotoluidine and closely related to lignocaine. It was synthesised by Löfgren and used clinically by Eriksson and Gordh in 1959. It is a very stable compound but is rapidly metabolised in the liver, kidneys and lungs, partly by amidase, so that it is less cumulative and less toxic than lignocaine. One of the degradation products, o-toluidine, causes the oxidation of haemoglobin to methaemoglobin. If more than 600 mg of prilocaine is used, the methaemoglobinaemia will show as cyanosis if 1.5 gm per cent or more of the haemoglobin is circulating as methaemoglobin, but is of little clinical importance unless there is severe anaemia or circulatory impairment. There is an associated shift of the oxygen dissociation curve of the remaining haemoglobin which hinders oxygen liberation at tissue level. Methaemoglobin crosses the placenta and prilocaine is therefore better avoided for obstetric analgesia lest an already hypoxic fetus be exposed to further risk. Methaemoglobinaemia usually disappears spontaneously within 24 hours, but the methaemoglobin may be reduced if felt necessary by the intravenous injection of methylene blue 1 to 2 mg/kg.

Onset and duration of action of prilocaine in the extradural space are slightly longer than those of lignocaine. It has good penetrative powers and may be used in concentrations similar to those of lignocaine, although Bromage (1978c) has found that 3 per cent prilocaine without adrenaline is approximately equivalent to 2 per cent lignocaine with adrenaline in terms of speed of onset and efficiency of blockade. The addition of adrenaline improves the duration and quality of prilocaine analgesia but less impressively than with lignocaine. Prilocaine is therefore the agent of choice when the addition of adrenaline is inadvisable because of the patient's general condition, e.g. thyrotoxicosis, hypertension, during tricyclic antidepressant therapy, or where the local circulation is poor. Because of its low systemic toxicity, prilocaine is also the preferable analgesic agent when high dosage and strong concentration are required or when injection is into a vascular area such as the sacral extradural space.

Fisher and Bryce-Smith (1971), in a comparison of intradural agents, found that 5 per cent 'heavy' prilocaine solution produced very satisfactory conditions. The duration of useful analgesia was comparable with that of cinchocaine. Following this work, a commercial preparation of 5 per cent 'heavy' prilocaine was available for a limited time in Britain. At the time of going to press the only commercial preparation of prilocaine available is 0.5 per cent.

Mepivacaine hydrochloride

Mepivacaine (Carbocaine, Scandicaine, Meaverin) is a tertiary amine synthesised by Ekenstam in 1956. It is clinically comparable with lignocaine. Its pKa is 7.8 and 75 per cent of the drug is protein bound (Reynolds, 1970). Tucker et al (1970) estimated its protein binding capacity as less than that of bupivacaine but greater than that of lignocaine; its placental transfer is rapid. Solutions of mepivacaine are very stable and can be autoclaved. Without a vasoconstrictor, the solutions have a practically neutral reaction so the risk of metallic ion release when in contact with syringes, gallipots or cannulae is minimal. When a vasoconstrictor is added, the pH of the solution is reduced to 3.5 to 4.5 by the combination of the adrenaline and antioxidant, and caution should be observed. It does not cause methaemoglobin formation.

Mepivacaine is pharmacologically similar to lignocaine and provides a slightly longer duration of analgesia. Its penetrative powers are as efficient as those of lignocaine, and it causes less vasodilation (Reynolds, 1972). It was originally thought that the addition of adrenaline was unnecessary, but Tucker et al (1972), after studying plasma levels of mepivacaine, recommended the addition of adrenaline. In a randomised study of obstetric caudal analgesia, Gunther and Belville (1972) found significantly prolonged analgesia when adrenaline was used. It has a narrower safety margin than bupivacaine in extradural blockade (Reynolds, 1971) and is markedly cumulative (Moore et al 1968), giving rise to high fetal blood concentrations. Boyes (1975) states that the metabolism by the neonate is impaired, but within 24 hours of birth the excretion process is capable of eliminating the drug.

This agent can be used for all types of analgesia in doses and concentrations similar to those of lignocaine, but does not appear to have any advantage over lignocaine. It is not suitable for obstetric analgesia. A preparation with glucose having a specific gravity of 1.025 is available for intradural analgesia. Used thus, it is a satisfactory agent for operations not exceeding one and a half hours (Siker et al, 1966).

Bupivacaine hydrochloride BP

Bupivacaine (Marcain, Marcaine) was synthesised in 1957 by Ekenstam and his colleagues (Ekenstam et al, 1957) and used clinically by Telivuo in 1963 (Telivuo, 1963). It is derived from mepivacaine, is a very stable compound and may be autoclaved repeatedly. In clinical use 80 to 95 per cent is protein bound; neonatal plasma proteins have less capacity than those of the adult to bind bupivacaine (Mather et al, 1971). Bupivacaine is a highly lipid soluble substance and has a potency approximately four times that of lignocaine or mepivacaine. It is more protein bound and less cumulative than these two agents; it has a longer latency but is considerably longer lasting. It has a shorter onset of action and longer duration than amethocaine in extradural block (Bromage, 1969; Watt et al, 1970). Duration of effect, assessed as time elapsed before need of further analgesia, may be from 3 to 8 hours in the lumbar extradural space, 10 hours in the sacral extradural space, but only $1\frac{1}{2}$ to 2 hours in thoracic extradural analgesia, perhaps because of the small dosage required in this area. It appears to produce sensory analgesia more efficiently than motor block. Some workers believe that the addition of adrenaline increases its duration only marginally, in contrast to lignocaine in which the duration is markedly improved by the addition of 1:200 000 adrenaline. Bromage (1978d) has found that the addition of 1:200 000 adrenaline improves the quality of blockade. However, adding adrenaline is important for maintaining minimal blood levels of bupivacaine and decreasing the risk of systemic toxicity when a large dose is used, and particularly in a vascular site. The comparatively long duration of action is a valuable characteristic for postoperative analgesia, and when uncertainty exists regarding the starting time or duration of surgery.

Bupivacaine is particularly useful in obstetric analgesia because of the relatively low systemic toxicity to the mother and fetus; analgesia from extradural bupivacaine has a duration of 2 to 4 hours in the first stage of labour. Reynolds and Taylor (1971) suggest that because bupivacaine is unlikely to accumulate in the dosage required during the first stage, adrenaline is not necessary and offers no significant advantage. It may, however, help in the protection of the mother from systemic toxicity if higher doses of the drug (total dose exceeding 320 mg — Reynolds et al, 1973) are required at the end of labour, and the decreased maternal concentration will cause the fetus to be exposed to a lower plasma level than if plain bupivacaine is used for a final extradural dose just prior to delivery. Ghoneim and Pandya (1974) found that pethidine and other drugs cause displacement of bupivacaine from plasma proteins and may, therefore, possibly increase its toxicity. Acidosis increases the toxic effects of local analgesic agents on the central nervous system and bupivacaine causes no EEG changes until shortly before a convulsion occurs (Engelsson and Matousek, 1975). As mentioned earlier, some case reports have been described suggesting that severe cardiac depression, often leading to cardiac arrest, may occur soon after convulsions appear. It is possible that in clinical conditions where hypoxia and acidosis are present, the more potent agents such as bupivacaine and etidocaine are relatively more toxic to the heart than agents such as lignocaine (Albright, 1979; Covino, 1982; Tucker, 1982).

The maximum safe dose of bupivacaine is in the region of 2 mg/kg body weight, (25 to 30 ml of the 0.5 per cent solution in the average adult). The concentration range currently available is 0.25 per cent, 0.5 per cent and 0.75 per cent plain, 0.25 per cent with adrenaline 1:400 000 and 0.5 per cent with adrenaline 1:200 000. Bupivacaine with adrenaline has some sodium metabisulphite added by the manufacturer to decrease the possibility of oxidation of the adrenaline. 0.5 per cent and 0.75 per cent strengths are used in extradural block for surgical procedures. 0.5 per cent with adrenaline 1:200 000 gives satisfactory operating conditions in most cases but 0.75 per cent gives better motor block and slightly shortens latency of onset. 0.75 per cent bupivacaine with adrenaline 1:200 000 has the disadvantage in the postoperative phase in that patients may be unable to move their legs for some considerable time because of the profound motor block. The plain 0.75 per cent solution gives less motor block but good sensory analgesia except in the resistant segments of L.5 and S.1. Concentrations used in obstetrics range from 0.125 per cent to 0.5 per cent, and 0.25 per cent and 0.375 per cent are popular. When postoperative analgesia is required, 0.25 per cent to 0.3 per cent concentrations are useful, so that motor blockade is not produced. When bone surgery has taken place, 0.5 per cent concentration appears necessary to control postoperative pain, although this has the disadvantage of blocking some motor power, and the patient should be warned before the extradural block is given.

The carbonated form of bupivacaine does not unfortunately decrease the onset of action time or improve the quality of analgesia as is the case with the carbonated salts of lignocaine and prilocaine. Brown et al (1980) in a double blind trial comparing carbonated bupivacaine with bupivacaine hydrochloride in extradural anaesthesia concluded that the carbonated bupivacaine offered no advantage over the hydrochloride salt.

Several clinical trials using intradural bupivacaine have been undertaken over the last few years, involving some thousands of patients, with promising results. (Nolte et al, 1977; Farrar et al, 1979; Nolte and Stark, 1979; Stratmann et al, 1979; Chambers et al, 1981; Chambers et al, 1982b; Löfström et al, 1982; McClure, 1982; Nolte, 1982; Rubin, 1982; Tuominen et al, 1982; Ryan et al, 1983; Tattersall, 1983). 0.5 per cent plain bupivacaine intradurally gives very good results for surgery to the lower limbs or perineum (see Ch. 8). The central neural blockade produced is highly reliable and lasts between 2 to 4 hours. Minimal circulatory effects are usually produced.

However, when lower abdominal surgery is contemplated, the hyperbaric solution may be found necessary to reach the required height, and bupivacaine 0.5 per cent in 5 per cent to 8 per cent dextrose produces consistently good central neural blockade (Moore, 1980; Chambers et al, 1981). The use of 0.75 per cent bupivacaine in 8 per cent dextrose offers no additional advantage (Chambers et al, 1982a). Within the range 2 to 4 ml, increasing the volume of 0.5 per cent solution given does not produce any change in spread, but ensures a longer duration of action — an effect related to increased dosage. Added vasoconstrictors cannot be relied upon to produce a significant increase in duration in individual cases (Chambers et al, 1982a).

Ryan et al (1983) using plain bupivacaine 0.5 per cent found that 3.0 to 3.5 ml intradurally in the L.3–4 interspace in the sitting position, gave adequate analgesia for endoscopic prostatic resection or lower limb surgery. They recommend 4 ml for open prostatectomy or hip surgery, but suggest volumes of only 2 to 3 ml in frail patients or those over 70 years of age.

Nolte (1982) in a follow up of more than 3000 cases of intradural anaesthesia, found no neurological sequelae related to the use of bupivacaine.

Bupivacaine plain 0.5 per cent is freely available. Although its specific gravity at 37°C (0.998) is slightly less than that of cerebrospinal fluid (1.001), in practice it behaves as an isobaric solution in intradural analgesia and the patient can be tilted head down immediately after injection. It is autoclavable and free of preservative. A solution of hyperbaric bupivacaine 0.5 per cent with 8 per cent dextrose is under preparation in the United Kingdom.

Bupivacaine has currently established itself a place in the anaesthetists' armamentarium as a long-acting agent producing less motor than sensory block. The sensory block gives good analgesia. It serves a useful function in central neural blockade for general surgical, gynaecological and orthopaedic operations, for postoperative and post-traumatic analgesia, and is particularly useful for obstetric analgesia.

Etidocaine hydrochloride BP

Etidocaine (Duranest; W-19053) is a relatively new, potent, long-acting local analgesic agent which is chemically related to lignocaine. It is a stable compound and the plain solution may be autoclaved five times without decomposition; solutions with adrenaline should not be autoclaved more than twice because of the loss of potency of the adrenaline. Characteristics of etidocaine are its high lipid solubility and strong protein binding capacity. Clinically it has a very rapid onset and long duration of action, the latter being comparable to bupivacaine. Motor block is profound, but unfortunately sensory blockade is not, and analgesia is sometimes inadequate. During surgery under central neural blockade, traction on viscera may be felt, and in the postoperative phase, there may be undesirable immobility of the legs. Etidocaine could be a useful agent when profound muscular relaxation is required during surgery. It is not the drug of choice for obstetric analgesia where muscular activity is desirable as in vaginal delivery. However, clinical reports have not always been in complete agreement. Poppers (1975) found satisfactory analgesia with the 0.25 per cent and 0.5 per cent concentrations, accompanied by only minimal muscle relaxation. Galindo et al (1975) found that extradural etidocaine 1.5 per cent achieved excellent blockade for surgical anaesthesia and postoperative pain relief. They noted that it was effective in blocking spinal roots of large diameter which are particularly difficult to block, notably the 1st sacral segment.

Investigators have not always agreed about the role of adrenaline in relation to etidocaine (Bromage, 1978e). Some have felt that adrenaline 1:200 000 improves the quality of analgesia markedly, while others concluded that it had no effect apart from speeding the onset of motor blockade. Buckley et al (1978) found that the addition of adrenaline 1:200 000 did not significantly prolong the duration of analgesia but produced more motor block. Etidocaine 1.5 per cent gave longer duration of analgesia and more intense motor block than the 1 per cent solution.

Littlewood et al (1977) compared various concentrations of 10 ml of plain solutions of lignocaine, bupivacaine and etidocaine in a double blind trial as agents for extradural analgesia for labour pain relief. They found that increasing the drug concentration reduced the onset times and increased both the duration of analgesia and degree of motor block, but had little effect on dermatomal spread or on frequency of hypotension. Based on their results they classified the agents in relation to onset and duration of analgesia and degree of motor blockade. Of the agents and concentrations giving moderate duration of analgesia, i.e. approximately 1 hour, 1.5 per cent lignocaine had a moderate onset time with minimal motor block; 0.25 per cent and 0.375 per cent bupivacaine had slow onset times with minimal motor block, and 0.75 per cent etidocaine had a rapid onset with moderate motor block. Of the agents and concentrations giving long duration of analgesia, i.e. approximately $1\frac{1}{2}$ to 2 hours, bupivacaine 0.5 per cent and 0.75 per cent had moderate onset times and motor block, but etidocaine 1.0 per cent had a rapid onset time and intense motor block. The overall propensity of etidocaine to block motor fibres more than sensory fibres limits its clinical use.

Etidocaine appears to be twice as toxic as lignocaine when absorbed slowly from subcutaneous sites, but about four times as toxic as lignocaine when given by rapid intravenous injection. However, as mentioned earlier in this chapter, where hypoxia and acidosis exist clinically, the potent, longer acting drugs etidocaine and bupivacaine may be relatively more toxic to the cardiovascular system than lignocaine.

Etidocaine has been used in 0.25 per cent, 0.5 per cent, 0.75 per cent, 1 per cent and 1.5 per cent concentrations but because motor block is disproportionately severe compared with sensory block, this long-acting agent has become less popular and is gradually being withdrawn from use in some countries.

VASOCONSTRICTOR DRUGS

Vasoconstrictor drugs have been used in local analgesia since Braun introduced adrenaline in 1902 (Braun, 1903). When combined with a local analgesic agent, the vasoconstriction produced decreases the rate of absorption from the injected site thereby causing a slower rise in the plasma level of the analgesic agent, and consequently reducing potential systemic toxicity. By the same vasoconstrictive effect and decreased rate of absorption, the duration of effect of the agent is increased. The local vasoconstriction causes ischaemia of skin and tissues locally, aiding surgical vision, although it should be noted that adrenaline dilates those blood vessels which supply muscle.

Adrenaline BP (Epinephrine)

Adrenaline acid tartrate is synthesised for pharmaceutical purposes, and is available in ampoules containing 1 ml of 1:1000 solution. The ampoules may be autoclaved once or twice without appreciable loss of potency (Berry and West, 1944; Thomas, 1956). The solution is prone to oxidation and is decomposed by heat and sunlight. When adrenaline is commercially added to a local analgesic solution an anti-oxidant is also added and this imparts marked acidity to the adrenaline-local analgesic mixture. This increased acidity causes some discomfort on injection, and causes a slower onset of blockade from the acidified local analgesic agent containing adrenaline than from the near neutral solution to which adrenaline is added shortly before use (de Jong, 1970).

The total dose of adrenaline used should not exceed 0.5 mg (i.e. 0.5 ml of 1:1000 solution) and preferably in a concentration no greater than 1:200 000.

Adrenaline-local analgesic mixtures must not be used on patients taking tricyclic antidepressants as these inhibit the destruction of catecholamines and the cardiovascular effects of adrenaline may be potentiated. Tricyclic antidepressants should be withdrawn for three days preceding the use of adrenaline, or alternatively felypressin can be employed to produce a relatively ischaemic field, or a local analgesic of low toxicity such as prilocaine substituted, thus avoiding the need for a vasoconstrictor. It would be wise to avoid adrenaline in patients taking monoamine oxidase inhibitors.

Some anaesthetists prefer to maintain sleep with a volatile agent in patients who have had central neural blockade and the increased possibility of arrhythmias must be borne in mind when adrenaline has been added to the local analgesic agent.

Some workers use adrenaline with the local analgesic agent in intradural block. In the United States it has been common practice to add adrenaline to hyperbaric amethocaine to prolong the effects of the block. Chambers et al (1982a), in a series using either adrenaline or phenylephrine with hyperbaric bupivacaine, found that vasoconstrictors could not be relied upon to produce a significant and consistent increase in duration in individual cases.

Phenylephrine hydrochloride BP (Neophryn, Neosynephrine)

Phenylephrine may be used as a vasoconstrictor. It causes no cerebral stimulation or tachycardia. It may be used in conditions in which the beta effects of adrenaline are undesirable such as hyperthyroidism. Compared with adrenaline its vasoconstrictor activity is weak and it is therefore added as a dose of 0.25 to 0.5 ml of 1 per cent solution to the local analgesic preparation. It is more stable than adrenaline and, being metabolised more slowly, has a longer vasoconstrictor effect in equivalent dosage. If accidentally injected intravenously, dysrhythmias are unlikely to be produced. If added to a spinal analgesic solution the duration of analgesia will be prolonged (Meagher et al, 1966; Lund, 1971). It is sterilised by filtration.

VASOPRESSORS IN HYPOTENSION

In the authors' experience, pressor drugs are seldom required in central neural blockade, although workers in other centres formerly used them routinely. A considered dosage of local analgesic agent is used in respect to the age, general condition of the patient and height of block required. Varying volumes of fluid are given via a previously cannulated vein and the volume may range from 200 ml up to as much as 2 or 3 litres in the obstetric patient. It is a clinical impression that if approximately 200 ml of fluid is administered to the elderly hypertensive patient with labile blood pressure before sympathetic blockade has caused the blood pressure to fall, the drop will be considerably reduced. The ischaemia produced in the surgical field does not appear to be directly related to the decrease in the blood pressure.

If the arterial pressure falls below an unacceptable limit for the circumstances (e.g. systolic of 70 mmHg), the volume of fluid is increased, and if bradycardia associated with increased vagal tone is present, small increments (0.2 mg) of atropine are given intravenously. Other simple measures are elevation of the legs, and the administration of oxygen while increasing the flow of intravenous fluids.

On those occasions when the fall in arterial pressure is precipitous, and additional aid is required to restore control, it is advisable to have available a vasopressor drug with which the anaesthetist is familiar. Some anaesthetists of wide experience and repute give a vasopressor prophylactically, and have good reasons for so doing (see Ch. 4).

SYMPATHOMIMETIC AMINES

Sympathomimetic amines acting directly by stimulation of alpha and beta receptors, and indirectly by release of catecholamines:

Ephedrine BP

This is the active principle of ma huang, a herb that has been used by Chinese medicine men for 5000 years. Its adrenaline-like properties were described in 1917 and it was first used to control hypotension during spinal analgesia in 1927 (Ockerblad and Dillon, 1927). Its merits as a vasopressor for the treatment of excessive hypotension due to vasomotor sympathetic block following intradural or extradural analgesia have only recently been fully appreciated. The positive inotropic and chronotropic actions of ephedrine increase the cardiac output and venous return: the blood-pressure is raised but not as a result of peripheral vasoconstriction. These properties make ephedrine the vasopressor of choice when one is deemed to be required in obstetrics. However, animal work has shown (James et al, 1970) that occasionally correction of maternal hypotension is accompanied by a further reduction in placental blood flow, as opposed to the increase which usually takes place following ephedrine administration. Hence other methods such as alteration of the mother's position, elevation of legs and increased infusion of intravenous fluids should be the initial methods of choice.

Stimulation of the central nervous system is an important side-effect to note when ephedrine is given in a hypotensive state. Tachyphylaxis can occur which may be explained by its indirect action of release of catecholamine stores. It potentiates the effects of injected adrenaline or noradrenaline by its inhibitory effect on monoamine oxidase. It is contraindicated in patients taking monoamine oxidase inhibitors.

The intravenous dose is 5 to 30 mg. It can also be given intramuscularly.

Methylamphetamine (Methedrine, Pervitin)

Methylamphetamine was a useful vasopressor which had chronotropic and inotropic effects on the heart. Unfortunately it has suffered social abuse because of its cerebral stimulant effect and is now difficult to obtain. The dose is 5 to 10 mg intravenously. It can also be given intramuscularly.

The use of methylamphetamine is now discouraged.

Metaraminol bitartrate (Aramine)

Metaraminol does not stimulate the cerebral cortex. Reflex bradycardia produced may be counteracted by atropine. Administration to patients taking monoamine oxidase inhibitors may result in potentiated vasopressor action. It should be used cautiously in patients with severe heart disease. Intravenous dosage is 0.5 to 5 mg. It can be given by intravenous infusion.

Mephentermine sulphate BP (Mephine, Wyamine)

Mephentermine has anti-arrhythmic properties and it stimulates the cerebral cortex in a similar way to ephedrine. It should not be used with monoamine oxidase inhibitors, antihypertensive agents or tricyclic antidepressants. It should be given cautiously in patients with severe cardiovascular disease.

Intravenous dosage is 3 to 5 mg slowly; onset of action takes about four minutes. Intramuscular dosage is 20 to 35 mg.

SYMPATHOMIMETIC AGENTS ACTING PREDOMINANTLY ON ALPHA RECEPTORS

Phenylephrine hydrochloride BP

Used systemically, the blood-pressure is raised by direct action on the alpha adrenergic receptors producing constriction of the vessel walls. The vasoconstrictive property makes it suitable for addition to local analgesic agents, instead of adrenaline. The increase in blood-pressure from systemic use may cause a reflex bradycardia but may be counteracted by atropine if necessary. It should not be used in patients on monoamine oxidase inhibitors or tricyclic anti-depressants, or in haemorrhage or peripheral ischaemia because any vasoconstriction would be increased. Care is necessary where bradycardia or heart block pre-exist. It should not be given in severe myocardial or coronary disease or in obstetrics because of constriction of the uterine arteries and increased uterine tone (Schnider, 1966). Dosage is 0.5 mg intravenously or as an intravenous infusion, but if administered with a halogenated volatile anaesthetic the initial dose should not exceed 0.1 to 0.2 mg intravenously as it sensitises the heart to catecholamines (McIntyre, 1965).

Methoxamine hydrochloride BPC (Vasoxine)

Methoxamine is a potent vasopressor with a prolonged effect. The peripheral vasoconstriction is associated with increased afterload and cardiac work without any direct improvement of cardiac contractility. Because of the vasoconstrictor effect, particular care should be used in patients with hyperthyroidism, coronary or hypertensive heart disease. Delayed hypertensive effects have been observed. Like phenylephrine, methoxamine is not suitable for obstetric use. Special care should be taken in patients already on beta blockers. It does not stimulate the cerebral cortex. Intravenous dose is 2 mg, or 5 to 20 mg intramuscularly.

Noradrenaline acid tartrate BP (1-Arterenol, Norepinephrine, Levophed)

Noradrenaline is the neurohumoral transmitter for sympathetic nerve endings. It is a powerful stimulator of alpha receptors and is a potent vasoconstrictor, but dilates the coronary arteries. To restore or maintain vascular tone decreased by sympathetic block, a noradrenaline infusion of 2 to 4 μg/ml at a rate of 1 to 3 ml/min helps to replace inhibited catecholamine output. Noradrenaline solution is diluted and given in a 5 per cent dextrose or dextrose-saline solution into a large vein. It was used as a vasoconstrictor added to local analgesic agents, but lost popularity because of the irritant effect on the tissues.

SYMPATHOMIMETIC AMINES ACTING PREDOMINANTLY ON THE BETA RECEPTORS

Dopamine (Intropin)

This is a naturally occurring physiological derivative of noradrenaline, with beta adrenergic effects. Depending on the dose given it increases renal blood flow, improves cardiac contractility without increase in heart rate, and raises the blood-pressure. It is given as an infusion of 800 mg in 500 ml saline or dextrose-saline solutions into a large vein and the infusion rate should be controlled dependent on patient response.

Other agents

1. Atropine is a very useful agent when blood-pressure is low due to unopposed vagal tone with bradycardia. It is quickly available to the anaesthetist and 0.2 mg increments intravenously may raise the pressure to an acceptable limit without causing undue tachycardia or stimulating the cerebral cortex.

2. Ergotamine tartrate has been used for the prophylaxis and treatment of hypotension resulting from central neural block (Klingenström, 1960; Gordh, 1969). Gordh injects 0.125 mg intravenously and another 0.125 mg subcutaneously just before the block is given.

It is a wise precaution for the anaesthetist to become familiar with one or two vasopressors for use judiciously if the blood-pressure remains undesirably low in spite of the vascular volume being supplemented, bradycardia below 60 reversed and the legs elevated. The vasopressor should be initially given in minimal dosage, and repeated it necessary.

Intravenous fluids

The vasodilatation produced by the sympathetic block following central neural blockade is in proportion to the height of the block. The vasodilatation leads to a fall in central venous pressure and cardiac output unless fluids are given to augment the circulatory blood volume. Bromage (1983) suggests that blocks to T.10 require crystalloid infusion of 10 per cent blood volume and blocks to T.1 require crystalloid infusion of 30 per cent blood volume. Crystalloid fluids normally administered are isotonic saline, dextrose 5 per cent, dextrose 4 per cent with saline 0.18 per cent, or Hartmann's (compound sodium lactate) solution. Haemodilution has the advantage of producing some rheological improvement in flow and delivery of oxygen to the tissues (Replogle et al, 1967) by causing some reduction in the haematocrit. The authors have found Hartmann's solution to be a satisfactory fluid for routine use.

Plasma is available in limited supply as plasma protein fraction. If the patient is anaemic or there is appreciable blood loss, blood should be given.

Plasma volume expanders

Other plasma volume expanders may be used in conjunction with crystalloid infusions to prevent or combat hypotension produced by sympathetic block. Much experimental work has been done on the use of colloids and crystalloids and the individual clinical circumstances will influence decisions of which intravenous fluid to use (Horsey, 1982).

Dextran is a plasma substitute produced by bacterial action on sucrose. The renal threshold for dextran molecules is about 50 000 and the most appropriate molecular weight for dextran as a plasma volume expander is 70 000 to 110 000. Dextran preparations with an average molecular weight of 70 000 are the most suitable for clinical use as plasma or blood substitutes and are available in either 0.9 per cent saline or 5 per cent glucose. These preparations interfere with cross-matching and prolong the bleeding time; there is a small incidence of anaphylactoid reactions.

Vickers et al (1969) showed that dextran 70 was as effective as stored blood in maintaining blood volume for up to three days after surgery.

Gelatins

Gelatins are derived from animal collagen. Haemaccel (polygeline) is a urea-linked gelatin with a high calcium content; administration may cause release of histamine (Ring and Messmer, 1977) which is possibly related to the rate of infusion. It has been suggested (Horsey, 1982) that because of the possibility of anaphylactoid reactions the use of gelatin solutions is contraindicated for the treatment of the 'relative' hypovolaemia produced by the sympathetic block of central neural blockade. Gelofusine is a succinylated gelatin, sometimes referred to as 'modified fluid gelatin'.

Hydroxyethyl starch has been used as a plasma expander but is antigenic and has found little clinical application to date. Human serum albumin is a safe colloid solution but its use is limited by availability and expense.

SEDATIVE DRUGS — USED IN ASSOCIATION WITH CENTRAL NEURAL BLOCKADE

Patients for central neural blockade should usually be sedated so that when the injection is given, the patient is free from anxiety, pain is minimal and there is preferably amnesia for the medical procedures undertaken. Obstetric analgesia requires modification of these aims, as the well-being of the fetus limits the drugs and dosage that can be given.

Benzodiazepines

These tend to be anxiolytic in low dosage and hypnotic in high dosage. They have no analgesic effect. Hypnotic drugs suitable for oral sedation the previous evening or same day, are temazepam (Normison, Euhypnos) 10 mg; flurazepam (Dalmane) 15 to 30 mg, or nitrazepam (Mogadon) 5 to 10 mg.

Lorazepam (Ativan)

Lorazepam is a useful drug which can be given orally, intramuscularly or intravenously. It may be prescribed in 1 to 2 mg doses, orally, six hourly during the day preceding operation as an anxiolytic without causing undue drowsiness, or in a larger dose, 2 to 5 mg as the main premedication prior to surgery. The intravenous route (dosage 2 to 4 mg) may take up to 40 minutes before full effect is apparent (Dundee et al, 1979) and amnesia is delayed. Intramuscular absorption is slow, and as rapid an effect may be obtained by oral administration. It is metabolised by a simple one step process to a pharmacologically inactive glucuronide. It is compatible with a wide range of other drugs and has minimal effect on blood-pressure and respiration.

Diazepam (Valium)

Diazepam, given either orally (2 to 5 mg) or intravenously, is a useful sedative, although intravenous injection (dosage approx 5 to 10 mg) may be painful and can result in superficial venous thrombosis. Diazepam is metabolised to n-desmethyldiazepam which has a prolonged hypnotic effect (Dundee, 1983), although this is probably not so important with single doses. The hypnotic action of the metabolite can cause difficulties in use with young children or the elderly. Diazepam administered rectally acts rapidly and can be useful for children; suppositories are available containing 5 mg or 10 mg diazepam. *Diazemuls* is an emulsion of diazepam in soya bean oil and is less likely to cause local pain or thrombosis. It is commercially prepared in 2 ml ampoules containing 10 mg diazepam. The cost is higher than an equivalent dose of the standard preparation of diazepam.

Midazolam (Hypnovel)

Midazolam is an imidazole benzodiazepine. It is produced as a non-viscid solution which has hypnotic, anxiolytic, muscle relaxant and anticonvulsant activity. Midazolam is soluble in water below a pH of 4; the commercial solution is buffered at pH 3.5 and should not be mixed with other drugs (Dundee, 1983). It is administered intravenously, dosage 2.5 to 10 mg and only occasionally causes pain or thrombophlebitis. It has a rapid onset of action (30 to 100 seconds) and the effect is more intense than equivalent doses of diazepam. Amnesia produced is anterograde and appears to be transient, possibly lasting only a matter of minutes following intravenous injection, although Al-Khudhairi et al (1982) found that midazolam provided much better amnesia than diazepam.

Midazolam is rapidly cleared from plasma, it has a shorter half-life than equivalent doses of diazepam (approximately 1 to 2½ hours) (Dundee et al, 1980; Greenblatt et al, 1981) and there are no known metabolites which have an active hypnotic effect. It has a longer elimination half-life in the elderly who are also more susceptible to its effects. Cardiovascular studies suggest that midazolam may have a slightly greater margin of safety than diazepam in poor-risk patients (Dundee, 1983). Charuchinda and Srisupinanonta (1983) found that midazolam produced no significant alteration in heart rate or blood-pressure even in patients with impending shock. Ounkasem and Chareonthaitawee (1983) noted that induction time with midazolam is nearly twice as long as that associated with thiopentone, but midazolam has less effect on blood-pressure. Greenblatt et al (1981) suggest that midazolam may be effective orally as less than 50 per cent of the dose is removed by first-pass hepatic extraction.

Chlormethiazole (Heminevrin, Hemineurin)

Chlormethiazole is a powerful sedative, hypnotic and anticonvulsant derived from the thiazole portion of thiamine hydrochloride, vitamin B_1. It has been used in the treatment of status epilepticus, of pre-eclampsia in obstetrics, and in the management of alcohol withdrawal symptoms, including delirium tremens. Schweitzer (1978) used it by infusion as supplementary sedation during surgery under extradural block. It was found to have no analgesic effect, and its lack of cardiovascular and respiratory depression make it suitable for use in the elderly. Wilson et al (1969) used an intravenous infusion in fit volunteers and found that both induction of light anaesthesia and maintenance were easy, and that the recovery period was short and uneventful. An increase in heart rate was noted, but cardiac output was maintained at the pre-induction level. It can be given as an intravenous infusion, 4 g to 500 ml of glucose solution at an initial rate of 20 ml/min. Before sedation is produced a tingling sensation may be experienced in the nose, possibly accompanied by sneezing (Rogers et al, 1981).

Di-isopropylphenol (Disoprofol; Diprivan)

This recently evaluated anaesthetic agent rapidly induces anaesthesia, has a short elimination half-life and is non-cumulative. It has no appreciable effect on the cardiovascular system and these properties suggest it may be a good agent for continuous infusion anaesthesia (O'Callaghan et al, 1982). It occasionally causes pain on injection and unfortunately it is insoluble in water.

Althesin

Althesin, a combination of alphaxalone and the steroid alphadolone acetate, produces rapid induction of anaesthesia and enables recovery to be quick. It has been used for continuous intravenous infusion. Unfortunately it is not water soluble and is marketed with cremophor EL as the vehicle. It has been withdrawn from the market.

Etomidate (Hypnomidate)

Etomidate is a non-barbiturate, carboxylated imidazole, with a short duration of action. It is non-cumulative, has minimal cardiovascular and respiratory effects and recovery is rapid. Etomidate, usually combined with a narcotic, has been used for continuous intravenous infusion anaesthesia. There is recent evidence that when it is used for prolonged sedation, such as in intensive therapy units, there is suppression of adrenocortical function and it should not be used for such procedures. There are two preparations of etomidate marketed, the alcohol concentrate being the one used for infusion techniques. It has caused pain and venous thrombosis.

Narcotic analgesics

Narcotic analgesics of the anaesthetist's choice may be given as premedication. Pethidine, morphine, papaveretum, diamorphine or phenoperidine may be used either intramuscularly one hour beforehand or as intravenous supplements if necessary prior to the administration of blockade. The addition of hyoscine will aid amnesia. Small, and if necessary, repeated doses given intravenously are often useful to 'smooth out' the effects of other sedative drugs, for example diamorphine 1 mg.

REFERENCES

Albright, G. A. (1979) Cardiac arrest following regional anesthesia with etidocaine or bupivacaine. *Anesthesiology*, **51**, 285.

Al-Khudhairi, D., Whitwam, J. G. & McCloy, R. F. (1982) Midazolam and diazepam for gastroscopy. *Anaesthesia*, **37**, 1002.

Ansbro, F. P., Latteri, F. S. & Bodell, B. (1953) Continuous segmental thoracolumbar epidural block. *Anesthesia and Analgesia*, **32**, 73.

Berry, H. & West, G. B. (1944) The stability of adrenaline solutions. *Quarterly Journal of Pharmacology*, **17**, 242.

Boyes, R. N (1975) A review of the metabolism of amide local anaesthetic agents. *British Journal of Anaesthesia*, **47**, 225.

Braun, H. (1903) Über der Bedeutung des Adrenalin für Chirurg. *Münchener Medizinische Wochenschrift*, **50**, 352.

Braun, H. (1905) Über einige neu örtliche Anaesthesists. *Deutsche Medizinische Wochenschrift*, **31**, 1667.

Bromage, P. R. (1965) A comparison of the hydrochloride and carbon dioxide salts of lignocaine and prilocaine in epidural analgesia. *Acta Anaesthesiologica Scandinavica* Suppl., **16**, 55.

Bromage, P. R. (1969) A comparison of bupivacaine and tetracaine in epidural analgesia for surgery. *Canadian Anaesthetists' Society Journal*, **16**, 37.

Bromage, P. R. (1978a) *Epidural Analgesia*, ch. 9, p. 293. Philadelphia: Saunders.

Bromage, P. R. (1978b) *Epidural Analgesia*, ch. 9, p. 297. Philadelphia: Saunders.

Bromage, P. R. (1978c) *Epidural Analgesia*, ch. 9, p. 299. Philadelphia: Saunders.

Bromage, P. R. (1978d) *Epidural Analgesia*, ch. 9, p. 303. Philadelphia: Saunders.

Bromage, P. R. (1978e) *Epidural Analgesia*, ch. 9, p. 312. Philadelphia: Saunders.

Bromage, P. R. (1983) New aspects of physiology and pharmacology of regional anesthesia. (Abstracts) *Third Asean Congress of Anesthesiologists* (Bangkok), p. 39.

Bromage, P. R. & Gertel, M. (1970) An evaluation of two new local anaesthetics for major conduction blockade. *Canadian Anaesthetists' Society Journal*, **17**, 557.

Bromage, P. R., Pettigrew, R. T. & Crowell, D. E. (1969) Tachyphylaxis in epidural analgesia. I. Augmentation and decay of local anesthesia. *Journal of Clinical Pharmacology*, **9**, 30.

Bromage, P. R., Burfoot, M. F., Crowell, D. E. & Pettigrew, R. T. (1964) Quality of epidural blockade. I. Influence of physical factors. *British Journal of Anaesthesia*, **36**, 342.

Bromage, P. R., Burfoot, M. F., Crowell, D. E. & Truant, A. P. (1967) Quality of epidural blockade. III. Carbonated local anaesthetic solutions. *British Journal of Anaesthesia*, **39**, 197.

Brown, D. T., Beamish, D. & Wildsmith, J. A. W. (1981) Allergic reaction to amide local anaesthetic. *British Journal of Anaesthesia*, **53**, 435.

Brown, D. T., Morison, D. H., Covino, B. G. & Scott, D. B. (1980) Comparison of carbonated bupivacaine and bupivacaine hydrochloride for extradural anaesthesia. *British Journal of Anaesthesia*, **52**, 419.

Buckley, F. P., Littlewood, D. G., Covino, B. G. & Scott, D. B. (1978) Effects of adrenaline and the concentration of solution on extradural block with etidocaine. *British Journal of Anaesthesia*, **50**, 171.

Catchlove, R. F. H. (1973) Potentiation of two different local anaesthetics by carbon dioxide. *British Journal of Anaesthesia*, **45**, 471.

Chambers, W. A., Edstrom, H. H. & Scott, D. B. (1981) Effect of baricity on spinal anaesthesia with bupivacaine. *British Journal of Anaesthesia*, **53**, 279.

Chambers, W. A., Littlewood, D. G. & Scott, D. B. (1982a) Spinal anesthesia with hyperbaric bupivacaine: effect of added vasoconstrictors. *Anesthesia and Analgesia*, **61**, 49.

Chambers, W. A., Littlewood, D. G., Edstrom, H. H. & Scott, D. B. (1982b)

Spinal anaesthesia with hyperbaric bupivacaine: effect of dose and volume administered. *British Journal of Anaesthesia*, **54**, 75.
Charuchinda, P. & Srisupinanonta, S. (1983) Comparative study of midazolam to thiopentone. (Abstracts) *Third Asean Congress of Anesthesiologists* (Bangkok), p. 176.
Cousins, M. J. & Bromage, P. R. (1971) A comparison of the hydrochloride and carbonated salts of lignocaine for caudal analgesia in outpatients. *British Journal of Anaesthesia*, **43**, 1149.
Cousins, M. J. & Mather, L. E. (1980) Clinical pharmacology of local anaesthetics. *Anaesthesia and Intensive Care*, **8**, 270.
Covino, B. G. (1982) New developments in the field of local anaesthetics and the scientific base for their clinical use. *Acta Anaesthesiologica Scandinavica*, **26**, 242–249.
Covino, B. G., Marx, G. F., Finster, M. & Zsigmond, E. K. (1980) Editorial: prolonged sensory/motor deficits following inadvertent spinal anesthesia. *Anesthesia and Analgesia*, **59**, 399.
de Jong, R. H. (1970) *Physiology and Pharmacology of Local Anesthesia*, p. 82. Springfield: Thomas.
Dundee, J. W. (1983) Updating the benzodiazepines. VII. *S.A.A.D. Digest*, **5**, 169.
Dundee, J. W., Lilburn, J. K., Nair, S. G. & George, K. A. (1977) Studies of drugs given before anaesthesia. XXVI. Lorazepam. *British Journal of Anaesthesia*, **49**, 1047.
Dundee, J. W., Samuel, I. O., Toner, W. & Howard, P. J. (1980) Midazolam: a water soluble benzodiazepine. *Anaesthesia*, **35**, 454.
Dundee, J. W., McGowan, W., Lilburn, J. K., McKay, A. C. & Hegarty, J. E. (1979) Comparison of the actions of diazepam and lorazepam. *British Journal of Anaesthesia*, **51**, 439.
Einhorn, A. (1905) Synthesised p-aminol-benzoyl-diethylamino-ethanol hydrochloride. *Deutsche Medizinische Wochenschrift*, **31**, 1668.
Eisele, J. H. & Reitan, J. A. (1971) Scleroderma; Raynaud's phenomenon — local anesthetics: prolonged effect of lidocaine. *Anesthesiology*, **34**, 386.
Eisleb, O. (1931) Über ein neues Lokalanestheticum der Novokainreihe (Pantokain). *Archives of Experimental Pathology and Pharmacology*, **160**, 53.
Ekenstam, B., Egner, B. & Pettersson, G. (1957) Local anaesthetics No. 1: N: alkyl pyrrolidine and N: alkyl piperidine carboxylic acid amides. VII. *Acta Chemica Scandinavica*, **2**, 1183.
Engelsson, S. & Matousek M. (1975) Central nervous system effects of local anaesthetic agents. *British Journal of Anaesthesia*, **47**, 241.
Eriksson, E. & Gordh, T. (1959) Clinical trials of a new local anaesthetic. *Acta Anaesthesiologica Scandinavica* Suppl., **2**, 81.
Farrar, M. D., Nolte, H. & Meyer, J. (1979) Spinal subarachnoid anaesthesia with bupivacaine. *Anaesthesia*, **34**, 396.
Fisher, A. & Bryce-Smith, R. (1971) Spinal analgesic agents. A comparison of cinchocaine, lignocaine and prilocaine. *Anaesthesia*, **26**, 324.
Flowerdew, R. M. (1982) Chloroprocaine. *Anaesthesia*, **37**, 349.
Fourneau, E. (1904) Stovaine: anaesthétique locale. *Bulletin de la Société de Pharmacologie* (Paris), **10**, 141.
Galindo, A., Hernandez, J., Benavides, O., Oretegon de Muroz, S. & Bonica, J. J. (1975) Quality of spinal extradural anaesthesia: the influence of spinal nerve root diameter. *British Journal of Anaesthesia*, **47**, 41.
Ghoneim, M. M. & Pandya, H. (1974) Plasma protein binding of bupivacaine and its interaction with other drugs in man. *British Journal of Anaesthesia*, **46**, 435.
Gordh, T. (1949) Xylocain — new local analgesic. *Anaesthesia*, **4**, 4.
Gordh, T. (1969) *Illustrated Handbook in Local Anaesthesia*, p. 112. London: Lloyd-Luke.

Greenblatt, D. J., Looviskar, A., Ocho, H. R. & Lauven, P. M. (1981) Automated gas chromatography for studies of midazolam pharmacokinetics. *Anesthesiology*, **55**, 176.

Gunther, R. E. & Belville, J. W. (1972) Obstetric caudal analgesia: a randomized study comparing 1 per cent mepivacaine with 1 per cent mepivacaine and epinephrine. *Anesthesiology*, **37**, 288.

Hemmings, C. T. Weeks, S. K. & Smith, J. B. (1983) Epidural anaesthesia for Caesarean section: lidocaine HCl versus lidocaine CO_2. *Canadian Anaesthetists' Society Journal*, **30**, S.84.

Horsey, P. J. (1982) Blood transfusion. In Atkinson, R. S. & Langton Hewer, C. (eds) *Recent Advances in Anaesthesia and Analgesia*, 14, p. 95. Edinburgh: Churchill Livingstone.

James, F. M., Greiss, F. C. & Kemp, R. A. (1970) An evaluation of vasopressor therapy for maternal hypotension during spinal anesthesia. *Anesthesiology*, **33**, 25.

Klingenström, P. (1960) The effects of ergotamine on blood pressure, especially in spinal anaesthesia. *Acta Anaesthesiologica Scandinavica* Suppl., **4**.

Koller, C. (1884a) Über die Verwendung des Cocain zur Anaesthesierung am Auge. *Wiener Medizinische Wochenschrift*, **34**, 1276, 1309.

Koller, C. (1884b) Vorlaufige Mitteilung über lokale Anaesthesierung am Auge. Bericht über die 16 Versammlung der ophthalmologischen Gesselschaft. Heidelberg. *Beilageheft zu klinische Monatsblatter für Augenkeilkunde*, **60**.

Littlewood, D. G., Scott, D. B., Wilson, J. & Covino, B. G. (1977) Comparative anaesthetic properties of various local anaesthetic agents in extradural block for labour. *British Journal of Anaesthesia*, **49**, 75.

Liu, P. L., Feldman, H. S., Giasi, R., Patterson, M. K. & Covino, B. G. (1983) Comparative central nervous system toxicity of lidocaine, etidocaine, bupivacaine and tetracaine in awake dogs following rapid I.V. administration. *Anesthesia and Analgesia*, **62**, 375.

Löfström, J. B., Bengtsson, M. & Edström, H. (1982) Bupivacaine in spinal anaesthesia. *Proceedings of the European Society of Regional Anaesthesia* (Edinburgh), p. 32.

Lund, P. C. (1971) *Principles and Practice of Spinal Anesthesia*, p. 210. Springfield: Thomas.

Marx, G. F. & Finster, M. (1982) Chloroprocaine. *Anaesthesia*, **37**, 349.

Mather, L. E., Long., G. J. & Thomas, J. (1971) The binding of bupivacaine to maternal and foetal plasma proteins. *Journal of Pharmacy and Pharmacology*, **23**, 359.

McLeskey, C. H. (1981) Allergic reaction to an amide local anaesthetic. *British Journal of Anaesthesia*, **53**, 1105.

McClure, J. H. (1982) Spinal anaesthesia: effects of baricity and posture. *Proceedings of the European Society of Regional Anaesthesia*, (Edinburgh), p. 22.

McIntyre, J. W. R. (1965) Effects of phenylephrine during halothane anaesthesia in man. *Canadian Anaesthetists' Society Journal*, **12**, 634.

Meagher, R. P., Moore, D. C. & De Vries, J. C. (1966) Phenylephrine: the most effective potentiator of tetracaine spinal anesthesia. *Anesthesia and Analgesia*, **45**, 134.

Moore, D. C. (1980) Spinal anesthesia: bupivacaine compared with tetracaine. *Anesthesia and Analgesia*, **59**, 743.

Moore, D. C., Crawford, R. D. & Scurlock, J. E. (1980) Severe hypoxia and acidosis following local anesthetic induced convulsions. *Anesthesiology*, **53**, 529.

Moore, D. C., Bridenbaugh, L. D., Bagdi, P. A. & Bridenbaugh, P. O. (1968) Accumulation of mepivacaine hydrochloride during caudal block. *Anesthesiology*, **29**, 585.

Moore, D. C., Spierdijk, J., Van Kleef, J. D., Coleman, R. L. & Love, G. F. (1982) Chloroprocaine neurotoxicity: four additional cases. *Anesthesia and Analgesia*, **61**, 155.

Nolte, H. (1982) Bupivacaine in spinal anaesthesia. *Proceedings of the European Society of Regional Anaesthesia* (Edinburgh), p. 30.

Nolte, H. & Stark, P. (1979) Die Dosis-Wirkungsrelation des isobaren bupivacain zur Spinalanaesthesie. *Regional Anaesthesia*, 2, 1.

Nolte, H., Schikor, K., Gergs, P., Meyer, J. & Stark, P. (1977) Zur Frage der Spinalanaesthesie mit isobaren Bupivacain, 0.5 per cent *Der Anaesthesist*, 26c, 33.

O'Callaghan, A. C., Normandale, J. P., Grundy, E. M., Lumley, J. & Morgan, M. (1982) Continuous intravenous infusion of disoprofol (ICI 36868, Diprivan). Comparison with Althesin to cover surgery under local analgesia. *Anaesthesia*, 37, 295.

Ockerblad, N. F. & Dillon, T. G. (1927) The use of ephedrine in spinal anesthesia. *Journal of the American Medical Association*, 88, 1135.

Ounkasem, K. & Chareonthaitawee, P. (1983) Midazolam as an induction agent. (Abstracts) *Third Asean Congress of Anesthesiologists* (Bangkok), p. 177.

Poppers, P. J. (1975) Evaluation of local anaesthetic agents for regional anaesthesia in obstetrics. *British Journal of Anaesthesia*, 47, 325.

Ravindran, R. S., Bond, V. K., Tasch, M. D., Gupta, C. D. & Luerssen, T. G. (1980) Prolonged neural blockade following regional analgesia with 2-chloroprocaine. *Anesthesia and Analgesia*, 59, 447.

Reisner, L. S., Hochman, B. N., Plumer, M. H. (1980) Persistent neurological deficit and adhesive arachnoiditis following intrathecal 2-chloroprocaine injection. *Anesthesia and Analgesia*, 59, 452.

Replogle, R. L., Meiselman H. J. & Merrill, E. W. (1967) Clinical implications of blood rheology studies. *Circulation*, 36, 148.

Reynolds, F. (1970) Systemic toxicity of local analgesic drugs, with special reference to bupivacaine. *MD Thesis, University of London*.

Reynolds, F. (1971) A comparison of the potential toxicity of bupivacaine, lignocaine and mepivacaine during epidural blockade for surgery. *British Journal of Anaesthesia*, 43, 567.

Reynolds, F. (1972) In Wylie, W. D. & Churchill-Davidson, H. C. (eds) *A Practice of Anaesthesia* 3rd edn. London: Lloyd-Luke.

Reynolds, F. & Taylor, G. (1971) Plasma concentrations of bupivacaine during continuous epidural analgesia in labour: the effect of adrenaline. *British Journal of Anaesthesia*, 43, 436.

Reynolds, F., Hargrove, R. L. & Wyman, J. B. (1973) Maternal and fetal plasma concentrations of bupivacaine after epidural block. *British Journal of Anaesthesia*, 45, 1049.

Ring, J. & Messmer, K. (1977) Incidence and severity of anaphylactoid reactions to colloid volume substitutes. *Lancet*, 1, 466.

Rogers, H. J., Spector, R. G. & Trounce, J. R. (1981) Chlormethiazole (Heminevrin). *A Textbook of Clinical Pharmacology*, p. 203. London: Hodder & Stoughton.

Rubin, A. P. (1982) Bupivacaine in spinal anaesthesia. *Proceedings of the European Society of Regional Anaesthesia* (Edinburgh), p. 28.

Ryan, D. W., Pridie, A. K. & Copeland, P. F. (1983) Plain bupivacaine 0.5 per cent: a preliminary evaluation as a spinal anaesthetic agent. *Annals of the Royal College of Surgeons*, 65, 40.

Schnider, S. M. (1966) New and interesting aspects of obstetric conduction anaesthesia. *Acta Anaesthesiologica Scandinavica* Suppl., 25, 377.

Schnider, S. M. (1982) Neurotoxicity of local anaesthetics. *Proceedings of the European Society of Regional Anaesthesia* (Edinburgh), p. 64.

Schulte-Steinberg, O., Hartmuth, J. & Schutt, L. (1970) Carbon dioxide salts of lignocaine in brachial plexus block. *Anaesthesia*, 25, 191.

Schweitzer, S. A. (1978) Chlormethiazole (Heminevrin) infusion as supplemental sedation during epidural block. *Anaesthesia and Intensive Care*, 6, 248.

Scott, D. B. (1981) Toxicity caused by local anaesthetic drugs. Editorial. *British*

Journal of Anaesthesia, **53**, 553.
Siker, E. S., Wolfson, B., Stewart, W. D., Pavilack, P. & Pappas, M. T. (1966) Mepivacaine for spinal anesthesia: effects of changes in concentration of baricity. *Anesthesia and Analgesia*, **45**, 191.
Soderman, M. & Duke, P. C. (1983) Stability of carbonated lidocaine. III. *Canadian Anaesthetists' Society Journal*, **30**, S.71.
Stratmann, D., Götte, A., Meyer-Hamme, K. & Watermann, W. F. (1979) Spinal anesthesia using bupivacaine — clinical experience of more than 6000 cases. *Regional Anesthesia*, **2**, 49.
Sung, C. Y. & Truant, A. P. (1954) The physiological disposition of lidocaine and its comparison in some respects with procaine. *Journal of Pharmacology and Experimental Therapeutics*, **112**, 432.
Tattersall, M. P. (1983) Isobaric bupivacaine and hyperbaric amethocaine for spinal analgesia. A clinical comparison. *Anaesthesia*, **38**, 115.
Telivuo, L. (1963) A new long-acting local anaesthetic solution for pain relief after thoracotomy. *Annales Chirurgiae et Gynaecologiae Fenniae*, **52**, 513.
Thomas, D. V. (1956) Sterilization of epinephrine. *Anesthesiology*, **17**, 752.
Tucker, G. T. (1982) Clinical pharmacology of local anaesthetics. *Proceedings of the 6th European Congress of Anaesthesiology* (London), p. 44.
Tucker, G.T., Boyes, R. N., Bridenbaugh, M. D. & Moore, D. C. (1970) Binding of anilide type local anesthetics in human plasma. I. Relationships between binding, physicochemical properties and anaesthetic activity. *Anesthesiology*, **33**, 287.
Tucker, G. T., Moore, D. C., Bridenbaugh, P. O., Bridenbaugh, L. D. & Thompson, G. F. (1972) Systemic absorption of mepivacaine in commonly used regional block procedures. *Anesthesiology*, **37**, 277.
Tuominen, M., Kalso, E. & Rosenberg, P. H. (1982) Effects of posture on the spread of spinal anaesthesia with isobaric 0.75 per cent or 0.5 per cent bupivacaine. *British Journal of Anaesthesia*, **54**, 313.
Uhlmann, F. (1929) Uber Percain ein neues Lokalanaestheticum. *Narkose und Anaesthesie*, **6**, 168.
Vickers, M. D., Heath, M. L. & Dunlap, D. (1969) A comparison of Macrodex and stored blood as replacement for blood loss during planned surgery. I. Blood volume maintenance. *British Journal of Anaesthesia*, **41**, 677.
Watt, M. J., Akhtar, M. & Atkinson, R. S. (1970) Clinical comparison of bupivacaine and amethocaine. Onset and duration in extradural blockade. *Anaesthesia*, **25**, 24.
Whittet, T. D. (1954) The effect of autoclaving on ampoules of local analgesics. *Anaesthesia*, **9**, 271.
Wilson, J., Stephen, G. W. & Scott, D. B. (1969) A study of the cardiovascular effects of chlormethiazole. *British Journal of Anaesthesia*, **41**, 840.
Wüst, H. J., Liebau, W. & Richter, O. (1979) Tachyphylaxis in continuous epidural anaesthesia with bupivacaine 0.125 per cent and 0.25 per cent. *Anaesthesia*, **34**, 397.
Zaidi, S. & Healy, T. E. J. (1977) A comparison of the antibacterial properties of six local analgesic agents. *Anaesthesia*, **32**, 69.

6

Equipment

With the methods of sterilisation formerly in vogue, it is surprising that the sequelae to spinal analgesia were not both more serious and more common than they appear to have been. Meningeal infection is a grave complication of spinal analgesia and, except in the rare case of haematogenous infection from the patient's own body (Crawford, 1975), responsibility for it must be accepted by the anaesthetist if it occurs, as being due either to personal failure in carrying out a satisfactory aseptic technique, or to condoning faulty preparation of needles, syringes, etc. Many different ways of ensuring asepsis have been described. The optimum technique would reduce to a minimum loopholes for the introduction of noxious agents into the theca, and yet at the same time be simple enough to be understood by those playing their part in carrying it out, and straightforward enough not to invite slipshod performance.

If sepsis could be eliminated, one of the great hazards of spinal analgesia would disappear; and sepsis can be eliminated by the exercise of a reasonable amount of care, commonsense, and discipline. Obvious potential sources of infection are the patient's skin, the operator, and the syringes, needles and drugs; and the problem can conveniently be considered under these three headings. The means of avoiding infection described here have given satisfactory results for many years. Scrupulous attention to asepsis is necessary whether the contemplated block is intradural or extradural. In the case of the latter, accidental dural puncture is always a possibility, while the effects of extradural infection, lumbar or sacral, can also be dangerous to the patient.

The patient's skin (Lowbury et al, 1981)

The skin is prepared immediately before lumbar puncture (Fig. 6.1). The patient is placed in position and the back widely cleared of clothes, towels and bandages. A germicidal solution such

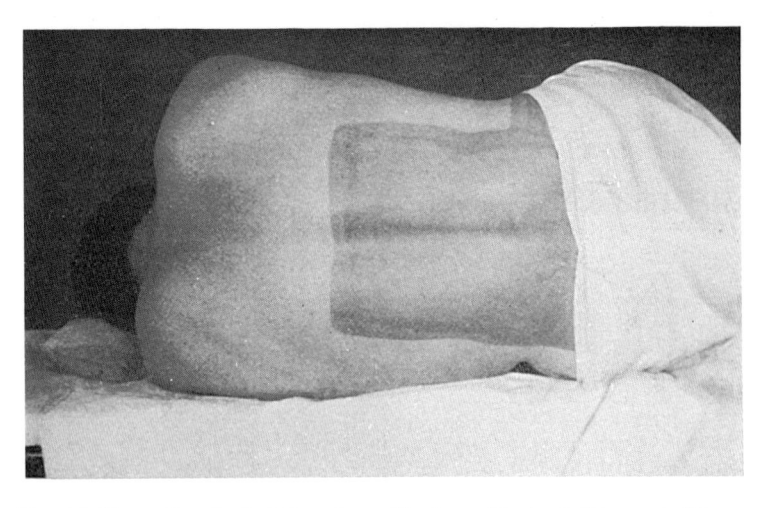

Fig. 6.1 The outline clearly defines the sterilised area. The level of the crest of the ilium is painted also. A line dropped from this passes between the spinous processes of the 4th and 5th lumbar vertebrae, or through the 4th process.

as 0.5 per cent chlorhexidine in 50 per cent alcohol (Beeuwkes and Vijver, 1959) is applied, by a sterile wool swab, first to the site of puncture, and then over an area extending for about six inches on either side of the lumbar and lower thoracic spines. The intended point of entry of the spinal needle is localised by touch and the point of an intradermal needle is placed in the skin, after which the prepared area is repainted and the fingers should not subsequently come into contact with the skin near the point of entry. The addition of dye to the antiseptic solution enables the anaesthetist to see at a glance the area of skin he has painted. A sterile towel is placed so that the anaesthetist can palpate the iliac crest through it, but any attempt at draping the lumbar area is deliberately avoided, since an unclipped towel might move and its unsterile undersurface spread contamination to the prepared area. Moreover, complete towelling prevents an overall view of the vertebral column and makes accurate spinal puncture more difficult.

The operator

Nose and mouth are covered with a mask, and a cap and a sterile gown should be worn. The hands should be prepared and gloved as for a surgical operation, and maintained sterile, but the application of gloves solely as a ritual, with little consideration as to whether they subsequently become contaminated or not, is much to be condemned. Strict attention is paid to what is virtually a 'no touch' technique. Care is taken to keep the fingers well away from the nozzle of the syringe, and fingering the openings at either end of the needle can be avoided, for example, by using a needle with light metal flanges (Macintosh, 1948), as illustrated in Figure 7.13. On the rare occasions when the shaft of a long needle has to be steadied during insertion, it is held in a sterile swab.

Syringes needles and drugs

From experience as onlookers at various hospitals, even those in which admirable facilities for sterilising exist, we have formed the opinion that asepsis in spinal analgesia is most likely to break down through faulty sterilisation of apparatus and drugs. Here are some examples of risks to which the patient is quite needlessly exposed:

1. Syringes and needles are 'sterilised' by methods not above suspicion, e.g. by immersion in chemical solutions.

2. Syringes and needles are rinsed out with so-labelled 'sterile distilled water' from a flask which has already been opened for some time, or the rinsing water is poured from a flask, the outlet of which quite obviously cannot be sterile.

3. An intradermal weal is made with local analgesic drawn from a rubber-stoppered stock bottle, after which the spinal needle is passed through this now possibly infected area.

4. An assistant is asked to open, with a non-sterile file, an ampoule of the local analgesic to be injected intradurally; and it is taken for granted that the solution remains uncontaminated by filings or small fragments of glass or plastic material (Seltzer et al, 1977).

5. The anaesthetist, if stressed by shortage of time or other difficulty, may allow the sweat from his forehead to contaminate his hands, syringe or needles. A cynic has stated that the sweat of a house officer is infected, that of a registrar is sterile, while the sweat of a consultant is actually antiseptic; we would not dispute the first clause!

None of the above risks is justified, for it should be an easy matter to sterilise every instrument and drug used in giving a spinal analgesic.

We cannot too strongly recommend that accepted methods of sterilisation be used in hospital practice. All the items necessary for performance of the block should be included in the pack, and when this is not possible ampoules and needles must be sterilised in such a way that a separate sterile pack can be emptied on to the anaesthetist's sterile tray. The outside of the ampoule must be sterile as well as the contents. Amethocaine in 2 per cent solution is the only commonly used local analgesic drug with antibacterial properties (Zaidi and Healy, 1977).

The following items are recommended for inclusion in a sterile pack:

4 or more spinal needles with stilettes (e.g. gauge 18, 22, 25).
1 × 10 ml glass syringe with metal or ceramic piston.
1 × 5 ml syringe.
1 × 2 ml syringe.
Ampoules of local analgesic solution, including any used for the skin weal.
Ampoules of adrenaline solution (1:1000).
1 spinal introducer, e.g. Sise.
1 file.
1 swab holder.
3 or 4 swabs of cotton wool.
Selection of hypodermic needles, sizes 21, 23, 25 gauge.
Metal gallipots (and antiseptic solution, if working alone).
Sterile towels.
Extradural space indicator, if used (e.g. Macintosh balloon).
Bacterial filter (Fig. 6.4).
Extradural catheters made from nylon and Teflon (Fig. 6.4).
Insulin syringe for the accurate measurement of the small volume of adrenaline solution required.

All the items can be packed in a drum or linen roll. Autoclaving used to be carried out by steam at 20 lb/in^2 for 30 minutes when the temperature of saturated steam is 126°C. The commonly used local analgesic solutions can be sterilised up to five times by using this technique (Whittet, 1954), which does not interfere with their analgesic potency. Too frequent autoclaving, however, may cause caramelisation of any contained glucose. Modern developments in sterilising technique have introduced variations in the method and hospital pharmacy departments will advise on individual circumstances.

The syringes should be of high quality. The piston must move freely within the barrel and must not stick, otherwise the subtle difference associated with the loss of resistance when locating the extradural space may be missed. For this reason we find plastic syringes unsatisfactory. The authors prefer a 10 ml glass syringe with metal or ceramic piston for location of the extradural space, and a 2 or 5 ml syringe for intradural injection.

Disposable sets are now available consisting of a plastic tray with small containers, syringes, needles, forceps, ampoules of local analgesic solution, etc. all sterilised by gamma radiation. Although expensive, these have proved to be extremely satisfactory (Bridenbaugh et al, 1967) but the plastic gallipots they contain have some disadvantages as they may be contaminated with small particles of plastic material, which could cause harm on injection (Seltzer et al, 1977).

Sterilisation 'in the field'

Exceptional circumstances may justify the acceptance of less absolute methods of sterilising instruments. The single-handed medical officer of a ship may consider an operation less hazardous under spinal analgesia given by himself, with a syringe prepared by boiling, than under general anaesthesia given by a lay anaesthetist.

All non-sporing and many sporing organisms are killed by boiling for five minutes (Lowbury et al, 1981). Sterner measures are however required to deal with the hepatitis B antigen. If sterilisation by boiling is to be adopted, syringes and needles should first be washed until perfectly clean, as organisms in pus or inspissated mucus have greatly increased resistance to boiling. The instruments are placed in a pan of warm water, brought to the boil and left for 5 to 10 minutes. The pan, still containing sufficient water to cover the instruments, is then removed from the source of heat, protected by a sterile towel, and allowed to cool.

The instruments should be boiled as near the time of operation as is practicable; and they should not be removed from the water until they are to be used for lumbar puncture. The fault to be found with boiling as a means of sterilisation is not so much the inadequacy of boiling as the ease with which contamination tends to be introduced afterwards, e.g. from cooling by addition of 'sterile' water, or storing in 'sterile' water, or handling. Attention is drawn particularly to the warning on page 315 of the danger of storing spinal analgesic solutions in spirit or other antiseptics.

Should it be desired to rinse the syringes before using, this can be done with the spinal analgesic solution itself which can then be discarded, or with sterile distilled water from ampoules.

Needles

Lumbar puncture needles are of several types and, in addition, vary in gauge and length (Fig. 6.2). There is the ordinary needle with an orifice at its tip and a short bevel to prevent part of the solution being injected into the extradural space (Fig. 7.21). Usual sizes are 20 to 25 gauge. The Tuohy needle has a relatively blunt point and lateral opening at its tip (Tuohy, 1945) (Fig. 6.3b) Usual sizes are 16 to 18 gauge, thin wall.

When a fine gauge needle is inserted it tends to deviate from the direction of the bevel although less when the stilette is still in situ (Drummond and Scott, 1980).

There is, in addition, a variety of other needles available but seldom used in the UK. They include the pencil pointed Whitacre needle designed to reduce the incidence of headache (Hart and Whitacre, 1951) (Fig. 6.3a) and the Quincke needle with a cutting bevel of medium length (Quincke, 1891) (Fig. 6.3c). (For a

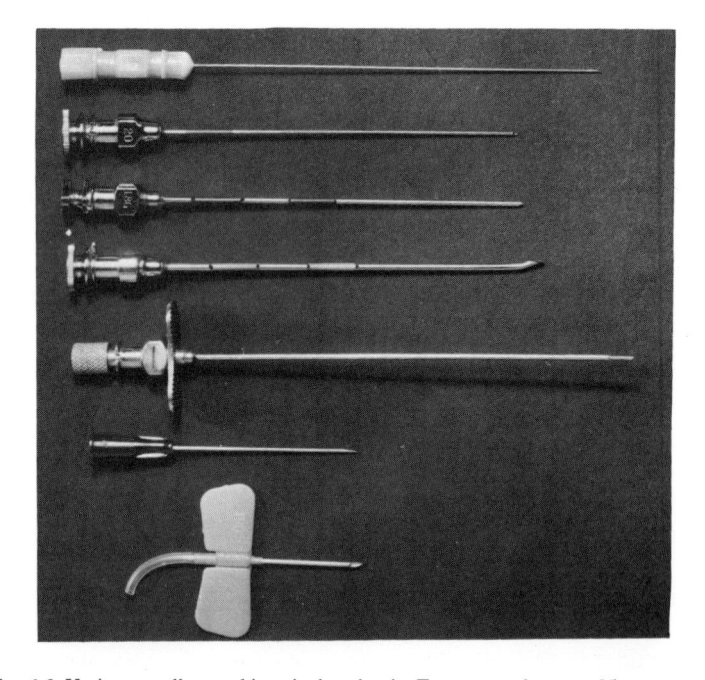

Fig. 6.2 Various needles used in spinal analgesia. From top to bottom: 25 gauge needle (disposable); 20 gauge needle; 18 gauge needle with centimetre markings; 16 gauge Tuohy needle; Macintosh spring-loaded needle; no. 1 disposable needle for sacral block; 19 gauge Butterfly needle for use as an introducer.

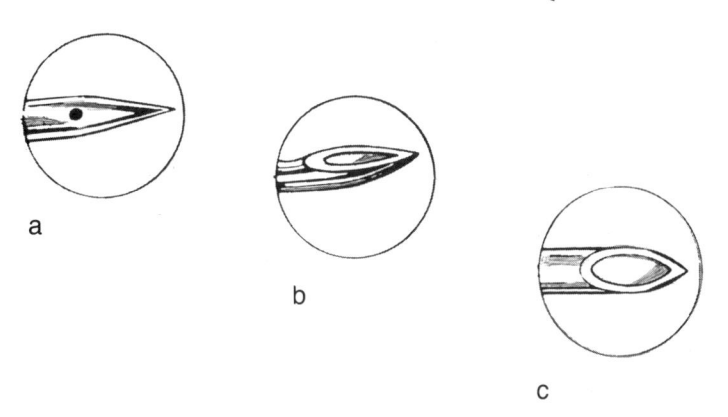

Fig. 6.3 Some needle points. (a) Whitacre pencil point; (b) Tuohy point; (c) Quincke point.

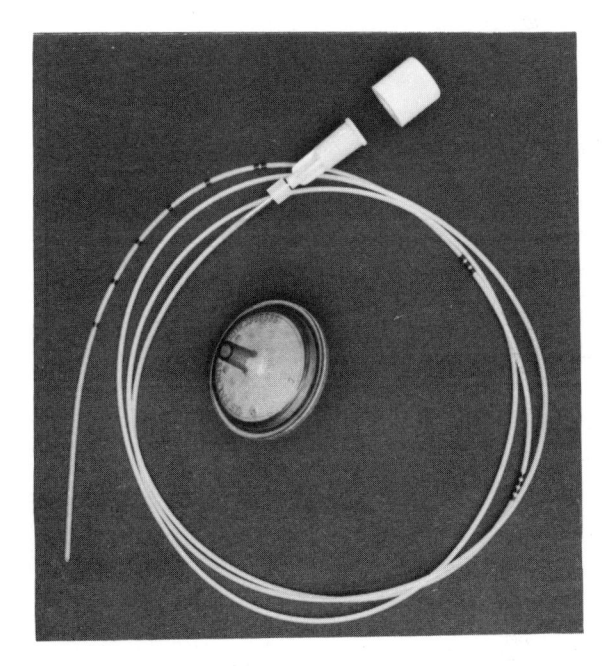

Fig. 6.4 Extradural catheter and filter.

description of a large number of other varieties see *Principles and Practice of Spinal Anesthesia* by P. C. Lund (1971), Springfield: Thomas.)

For intradural block the use of a fine needle, ranging from 20 to 25 gauge and measuring 10 cm (3½ inches), has many advantages.

However, the finer needles are more difficult to insert. One convenient method is to introduce a 20 gauge needle, 7.5 cm long, into the extradural space (using a suitable test for its introduction) and then to insert the finer but longer needle through it into the theca (Slattery et al, 1980). The point of the finer needle must extend 1 cm beyond the point of the larger needle when it is in place.

REFERENCES

Beeuwkes, H. & Vijver, A. E. D. (1959) Disinfection in anaesthesia. *British Journal of Anaesthesia*, **31**, 363.

Bridenbaugh, L. D., Moore, D. C. & DeVries, J. C. (1967) Sterile, convenient, economical, disposable spinal anesthesia trays — fact or fancy? *Anesthesia and Analgesia*, **42**, 191.

Crawford, J. S. (1975) Pathology in the extradural space. *British Journal of Anaesthesia*, **47**, 417.

Drummond, G. B. & Scott, D. H. T. (1980) Deflection of spinal needles by bevel. *Anaesthesia*, **35**, 854.

Hart, J. R. & Whitacre, R. J. (1951) Pencil-point and the prevention of post-spinal headaches. *Journal of the American Medical Association*, **147**, 657.

Lowbury, E. J. L., Ayliffe, G. A. J., Geddes, A. M. & Williams, J. D. (1981) *Control of Hospital Infections*, p. 73, 2nd ed. London: Chapman and Hall.

Macintosh, R. R. (1948) A spinal needle. *Lancet*, **2**, 612.

Quincke, H. I. (1891) Die Lumbalpunktion des Hydrocephalus. *Berliner Klinische Wochenschrift*, **28**, 929.

Seltzer, J. L., Porretta, J. C. & Jackson, B. G. (1977) Plaster particulate contamination in medicine cups. *Anesthesiology*, **47**, 378.

Slattery, P. J., Rosen, M. & Rees, G. A. D. (1980) An aid to identification of the subarachnoid space with a 25G needle. *Anaesthesia*, **35**, 391.

Tuohy, E. B. (1945) The use of continuous spinal anesthesia — utilising the urethral catheter technique. *Journal of the American Medical Association*, **128**, 262.

Whittet, T. D. (1954) The effects of autoclaving on ampoules of local analgesics. *Anaesthesia*, **9**, 274.

Zaidi, S. & Healy, T. E. J. (1977) A comparison of the antibacterial properties of six local analgesic agents. *Anaesthesia*, **32**, 69.

7

Technique of lumbar puncture

Lumbar puncture is used in neurological diagnosis to obtain specimens of cerebrospinal fluid, to inject radio-opaque dyes for radiography, to inject air for air-encephalography, for treatment, e.g. the injection of a chemotherapeutic agent, and for intradural spinal analgesia. When performed with skill by an experienced worker it need be neither painful nor dangerous.

Position of patient

In any manoeuvre in which direction is important, the eye should be on the same planes, vertical and horizontal, as the tools being used. During lumbar puncture, therefore, the eye should be behind the hub of the needle looking along the line of the shaft. It is also

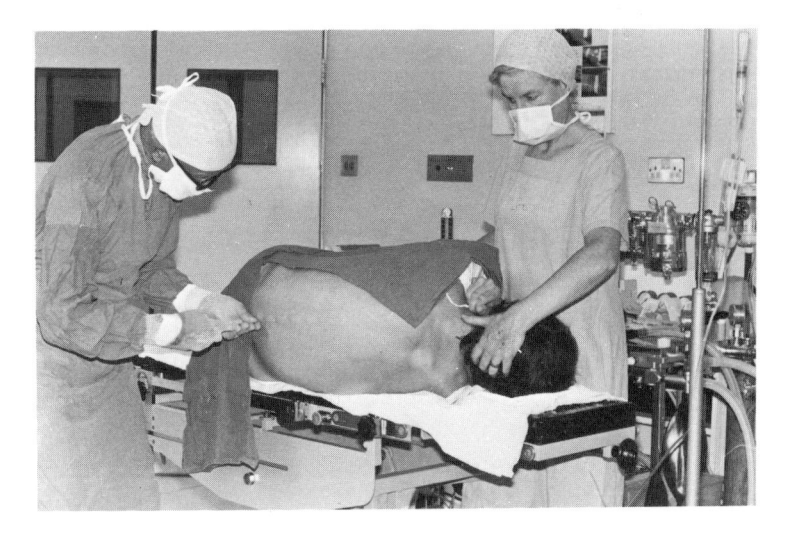

Fig. 7.1 The technique of lumbar puncture.

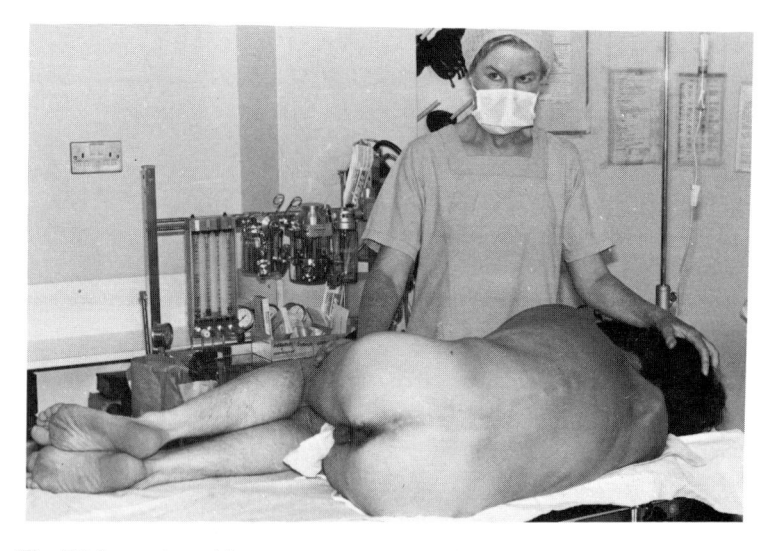

Fig. 7.2 Incorrect position.

convenient if the horizontal position of the needle can be checked to ensure that it enters the theca in the mid-line (the sagittal plane), if this approach is intended.

While one anaesthetist may feel that he has more control in the standing position, another may prefer to sit down for the job. This serves the treble purpose of making him comfortable, steadying his movements and bringing his eye nearer the horizontal plane of the field of operation. Some find lumbar puncture easier with the patient sitting up (Fig. 7.3), and the logical explanation is that in this position the site of puncture is higher off the table and more nearly on a level with the anaesthetist's eye, which is therefore better placed for accurate corrections to be made to the direction of the needle. For intradural block the smallest gauge needle which can be conveniently used should be employed, ranging from 21 to 26 gauge, 10 cm in length (3½ inches). It is often worthwhile using a larger needle, both as an introducer and also to locate the extradural space before proceeding to intradural puncture; the narrower but longer needle can then be inserted through the wider, shorter 20 gauge needle which should be 7.5 cm in length (Slattery et al, 1980).

The needle aims at penetrating the ligamentum flavum, for once this is done, lumbar puncture is virtually over. Whether the patient is lying down or sitting up is immaterial. What *is* important is that

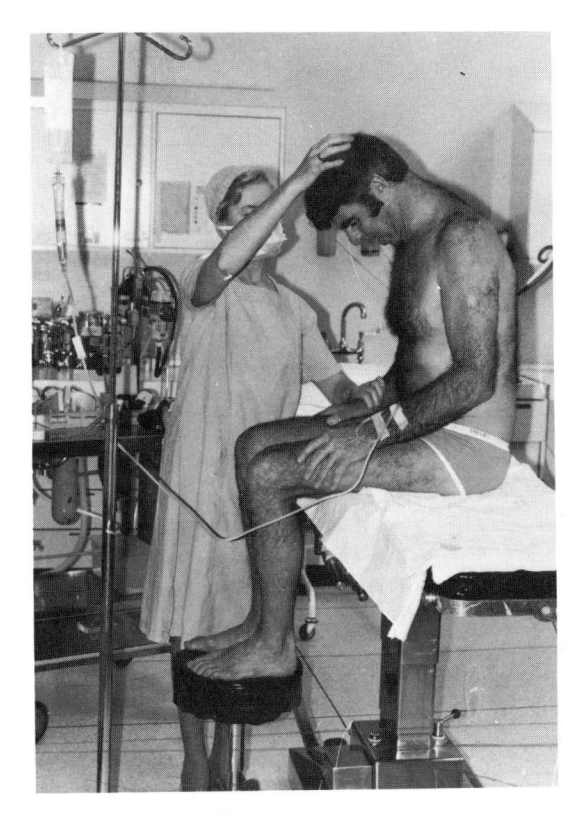

Fig. 7.3 Lumbar injection in the sitting position.

the lumbar vertebrae should be flexed on each other as far as possible; for in flexion the inferior articular processes of the upper vertebra ride up on the superior articular processes of the lower, the ligamenta flava are stretched and the interlaminar spaces are increased (Fig. 7.9B). In other words, flexion of the lumbar vertebrae increases the size of the target at which the needle aims.

Flexion of the thighs on the spine does not necessarily cause flexion of the lumbar vertebrae. It is not sufficient to tell the patient when sitting to 'bend well forwards', or when lying down, to 'draw your knees up to your chin'. A better position results from instructions such as 'try to arch your back like a cat', 'try to roll your head into your lap', or, with a finger-tip on the lumbar area, 'I want you to push out this part of your back'. Spinal analgesia should, whenever possible, be given with the patient on the operating table, but if this is not possible and the trolley sags the raised edge makes it difficult to carry out lumbar puncture with the patient lying down; he should therefore sit up so that the needle can be introduced in the proper plane. If the trolley is flat and firm, the patient can lie down. The performance of lumbar puncture in the patient's bed is undesirable, especially if regional analgesia is proposed. The assistant should concentrate on flexing the lumbar vertebrae. If the patient is sitting, the thighs are already flexed, so that all that is necessary is to flex the neck well towards the lap (Fig. 7.3). When the patient is lying down, flexion of the lumbar vertebrae is encouraged by an assistant firmly flexing the neck, and raising the knees to meet the downcoming head. During this manoeuvre there is a tendency for the assistant's mouth, nose and hair to project immediately over the area to be kept sterile; this is obviously undesirable, so that the puncture is not commenced till the assistant's head is well out of harm's way (Fig. 7.1). It is desirable that the patient's shoulders should be kept level with each other, the line joining them being vertical; a certain amount of rotation of the thoracic vertebrae does not matter, since the disposition of the articular facets on the processes of the *lumbar* vertebrae prevents rotation taking place there (Fig. 7.5).

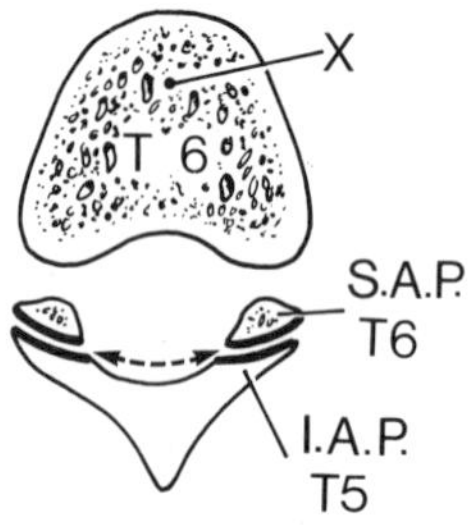

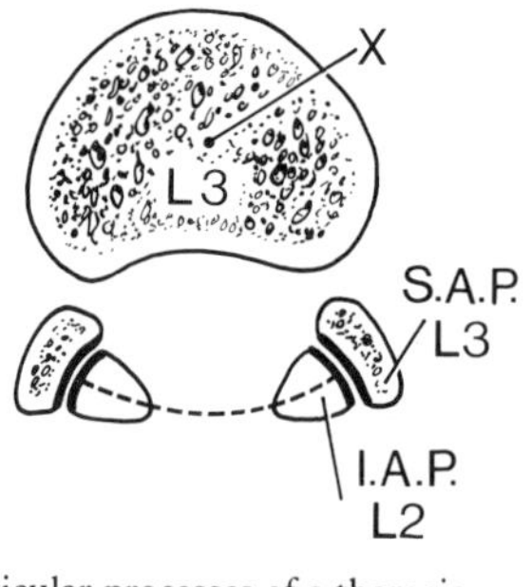

Fig. 7.4 (left) The disposition of the facets on the articular processes of a thoracic vertebra allow rotation of one vertebra on another. If X is the centre of rotation the circumference of a circle lies in the same plane as the articular surfaces of the processes, **Fig. 7.5** (right). In the lumbar region, however, the circumference of a circle drawn from X passes at right angles to the plane between the facets of the articular processes of two vertebrae: rotation cannot take place. (After Frazer, 1940).

Site of puncture

An appropriate site for lumbar puncture is easy to estimate, for a line joining the highest points of the two iliac crests passes just below the 4th lumbar spine (Tuffier's line) in most patients (Fig. 7.11). The precise level is a matter of indifference provided it is below L.2, the level at which the cord terminates. Other useful landmarks are the vertebra prominens (C.7) and the angle of the scapula which, with the arms to the side, is on the level of the spine of T.7. The distances between the lumbar spines may vary and the anaesthetist is well advised to choose the space where the gap is widest. The optimum point to make the skin puncture is easy to determine in the average patient in whom the spines are easily palpated, but an element of luck and guesswork enters into the calculation when the patient is obese enough for the landmarks to be obscured with a thick roll of fat. The identification of individual spinous processes in the elderly may be difficult, too, even though the patient is quite thin, as his supraspinous ligament is usually of bony firmness to the touch. Here the lumbar vertebrae are often practically fixed in a slightly extended position, the spinous processes are close together and the exploring fingers feel a uniform hard ridge in which it is difficult to locate an interspinous interval with confidence.

Median approach

By the time an interspinous space is identified and selected the anaesthetist will probably already have made up his mind whether to make a median puncture through the supraspinous ligament, or one immediately lateral to it, the so-called paramedian approach. If the former method is used in the patient lying on the side, the hips and shoulders should be maintained in the vertical plane and the needle inserted through a weal, midway between two spines, at right angles to the plane of the back in the mid-line. This median approach in the sagittal plane or the lateral approach can equally well be used in the sitting patient. The needle is cautiously advanced, strictly in the median or sagittal plane, either millimetre by millimetre, or continuously. Once the needle point enters the ligamentum flavum, the stylet can be removed so that a little further advance will result in the appearance of CSF, consequent on dural puncture. Some anaesthetists like to identify the extradural space, using for example the hanging drop test, or loss of resistance to air or fluid, before proceeding to dural puncture. If the 'loss of resistance' test is being used, the anaesthetist will be grasping a 10 ml syringe attached to the needle. A free flow of CSF is desirable, and for this the needle may require rotation into each of four quadrants, fractional advancement or withdrawal. The negative pressure from aspiration into a 2 ml syringe is sometimes necessary before a free flow is demonstrated, especially if a fine (e.g. 25 gauge) needle is being used, as CSF may be very timid about making its appearance. The present authors prefer the median approach (which is also suitable for thoracic block above T.4 or below T.9) but other workers, including the original author of this monograph (R.R.M.) favour the lateral or paramedian route.

The lateral or paramedian approach

Among the reasons for the choice of the paramedian approach are:
1. The occasional thickness and toughness of the supraspinous and interspinous ligaments seen in some old patients, which cause difficulty in insertion and which can easily bend or deflect a lumbar puncture needle, in the direction of the bevel (Drummond and Scott, 1980), especially a fine one used for intradural injection.
2. A small area of cystic degeneration may be present in the interspinous ligament, at a superficial level, which may give a false positive sign when loss of resistance tests are used (Sharrock, 1979).
3. With a median approach the angle of insertion is limited by the space available between the spinous processes, and must be roughly at a right angle to the dura. With a lateral approach the angle can be greater than a right angle, making it easier in extradural block, to glide the catheter up the extradural space, and so perhaps reducing the likelihood of damage to the dura by the tip of the catheter (Bonica, 1967; Carrie, 1971, 1977; Armitage, 1976, 1977; Chapman, 1977).
4. The paramedian approach does not require much flexion.

For the paramedian approach, which can also be used in the thoracic region between T.5 and T.9, an intradermal weal is raised with the smallest needle available at the level of the upper border of the lower spine and just lateral to the supraspinous ligament (Fig. 7.14). Now the small hypodermic needle is changed for a more robust one, and the tissues leading to the interlaminar space are generously infiltrated with 2 to 3 ml of local analgesic solution.

The anaesthetist now has a second minor decision to make — whether to use a lumbar puncture needle only, or to use a needle director as well if he proposes to puncture the dura with a fine 25 gauge needle (p. 179). The needle with its stylet in place is inserted through the skin weal and directed slightly upwards to miss the lamina of the lower vertebra, and slightly medially to compensate for

TECHNIQUE OF LUMBAR PUNCTURE 165

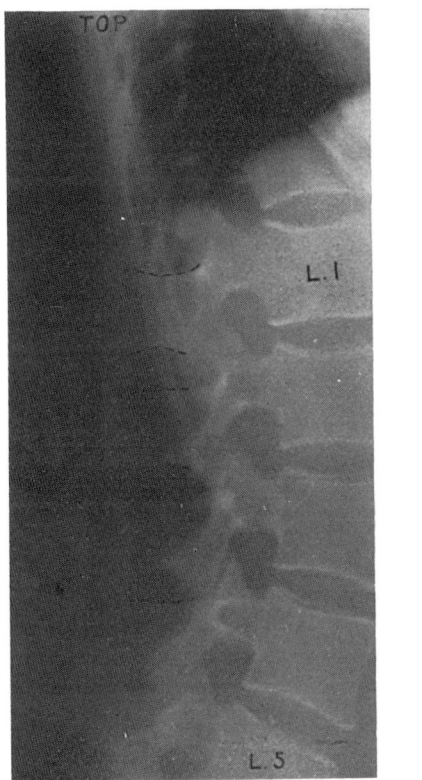

Fig. 7.6A

Fig. 7.7A

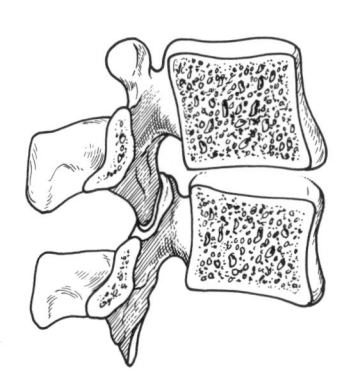

Fig. 7.6B
EXTENSION

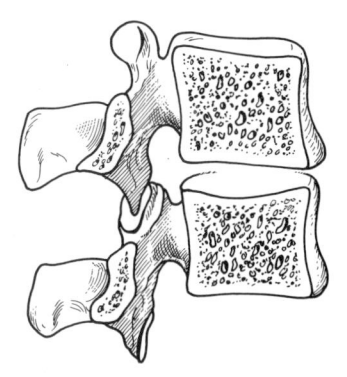

Fig. 7.7B
FLEXION

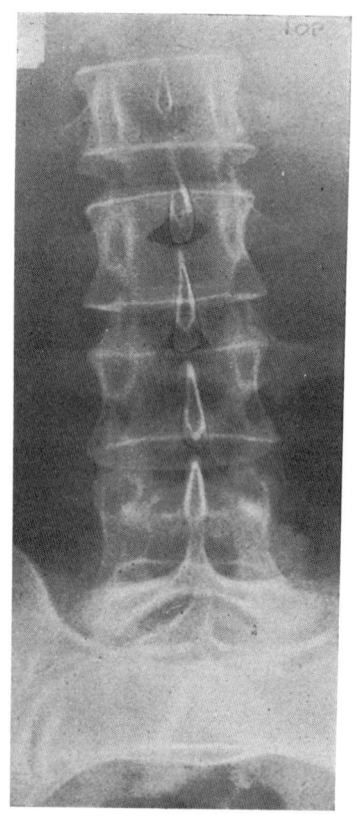

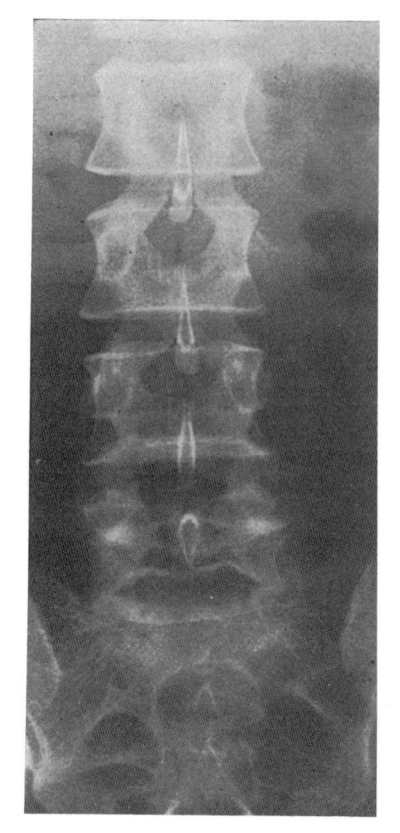

Fig. 7.8A

Fig. 7.9A

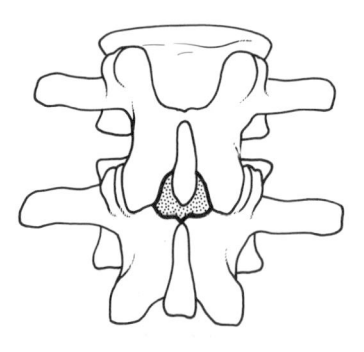

Fig. 7.8B
EXTENSION

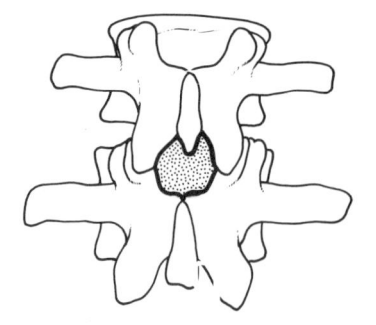

Fig. 7.9B
FLEXION

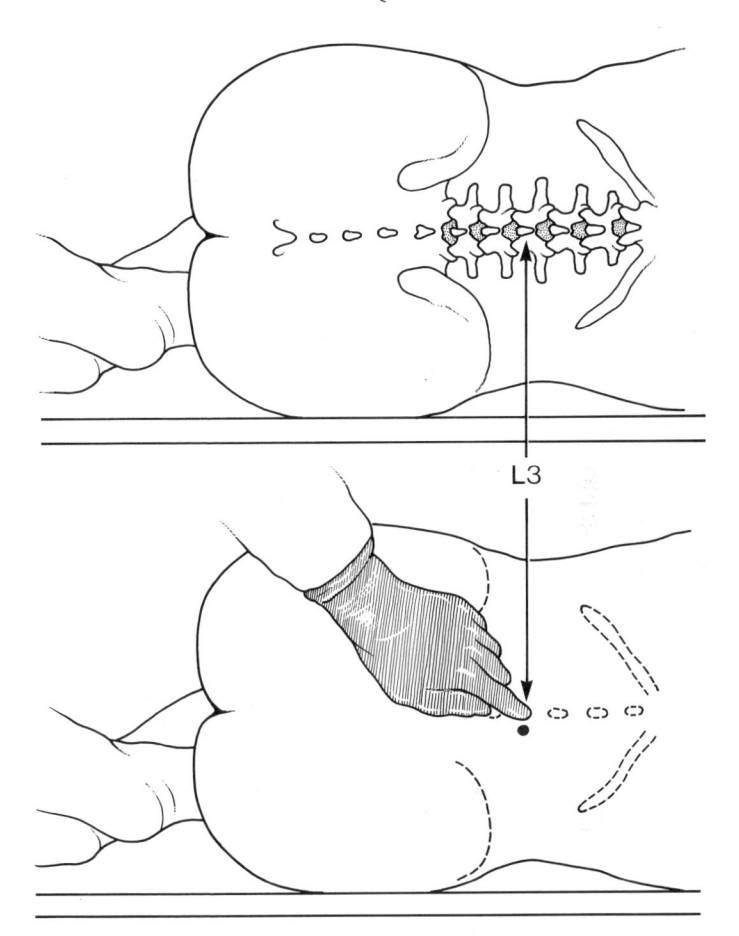

Fig. 7.10 Compare with Fig. 7.14.

the lateral start. The object is to encounter the ligamentum flavum in the centre of the interlaminar space. The needle passes through the skin, superficial fascia, a varying thickness of fat, and the lumbar aponeurosis into the lumbar muscles. In a thin patient these structures may not be identified separately by the needle, but in a robust subject the tough lumbar aponeurosis can generally be detected, and in an obese patient, too, the gradually advancing needle senses the difference in resistance between the fatty and fibrous tissue. The anaesthetist at this stage should have a mental picture of the underlying structures, so that in the event of bone

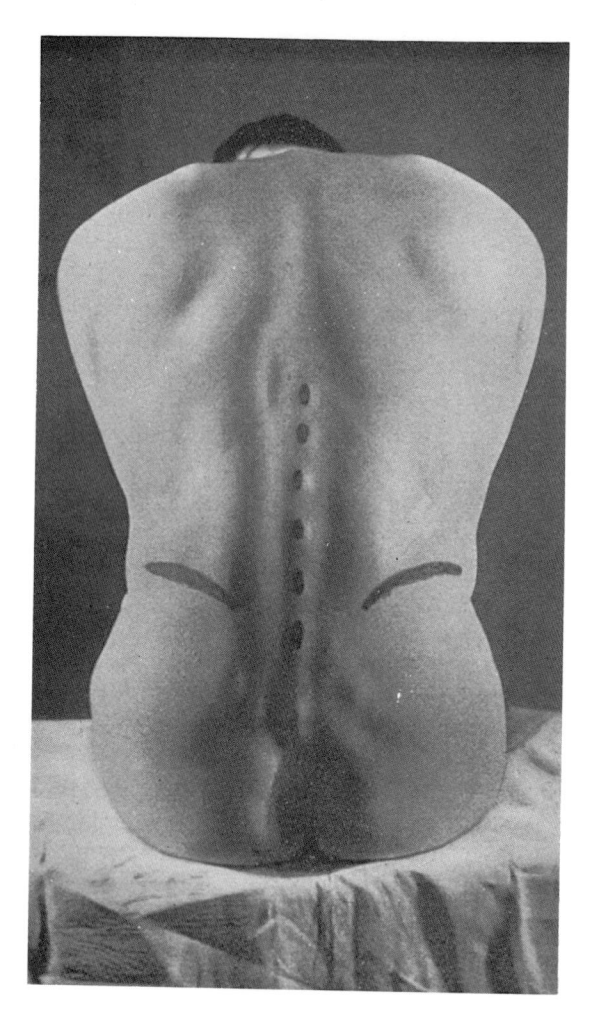

Fig. 7.11 The 12th thoracic and the five lumbar spinous processes are indicated. It was Tuffier who first advised that lumbar puncture should be carried out at the level of a line joining the iliac crests; for a time this was known as Tuffier's line.

being encountered (Fig. 7.15) the needle can be slightly withdrawn and appropriate correction made in its direction. It can be walked along the lamina with which it is probably making a contact, in a cephalo-median direction, until the more yielding yellow ligament is identified. The aperture of the Tuohy needle, if used for extradural block, should be pointed laterally to make dural puncture less likely. After the needle point has entered the yellow ligament, the

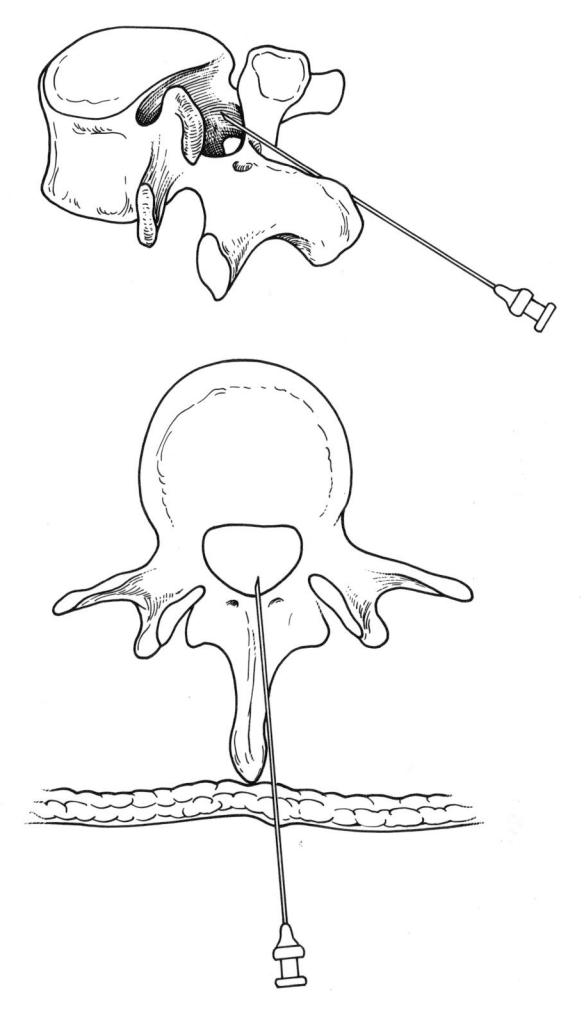

Fig. 7.12 The point of the needle is directed slightly upwards to steer clear of the upper margin of the lamina below, and slightly medially to compensate for its lateral start (if this approach is adopted).

extradural space (and the theca) can usually be entered easily. This is a convenient time to take out the stylet. The chances of the point of the needle now becoming blocked with tissue are very small, and if by any chance the dura is penetrated unexpectedly, a flow of cerebrospinal fluid through the fine needle will reveal the situation. The resistance of the ligamentum flavum can generally be appreciated, particularly in the robust male in whom it is strongly

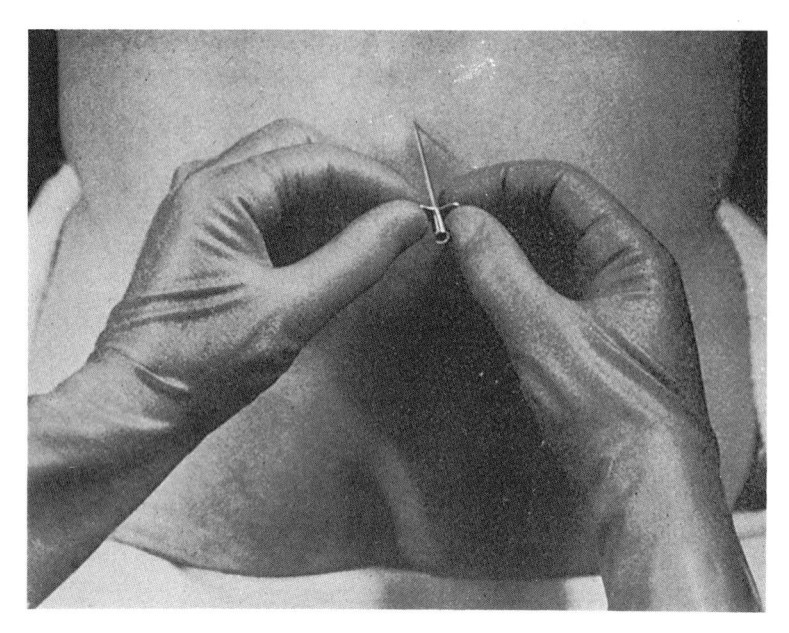

Fig. 7.13 The lateral or paramedian approach. Compare with Fig. 7.12.

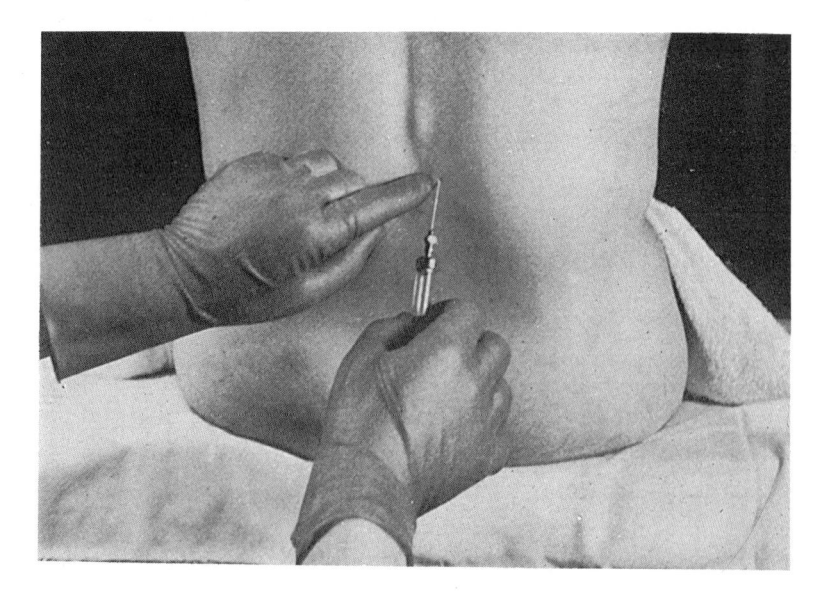

Fig. 7.14 A wide space between two lumbar spines is chosen, in this case L.2–3. The left index finger palpates the spine of L.3 and a hypodermic weal of local analgesic is raised immediately lateral to its upper border. Compare with Fig. 7.10.

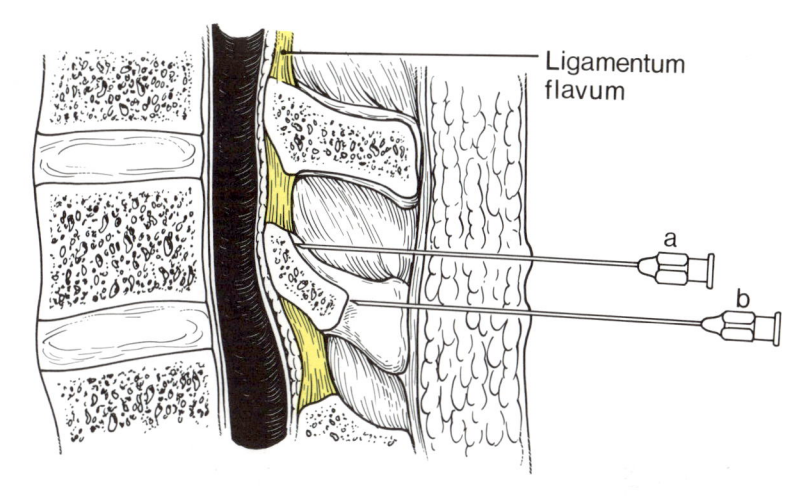

Fig. 7.15 The posterior surface of the lamina of a lumbar vertebra slopes downwards and backwards. If therefore the needle, slightly out of the median plane, encounters bone at a shallow depth, it is the lower border of the lamina on which it impinges; if the obstruction is deep, it is the upper border.

developed (Fig. 7.16). Once the ligamentum flavum (Fig. 7.17) is penetrated lumbar puncture, or the identification of the extradural space, is as good as done. The needle now lies within the extradural space and if pushed a little deeper almost inevitably pierces the dura. It is true that a needle somewhat ill directed may go through the ligamentum flavum and on its onward course fail to pierce the dura but touch it like a tangent to a circle. In these circumstances the point of the advancing needle may strike the nerve for that segment in the extradural space (Fig. 7.18) causing pain in the appropriate distribution. This shows that the point of the needle is too lateral and

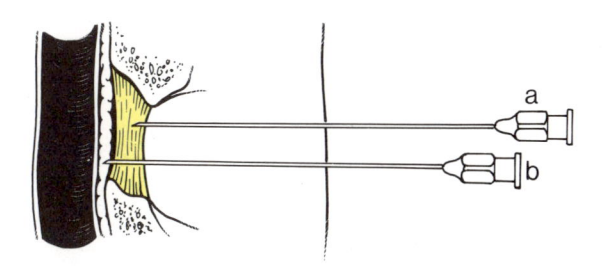

Fig. 7.16 The ligamentum flavum can often be recognised as the needle enters it (*a*), and in a powerful subject a second alteration in resistance may be detected as the needle passes through the distal side (*b*) to enter the extradural space.

172 LUMBAR PUNCTURE AND SPINAL ANALGESIA

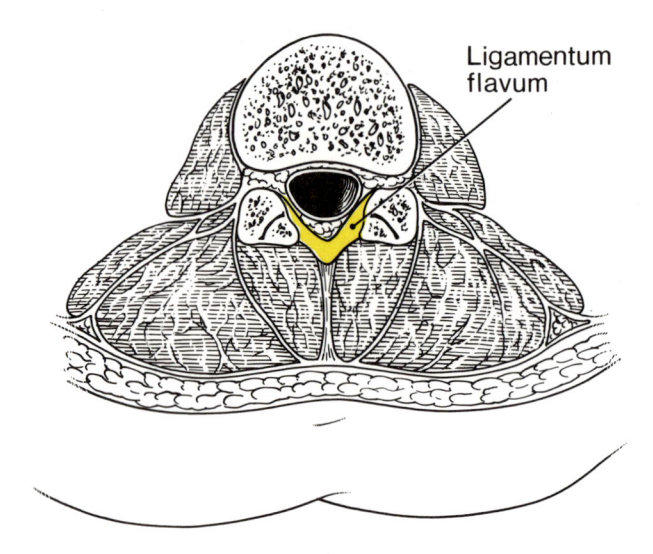

Fig. 7.17 The ligamentum flavum.

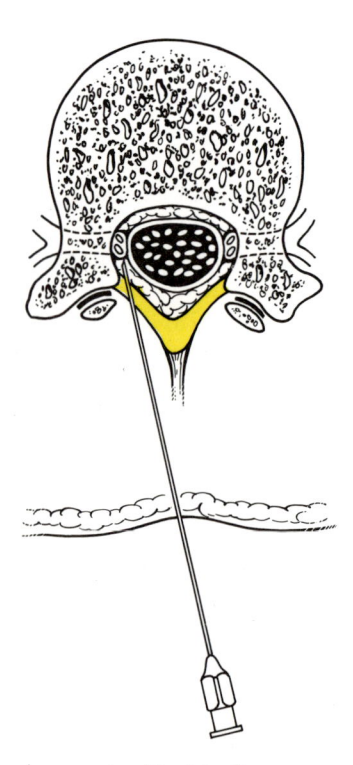

Fig. 7.18 The extradural space entered too laterally.

it may need to be withdrawn and reinserted strictly in the median plane. The side on which the pain is felt gives the clue to which side the needle has erred; and the necessary alteration in direction can generally be confirmed by looking along the line of the shaft. During an attempt at lumbar puncture, a shooting pain in the thigh unaccompanied by an issue of cerebrospinal fluid shows that the point of the needle has passed through the ligamentum flavum and that either it is in the position just discussed, or else though highly unlikely, that it has penetrated the dura and struck one of the constituent nerve roots of the cauda equina, but on account of blockage of the needle cerebrospinal fluid does not flow through it. Before piercing the dura the point of the needle inevitably passes through the extradural space. Lumbar puncture therefore affords the anaesthetist an admirable opportunity to practise identification of the space. This he can do by using one of the excellent methods which have been described in Chapter 9 (Dogliotti, 1933; Odom, 1936; Gutiérrez, 1942; Macintosh, 1950; Brooks, 1957; Salt, 1963; Atkinson et al, 1982).

The distance between the skin and the ligamentum flavum is determined partly by muscular development, but principally by the amount of fat in the subcutaneous tissue (Fig. 2.40). After a little experience the depth at which the extradural space will be encountered in any particular case can generally be estimated with considerable accuracy. It is usually between 3.5 and 5 cm but may be more if the needle is inserted at an angle, or if the patient is obese. The use of a marked needle (Lee, 1960), the first mark being 4 cm from the needle point, is a great help in estimating the depth of the point at any particular time. In a straightforward lumbar puncture the ligamentum flavum and the dura can usually be identified separately by the resistances they offer to the needle; this is made possible by the intervening layer of extradural fat which may be as deep as 1 cm in the median plane. But this is not always the case. Occasionally — particularly where the needle pierces the ligamentum flavum to one side of the median plane — resistance is felt only at one point, since the ligament and the dura are in actual contact in this situation (Fig. 7.19b).

In powerful men in whom the yellow ligament may be 1 cm thick, the needle can be felt to enter the ligament and after being pushed forwards some distance a second alteration in resistance is noted. This latter may give the impression that the dura has been pierced whereas it is caused by the point of the needle passing through the further side of the ligament into the extradural space (Fig. 7.16).

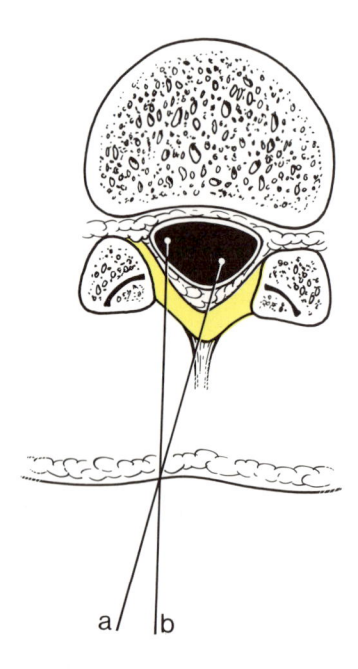

Fig. 7.19 Puncture of the dura.

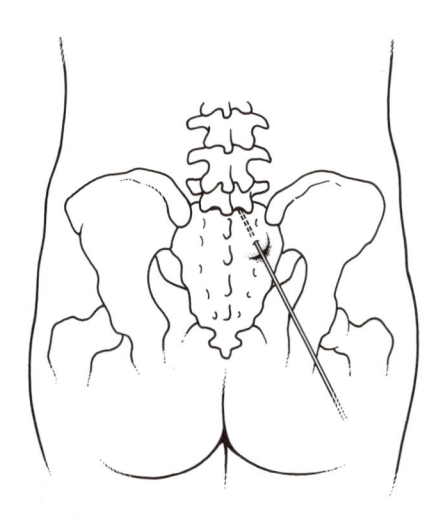

Fig. 7.20 The lumbo-sacral approach.

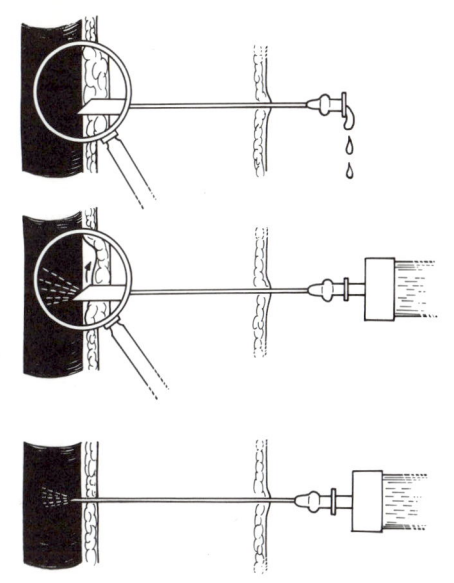

Fig. 7.21 The relationship of the bevel of the needle to the dura.

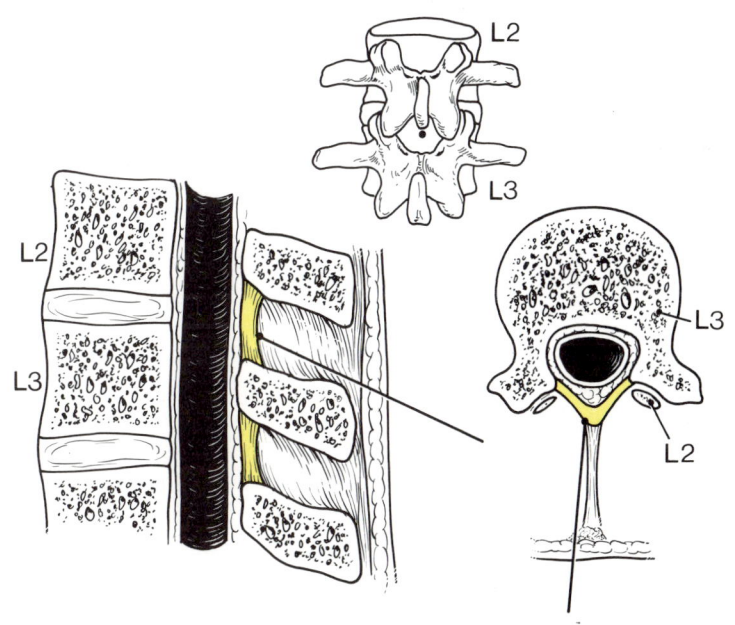

Fig. 7.22 Lateral (paramedian) approach: correct angulation of needle for lumbar puncture in an average subject.

The skin is punctured immediately to one side of the supraspinous ligament — in this case, the left side — and the needle is inclined medially enough to reach the median plane about 3 to 4 cm from the skin, and upwards enough for its slope to be slightly steeper than that of the upper margin of the spine. In the median approach, the skin is punctured over the supraspinous ligament and the needle advanced strictly in the sagittal plane.

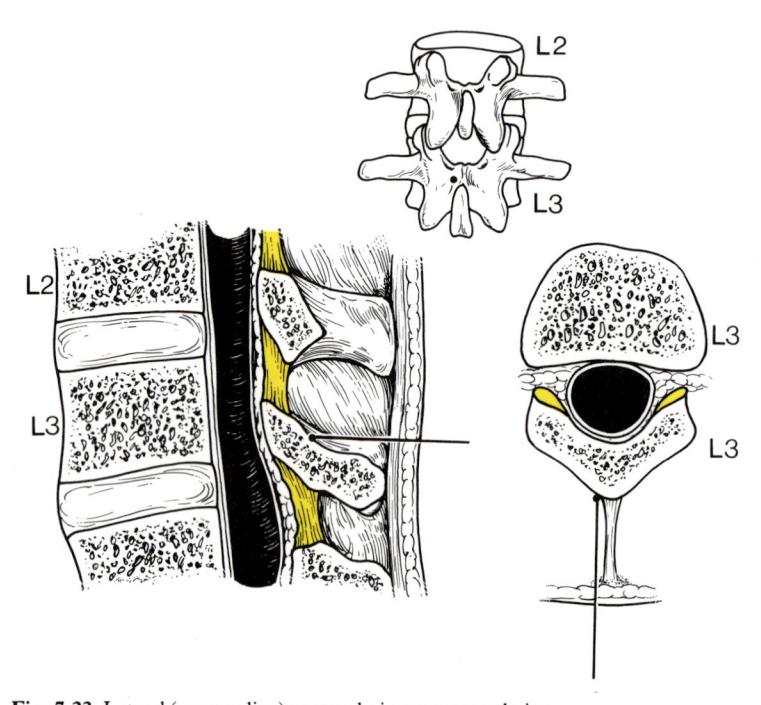

Fig. 7.23 Lateral (paramedian) approach: incorrect angulation.
The site of entry of the needle through the skin is good, but the point has not been directed upwards to miss the lamina of the lower vertebra. In fact, the needle has been thrust straight forwards and hits the left lamina just where it fuses with its opposite number to form the base of the spine, and below the limit of the attachment of the ligamentum flavum on the posterior aspect of the lamina.

When it occurs, this double alteration in resistance coupled with the absence of an issue of cerebrospinal fluid locates the point with considerable certainty in the extradural space; if now the needle is pushed on further, the resistance of the dura will be noted and when this is pierced cerebrospinal fluid will flow. If, using the lateral or paramedian approach, the needle is felt to enter the ligamentum flavum and immediately beyond is held up by bone, it shows that the point must be impinging on the upper boundary of the lamina of the lower vertebra, for only in this situation does ligamentum flavum overlie bone (Fig. 7.26). The needle should be partially withdrawn, the point directed slightly upwards and then pushed in again.

When cerebrospinal fluid appears, the needle should be slowly rotated through 360 degrees and pushed slightly onwards to ensure that the bevel lies wholly within the dura so that the greatest possible flow is obtained. If the dura is incompletely penetrated, any solution

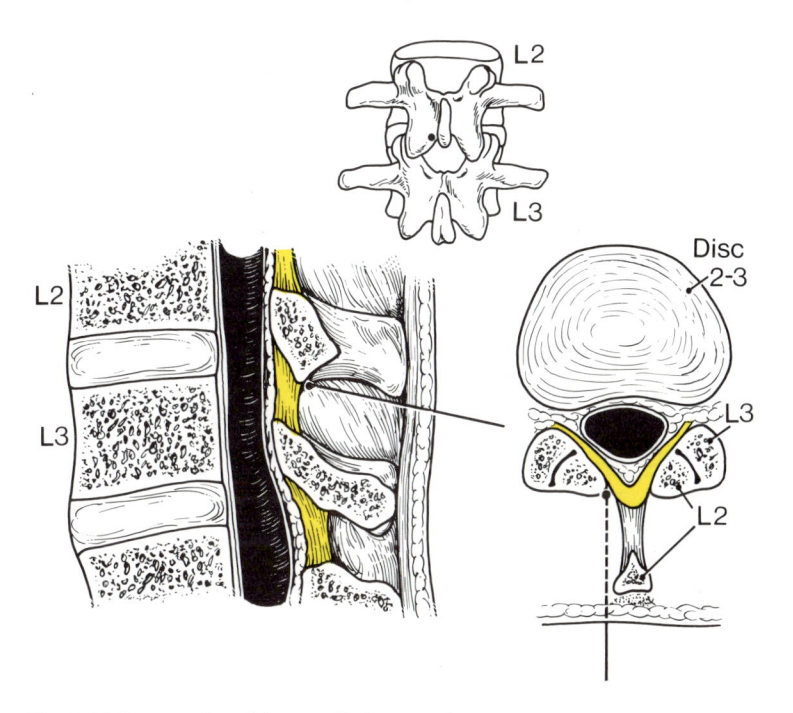

Fig. 7.24 Incorrect lateral (paramedian) approach.
The skin is penetrated to the left of the median plane and just below the lower margin of the spine of L.2. Even though the skin puncture is almost at the top of the gap between the two spines, the ligamentum flavum would have been pierced if the needle had been directed straight forwards and not slightly upwards, or if it had been inclined slightly medially.

injected will be deposited partly outside the dura (Fig. 7.21 centre). The bevel of the needle used for intradural injection should be as short as possible (Pitkin, 1927); with a long bevel, some of the solution may inadvertently be injected into the extradural space and its effect partly wasted.

A refinement of technique which may reduce the incidence of post-spinal headache is to see that the bevel of the lumbar puncture needle is directed laterally, so that it separates and does not divide the fibres of the dura which run longitudinally.

Occasionally, a patient maintained in the sitting position with his feet firmly placed on a stool during the lumbar puncture (see Fig. 7.3) will complain of faintness and may even sway forward or laterally and must be supported. This is usually blamed on a combination of discomfort, anxiety and the hypotensive effects of the drugs used for premedication.

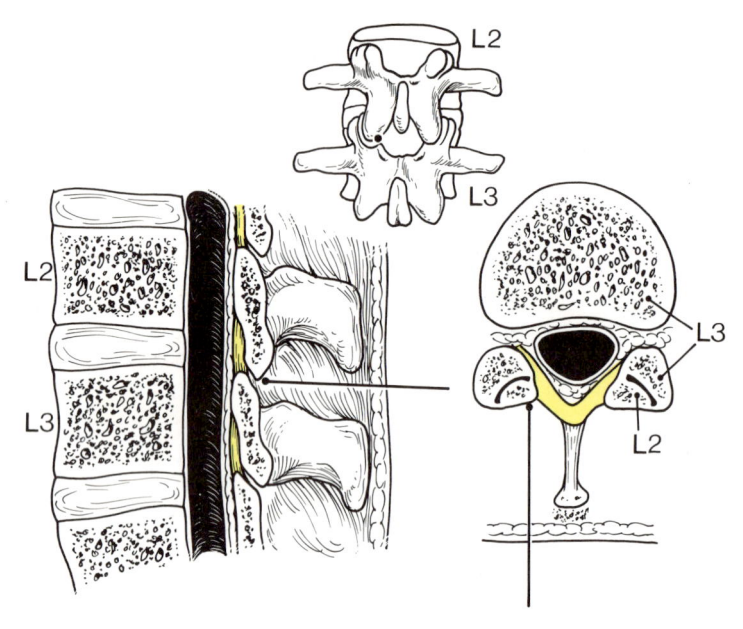

Fig. 7.25 Incorrect lateral (paramedian) approach.
The needle has pierced the skin just below the lower border of the spine of L.2, but allowance has correctly been made for this by keeping it in the horizontal plane. The error lies in the fact that although the skin is entered well to the left of the supraspinous ligament, the needle has been pushed straight ahead and strikes the inferior articular process. If the needle is withdrawn and directed slightly medially to compensate for the lateral start, lumbar puncture will present no difficulty.

Lumbo-sacral approach

If orthodox lumbar puncture presents difficulties, the dura may be reached by a needle directed through the space between the 5th lumbar vertebra and the sacrum. This cannot be reached from the mid-line because the spine of the 5th lumbar vertebra gets in the way. The patient is placed prone with a pillow under the hips and a weal is raised 1 cm medial and 1 cm inferior to the posterior superior iliac spine; this point is 1.5 cm lateral to the middle of the lumbo-sacral interspace, and from it a needle is advanced medially and towards the head, aiming to reach the mid-line at the lumbo-sacral junction, forming an angle of about 55 degrees with the skin, which is equal to the angle that the dorsal surface of the sacrum makes with the skin superficial to it at this point. The needle follows the course of the sacrum up to the lumbo-sacral space (Taylor, 1940), (see Fig. 7.20).

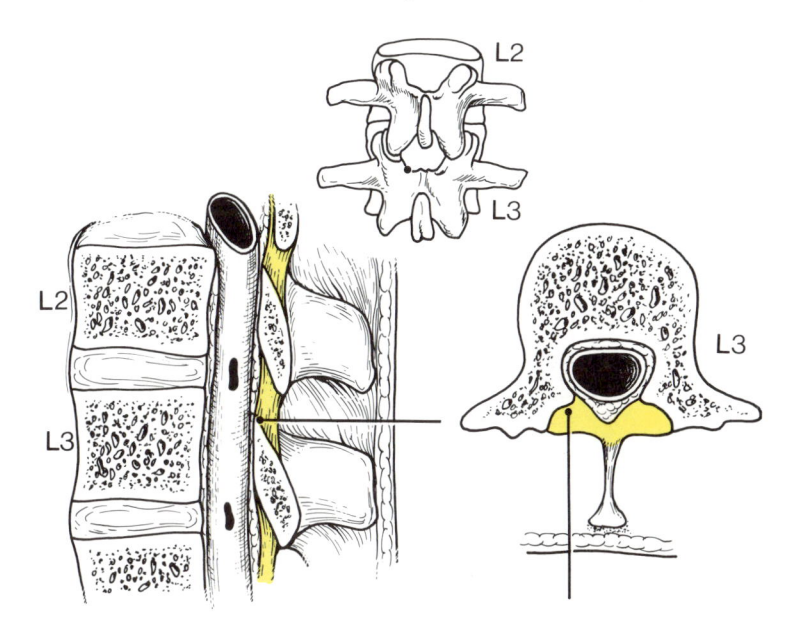

Fig. 7.26 Incorrect.
Here the needle pierces the skin at a level corresponding almost to the middle of the gap between the two spines, but too far to the left. The needle has been pushed directly ahead and hit the left pedicle of L.3, just where it becomes continuous with the lamina. If it had been directed slightly upwards and/or medially all would have been well. In any event the anaesthetist will probably feel the tip of the needle penetrate the ligamentum flavum before it is held up by bone. This is a sure sign that the needle is directed just too low, since the ligament is attached to the posterior aspect of the superior margin of the lamina of the lower vertebra. All that is necessary is partly to withdraw the needle, tilt it slightly upwards and reinsert.

The prone jack-knife position has been recommended for extradural injection. It is said to increase the distance between the ligamentum flavum and the dura (Mustafa et al, 1983).

Spinal needle director (Fig. 7.31)

A spinal needle director is a short, robust outer needle (e.g. 18 to 20 gauge) designed to be inserted through the skin so that an exceptionally fine inner needle, passed through its lumen, can be used for lumbar puncture without fear of bending. There is much to be said for a director. One was illustrated and described by Corning (Corning, 1894), as long ago as 1894, only three years after Quincke's classical description of the technique of lumbar puncture, but the article seems to have attracted no attention and we have been

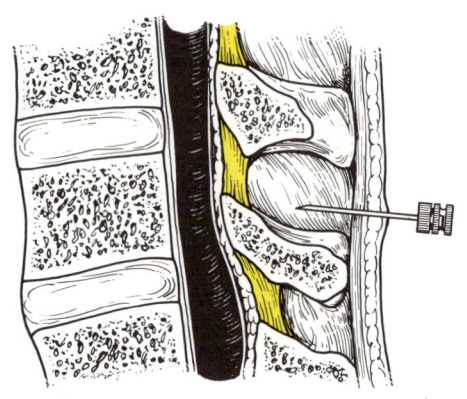

Fig. 7.27 One cause of error.

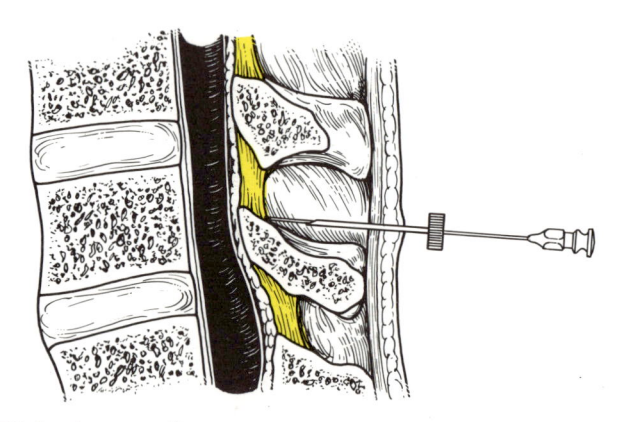

Fig. 7.28 Another cause of error.

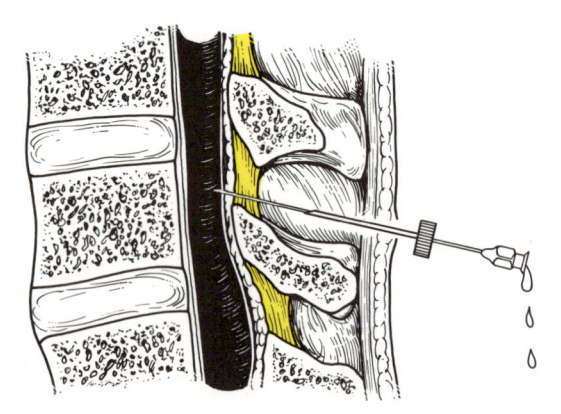

Fig. 7.29 Correct direction of needle.

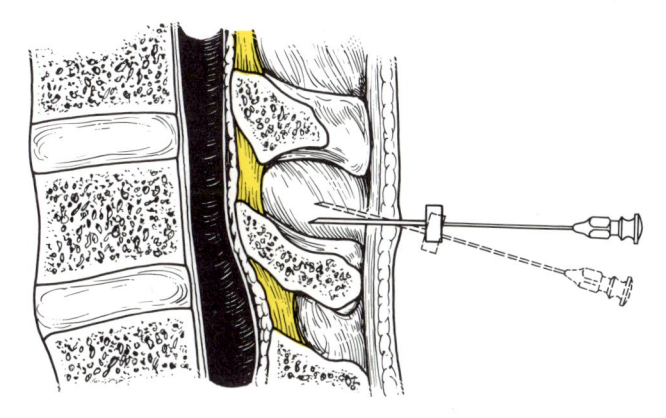

Fig. 7.30 Incorrect direction of needle.

unable to find anything further about this useful little piece of apparatus in the literature until 1928 when Sise (Sise, 1928), wrote about his introducer or director (Fig. 7.31).

A director is particularly useful when the anaesthetist aims at keeping to the median plane throughout, for the direction of the powerful director will not be deflected by the tough supra- and interspinous ligaments. A skin weal is raised and the director is thrust through the superficial resistant structures for about 2 to 3 cm towards the interlaminar space. Provided that the director is properly aligned, a fine lumbar puncture needle (e.g. 25 gauge) introduced through the lumen has now to overcome only the slight resistances offered by the ligamentum flavum and dura. The very fine

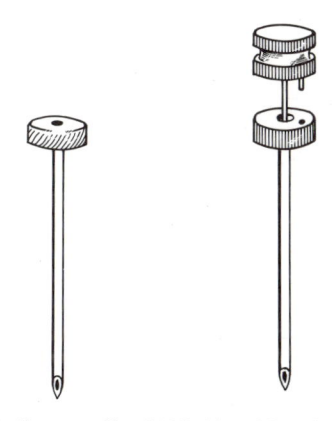

Fig. 7.31 Spinal needle directors. Sise (1928) (*a*) and Lundy (1942) (*b*).

lumbar puncture needle which a director makes practicable leaves only a very small hole in the dura through which seepage of cerebrospinal fluid subsequently can take place; for this reason many regard the use of a director as a prophylactic against post-lumbar puncture headache.

The director is probably an added safeguard against infection being carried to the subarachnoid space. It pierces the epidermis so that no part of the spinal needle subsequently directed through it comes into contact with the skin. Neither does the shaft of the needle have to be steadied by the operator's fingers as is the case when a fine needle is introduced without the support of a director.

Perhaps the greatest value of a director is in the elderly patient whose lumbar vertebrae are fixed slightly in extension and the size of whose interlaminar foramina are possibly still further reduced by osteoarthritis. Here on occasions, the needle seems to encounter bone in whichever direction it is thrust. If a director is not used, one frequently sees the anaesthetist repeatedly handling the skin over the spines to verify the landmarks, and the shaft of the needle when reinserting it. These manoeuvres, particularly in the presence of local haemorrhage, jeopardise asepsis and are to be discouraged. If a director is used, repeated attempts at dural puncture can be made without the anaesthetist touching the skin or the point or shaft of the needle; and if a little haemorrhage does take place through the needle, it can be withdrawn and replaced by a fresh one without making another skin puncture.

After a skin weal has been raised, the point of the director should not be pushed in for more than 2 to 3 cm through the skin, and it is important that this depth should not be exceeded in thin subjects because in these the dura can be surprisingly superficial. When the director is in place, the lumbar puncture needle is pushed on tentatively. If the director is skilfully or fortunately aimed, all is well and the needle passes uneventfully through the ligamentum flavum and extradural space into the dural sac. In this case the procedure has been as straightforward and easy as the textbook illustrations make it appear. If, however, bone is encountered (Fig. 7.28), the needle is withdrawn until it lies within the lumen of the director. The thumb and forefinger of the left hand now alter the aim of the director, and a fresh attempt at hitting the target is made by pushing in the lumbar puncture needle gently. Several attempts may be made without causing appreciable damage. A useful substitute for a director when a lumbar puncture needle of 22 or lesser gauge is to be used is a 19 gauge 'butterfly' intravenous needle with all but the last

2 mm of plastic tubing removed (Ariaraj, 1981).

If the patient coughs immediately after injection of the drug into the intradural space, the spread of analgesia is not necessarily increased (Dubelman and Forbes, 1979), although rapid injection causes turbulence and increased spread.

If, when performing an intradural block, the issuing CSF is definitely bloodstained, it is wise to pause for a few minutes; if blood is still then seen, the question of abandoning the block must be considered.

A frame has been described for the rare patient who is immovable but requires a lumbar puncture (Miranda, 1977).

A technique employing both continuous extradural and 'one-shot' intradural block has been described (Coates, 1982). First the extradural space is identified using either a straight, thin-walled 16 to 18 gauge or a Tuohy needle, and through this a 25 to 26 gauge spinal needle 1 cm longer is inserted into the theca and analgesic solution suitable for an intradural block injected. The fine spinal needle is now removed and a catheter is threaded into the extradural space, care being taken that it too does not pierce the dura. The patient thus receives a rapidly acting intradural block and can have postoperative pain relief by serial injections into the extradural space. Only one lumbar puncture is required. Brownridge uses two lumbar injections, one intradural the other extradural (Brownridge, 1981).

Contraindications to lumbar puncture

Raised intracranial pressure especially when this is due to a space-occupying lesion. The danger is the creation of a cerebellar pressure cone which could prove fatal. A unilateral space-occupying lesion may also result in herniation of brain substance through the tentorial falx. The introduction of computerised tomography has reduced the need for diagnostic lumbar puncture in strokes, infarction, haematoma, angiomas and in patients with suspected subarachnoid haemorrhage where it may do harm (Duffy, 1982, 1983; Pearce, 1982). Other neurologists would sanction lumbar puncture in certain patients with suspected subarachnoid bleeding (Teddy et al, 1983).

Relative contraindications include neighbouring skin infection, gross obesity, blood dyscrasias, patients on full anti-coagulant therapy, for fear of causing intra- or extradural bleeding, and a stiff and unyielding back from any cause.

Obvious infection of the skin of the back contraindicates lumbar puncture. Difficulty sometimes arises in deciding whether to give a spinal analgesic to a patient who already has a colostomy or a cystostomy, or is otherwise incontinent. On general principles a spinal analgesic should be avoided here, but on many occasions we have disregarded this counsel of perfection when we felt that the increased risk of sepsis was outweighed by the improved operating conditions offered by spinal analgesia for that particular case. No harm has resulted, probably because of meticulous care in preparing the site of puncture.

The myelogram

An early pioneer of contrast radiography of the central nervous system was Walter E. Dandy (1922) who injected air into the subarachnoid space for the diagnosis of spinal cord tumours. In 1918 he had already described pneumoencephalography (Dandy, 1918). About the same time the Swede Jacobeus insufflated air into the spinal canal (Jacobeus, 1921). Sicard and Forestier (1921) substituted iodised poppyseed oil for air in 1922. Myelography became popular after the publication in 1934 of the first description by Mixter and Barr (1934) of a herniated intervertebral disc and its surgical removal. Lipiodol was not the ideal contrast medium and gave place to Thorotrast (colloidal thorium dioxide) but this was abandoned because it proved irritating to the meninges and there was a risk of neoplasm. Other solutions included Abrodil (Arnell and Lindstrom, 1931), Pantopaque (Ramsey and Stain, 1944) and Conray, a water-soluble medium.

An anaesthetist is sometimes asked to inject a solution of a contrast medium into the intradural space by a colleague — orthopaedic surgeon, rheumatologist, oncologist or radiologist. This is a tribute to his skill and also to his realisation of the need for strict surgical cleanliness in the performance of such investigations. It is not quite so easy as it might appear and calls for a careful and meticulous technique if good X-ray pictures are to be obtained. Any contrast medium finding its way into the extradural space either due to inadvertent injection or to leakage from the intradural compartment will interfere with the radiographs and may complicate diagnosis.

A contrast medium sometimes used is iophendylate (Myodil). This is a viscous substance which should be warmed to blood heat before injection and requires the use of a lumbar puncture needle, not smaller in size than 20 gauge. The usual amount injected is between 5 and 10 ml. It is often replaced by lopamidol (Niopam) which is water-soluble. Metrizamide (Amipaque) is another water-soluble contrast medium which does not dissociate in solution. Iophendylate may cause spinal arachnoiditis, while a post-injection convulsion has been reported (Jones, 1980). Small volumes of CSF can be withdrawn and Pantopaque injected through a 24 g needle (Pulec, 1983); this reduces the incidence of lumbar puncture headache.

The lumbar puncture can be done in either the sitting or the lateral position and must be technically perfect. Cerebrospinal fluid must be seen to flow freely and must be capable of aspiration into a 2 ml syringe. The flow of only a few drops is not satisfactory. Sometimes the anaesthetist is asked to measure the pressure of CSF and this is done by connecting a sterile glass manometer to the lumbar puncture needle by a three-way tap and allowing the fluid to ascend the column. If the internal jugular vein in the neck is now compressed by an assistant, failure of the column to rise further is known as a positive Queckenstedt test and suggests the presence of an obstruction in the intradural space between the foramen magnum and the lumbar region in which the needle is inserted (Queckenstedt, 1916). One or more specimens of CSF may be needed for examination, and after they have been collected into sterile containers, the contrast medium is injected. After a short pause to allow the medium to spread away from the dural puncture, the syringe is disconnected and the needle withdrawn, taking care to see that no medium finds its way into the extradural space from the needle as it is extracted. Radiography follows.

An anaesthetist asked to make such an injection is advised to come to a clear understanding with the colleague asking him to do it, as to the responsibility for any untoward effects which may follow. The patient may already have signs or symptoms of disease in, or near the vicinity of the cord, while the effects of the injected contrast medium are not always benign.

Epidurography, using the non-ionic iodine containing contrast medium metrizamide may be preferred to myelography in the future (Hamilton, 1983) to diagnose the presence, level and degree of disc prolapse. In the absence of accidental dural tap it can be carried out on outpatients. It is said to be without the occasional untoward complications of intradural contrast techniques (Baker et al, 1978).

REFERENCES

Ariaraj, S. J. P. (1981) Butterfly indwelling needles used as spinal needle guides. *Anaesthesia*, **36**, 72.

Armitage, E. N. (1976) The paramedian approach to lumbar epidural analgesia. *Anaesthesia*, **31**, 1287.

Armitage, E. N. (1977) The paramedian approach to the epidural space. *Anaesthesia*, **32**, 672.

Arnell, S. & Lindstrom, F. (1931) Skiodan (Abrodil) for myelography. *Acta Radiologica Scandinavica*, **12**, 287.

Atkinson, R. S., Rushman, G. B. & Lee, J. A. (1982) *A Synopsis of Anaesthesia*, p. 762, 9th edn. Bristol: Wright.

Baker, R. A., Hillman, J. B., McLennan, J. E. et al (1978) Sequelae to metrizamide myelography in 200 examinations. *American Journal of Roentgenology*, **130**, 449.

Bonica, J. J. (1967) *Principals and Practice of Obstetric Analgesia and Anesthesia*, p. 633. Philadelphia: Davis.

Brooks, W. (1957) An epidural indicator. *Anaesthesia*, **12**, 227.

Brownridge, P. (1981) Epidural and subarachnoid analgesia for elective Caesarean section. *Anaesthesia*, **36**, 70.

Carrie, L. E. S. (1971) The approach to the extradural space. *Anaesthesia*, **26**, 252.

Carrie, L. E. S. (1977) The paramedian approach to the epidural space. *Anaesthesia*, **32**, 670.

Chapman, G. M. (1977) The paramedian approach to the epidural space. *Anaesthesia*, **32**, 671.

Coates, M. B. (1982) Combined subarachnoid and epidural techniques. *Anaesthesia*, **37**, 89.

Corning, J. L. (1894) *Pain in its Neuropathological and Anatomical Relations*, p. 247. Philadelphia.

Dandy, W. E. (1918) Ventriculography following the injection of air into the cerebral ventricles. *Annals of Surgery*, **68**, 5.

Dandy, W. E. (1922) Diagnosis and localisation of spinal cord tumours. *Bulletin of the Johns Hopkins Hospital*, **33**, 190.

Dogliotti, A. M. (1933) A new method of block anesthesia: segmental peridural spinal anesthesia. *American Journal of Surgery*, **20**, 107.

Drummond, G. B. & Scott, D. H. T. (1980) Deflection of spinal needles by bevel. *Anaesthesia*, **35**, 854.

Dubelman, A. M. & Forbes, A. R. (1979) Does cough increase the spread of subarachnoid analgesia? *Anesthesia and Analgesia*, **58**, 306.

Duffy, G. P. (1982) Correspondence. *British Medical Journal*, **285**, 1163.

Duffy, G. P. (1983) Correspondence. *British Medical Journal*, **286**, 143.

Frazer, J. E. (1940) *The Anatomy of the Human Skeleton*, p. 35, 4th edn. London: Churchill.

Gutiérrez, A. (1942) Revista de Cirujia Buenos Aires. *Anesthesia Metamerica Peridural*, **12**, 665.

Hamilton, G. (1983) Metrizamide epidurography. *Journal of the Irish Royal Colleges of Physicians and Surgeons*, **76**, 126.

Jacobeus, H. C. (1921) On insufflation of air into the spinal canal for diagnostic purposes in cases of tumour of the spinal cord. *Acta Medica Scandinavica*, **21**, 555.

Jones, D. F. (1980) Postoperative convulsion due to iophendylate (Myodil). *Anaesthesia*, **35**, 50.

Lee, J. A. (1960) A specially marked needle to facilitate extradural block. *Anaesthesia*, **15**, 186.

Lundy, J. S. (1942) *Clinical Anesthesia*, p. 257, Fig. 110(k). Philadelphia: Saunders.

Macintosh, R. R. (1950) Extradural space indicator. *Anaesthesia*, **5**, 98.

Miranda, D. R. (1977) Access for lumbar puncture in immovable patients. *British Journal of Anaesthesia*, **49**, 518.

Mixter, W. J. & Barr, J. S. (1934) Rupture of the intervertebral disc with involvement of the spinal canal. *New England Journal of Medicine*, **211**, 210.

Mustafa, K., Milliken, R. A. & Bizzarri, D. V. (1983) The advantage of the prone position approach to the lumbar epidural space. *Anesthesiology*, **58**, 464.

Odom, C. B. (1936) Epidural anesthesia. *American Journal of Surgery*, **34**, 547.

Pearce, J. M. S. (1982) Hazards of lumbar puncture. *British Medical Journal*, **285**, 1521.

Pitkin, G. P. (1927) Controllable spinal anesthesia. *Journal of the Medical Society of New Jersey*, **24**, 425.

Pulec, J. E. (1983) Correspondence. *Journal of the Royal Society of Medicine*, **76**, 84.

Queckenstedt, H. H. G. (1916) Zur Diagnose der Rückenmarkskompression. *Deutsche Zeitschrift für Nervenheilkunde*, **55**, 325.

Ramsey, G. H. S. & Stain, W. E. (1944) Pantopaque: a new contrast medium for myelography. *Radiology and Clinical Photography*, **20**, 25.

Salt, R. H. (1963) Identification of the extradural space. *Anaesthesia*, **18**, 404.

Sharrock, N. E. (1979) Recordings of, and anatomical explanations for false positive loss of resistance during lumbar extradural analgesia. *British Journal of Anaesthesia*, **51**, 253.

Sicard, J. A. & Forestier, J. (1921) Méthode générale d'exploration radiologique par l'huile iodée (lipiodol). *Bulletin et mémoires de la Sociéte de médecine de Paris* **46**, 463; (see also Shapiro, R. (1975) *Myelography*, 3rd edn. Chicago: Yearbook Publishing).

Sise, L. F. (1928) A device for facilitating the use of fine gauge lumbar puncture needles. *Journal of the American Medical Association*, **91**, 1186.

Slattery, P. J., Rosen, M. & Rees, G. A. D. (1980) Correspondence: an aid to identification of the subarachnoid space with a twenty-five gauge needle. *Anaesthesia*, **35**, 391.

Taylor, J. A. (1940) Lumbo-sacral subarachnoid tap. *Journal of Urology*, **43**, 561.

Teddy, P. J., Briggs, M. & Adams, C. B. T. (1983) Correspondence. *British Medical Journal*, **286**, 143.

8

Intradural analgesia (subarachnoid block)

In recent years there has been an increase in the practice of intradural block in Britain and other countries (Robertson et al, 1978; Crawford, 1979; Lanz et al, 1979; Moore, 1979). Commercially prepared hyperbaric solutions of local analgesic drugs have not always been easy to obtain in the UK and at the time of writing only two commercial preparations (mepivacaine 4 per cent and cinchocaine 0.5 per cent) are supplied here specifically for intradural analgesia. However, the ready availability of ampoules of plain 0.5 per cent bupivacaine without preservatives has stimulated interest in this agent. The solution is already used extensively for extradural analgesia both in surgery and obstetric practice while it withstands repeated sterilisation without deterioration.

Bupivacaine has been used for intradural block, both in its plain form and with the addition of glucose to make a hyperbaric solution, since it was first employed by Ekblom and Widman in 1966 (Ekblom and Widman, 1966). Recent studies have compared the mode of spread of these solutions within the intradural space with that of agents long established in clinical practice (Pflug et al, 1976; Brown et al, 1980; Wildsmith et al, 1981b). The results show that the traditional teaching based largely on the classic work of Arthur Barker (Barker, 1907, 1908a, 1908b) who used a glass spine, may have to be revised.

Although intradural block has been in clinical use for more than 85 years, and despite the many publications in the literature during this time, it must be accepted that the estimation of the spread of local analgesic solution in the intradural space, and consequently the extent of the block produced, remains more of an art than a science. The clinician has to consider not only the nature of the drug injected and the dose, but also the site of injection, the speed of injection, the specific gravity of the solution, the posture of the patient both during injection and afterwards, the volume of solution used, barbotage or its absence, the viscosity of the solution and finally the age, height and general condition of the patient. Some of the factors, especially the nature of the drug and its concentration, also influence the duration of the block.

Understanding the scientific basis underlying the spread of analgesic solutions within the intradural space is made difficult by the fact that not all workers have obtained the same results. Most of the recent work has been concerned with intradural block for operations on the hip joint, legs, groin and perineum, that is to a segmental level no higher than T.10. Upper abdominal surgery under intradural block has fallen out of favour in recent times and the anaesthetist who wishes to provide high spinal block for such procedures is probably best advised to keep to the well tried techniques using hyperbaric solutions of cinchocaine, amethocaine, lignocaine or mepivacaine or employ an extradural technique. The authors' long experience with 0.5 per cent cinchocaine made hyperbaric by the addition of 6 per cent glucose leads them to believe that this remains a most useful preparation, especially when prolonged action is desired. For operations lasting less than one hour, mepivacaine 4 per cent or lignocaine 5 per cent in hyperbaric solution provide an acceptable alternative.

Spread of local analgesic solution

If the site of operation is the leg or perineum, no difficulty arises about conveying the analgesic solution to the nerve roots to be rendered analgesic; the needle point already lies in their midst where they form the cauda equina just below the conus medullaris (see Fig. 8.1). A local analgesic injected here will necessarily produce analgesia below this level, just as would transection of the nerves.

If the field of operation is the upper abdomen, the problem arises as to how levels as high as T.4 can be blocked in the intradural space. Spinal puncture in the thoracic region is more difficult technically than in the lumbar region owing to the downward pointing thoracic spines, and also carries a possible risk of injury to the spinal cord itself. Orthodox lumbar puncture in the lumbar region allows injection of the analgesic drug at this level and the factors affecting spread to any desired level must then be considered.

Posture and baricity

The classic teaching that analgesic solutions for intradural injection should be hyper- or hypobaric and that spread within the intradural

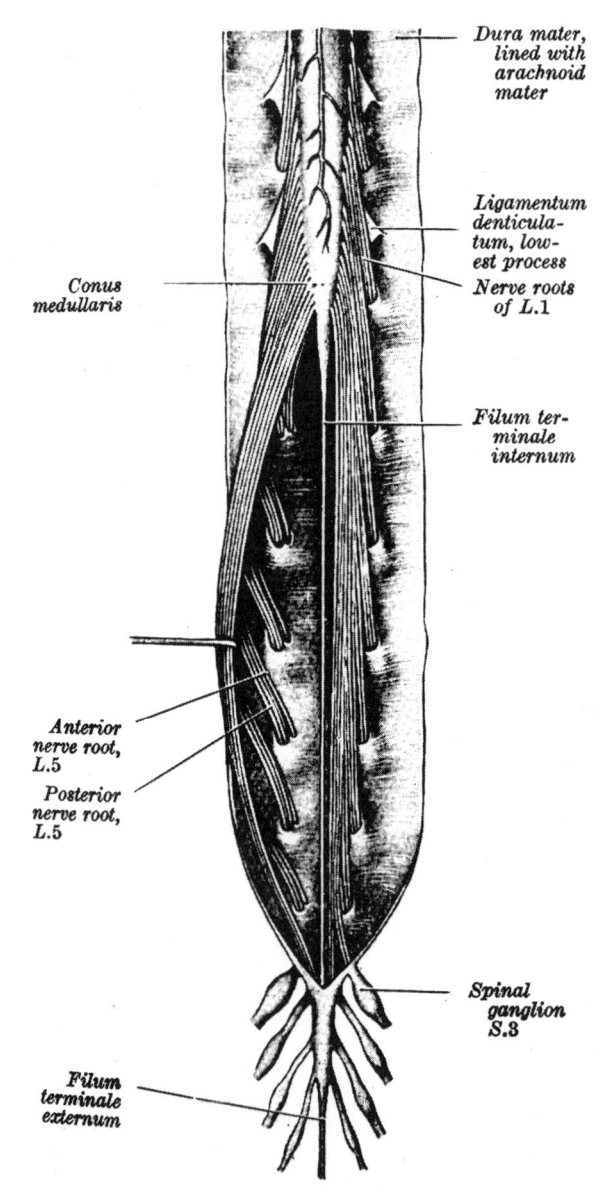

Fig. 8.1 The lower end of the spinal cord, the filum terminale and the cauda equina exposed from behind. The dura mater and the arachnoid mater have been opened and spread out. (Reproduced from *Gray's Anatomy*, 31st edn.)

space should be controlled by appropriate use of posture, bearing in mind the specific gravity of the cerebrospinal fluid and the injected fluid, has recently been questioned. A number of carefully constructed trials have shown that these factors are not so important as was once thought. For operations on the legs or perineum, it matters little whether the patient is sitting or in the lateral position since the needle point during injection is anyway amidst the nerve roots to be blocked. Nor does it matter whether the analgesic solution is hyperbaric or hypobaric. The difference between iso- and hypobaric solutions is not clinically significant and it is appropriate in modern times to consider two types of analgesic solution only — plain solutions and those made hyperbaric by the addition of glucose. Glucose has been used in various percentages, normally between 5 and 10 per cent, the more glucose added the more hyperbaric the resulting preparation.

Amethocaine and bupivacaine act in a similar way whether used in hyperbaric or plain solution (Brown et al, 1980; Chambers et al, 1981a; Wildsmith et al, 1981b; Tattersall, 1983), though the hyperbaric does tend to spread a few segments further in a cephalad direction than the plain solution if the patient is tilted head down (Sinclair et al, 1982). When 3 ml of the plain solution is injected, analgesia seldom extends above T.10 in the average patient, whereas the hyperbaric solutions in similar volume are likely to reach the mid-thoracic zone. A planned level, however, cannot be guaranteed and levels higher than expected may sometimes result. It is interesting to note that August Bier writing in 1898 mentioned the occasional capriciousness (launenhaft) of analgesic spread. This is by no means unknown today.

When it is desired to confine analgesia to the sacral nerves there is much to be said for giving the injection in the lateral position with head up tilt or with the patient sitting. For example, a small volume (0.6 ml) of hyperbaric cinchocaine can be trickled slowly down to reach the lower end of the dural sac. If the patient remains in the sitting position for about five minutes, the 4th and 5th sacral nerves only are blocked resulting in a very circumscribed area of analgesia around the anus, suitable for the operation of haemorrhoidectomy. With such a technique, block of the lumbar nerves, unnecessary for the operation and involving analgesia of a wide area of skin, can be avoided.

For abdominal operations, the classical teaching is to use gravity and posture to encourage hyperbaric solutions to reach segmental levels considerably higher than that of the lumbar puncture.

Although in some ways the intradural space is like the glass spine modelled for Barker (1907), being filled with fluid and the spinal cord, it is also broken up by nerve roots, the denticulate ligaments and fine trabeculae which attach the arachnoid to the pia mater. These may cause obstruction to the free flow of analgesic solution by forming baffles, with uneven distribution and occasional unexpected effects. Two important landmarks should be noticed in Figure 8.2. The summit of the lumbar convexity is the 3rd lumbar vertebra — the level at which lumbar puncture is commonly performed. The deepest point in the thoracic concavity is T.5–6, and at this level the spinal nerves which issue supply:

1. The uppermost sympathetic fibres in the anterior roots below T.4 which unite to form the splanchnic nerves.
2. The skin over the xiphisternum and below.
3. Motor nerves to the anterior abdominal wall.

If the nerves between the site of lumbar puncture and T.5–6 are anaesthetised, the whole of the abdominal wall will be rendered analgesic and the sympathetic nerve supply of the viscera will be interrupted (Fig. 2.33).

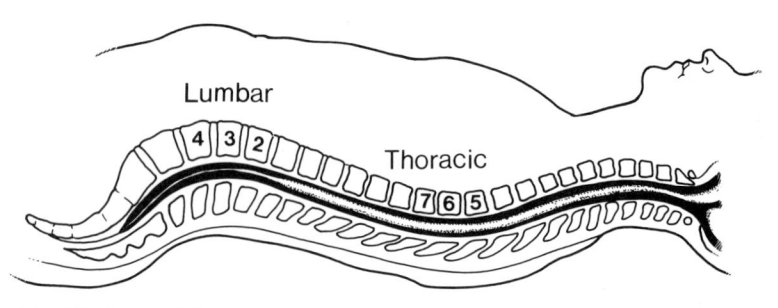

Fig. 8.2 Curves of the vertebral canal.

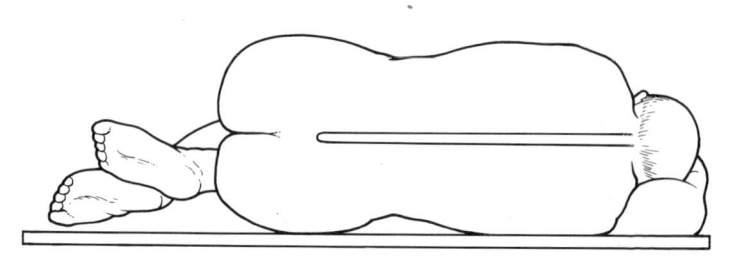

Fig. 8.3 When the average patient is in the lateral position ready for lumbar puncture, the vertebral column is more or less horizontal.

If lumbar puncture is made on an average patient (Fig. 8.2) lying on his side on a horizontal table, the injected 'heavy' fluid will at first lodge around the site of puncture. If the needle is now withdrawn, and the patient told to roll over on to his back, it will be found that the injected fluid remains for a very short time at the summit of the lumbar convexity, after which it may flow down the two slopes in different directions. That part of the solution which runs down into the sacral hollow is completely wasted as far as providing analgesia for abdominal surgery is concerned.

The technique of using a 'heavy' solution of a spinal analgesic for an abdominal operation is exceptionally easy. The patient lies on the side in which the incision is to be made, or on either side if the incision is to be mid-line. The whole table is now tilted (Fig. 8.7) until it is quite obvious to the observer's eye that the patient's vertebral column slopes downwards towards his head. In the case of the male with narrow hips and broad shoulders (Fig. 8.5), a considerable tilt of the table will be necessary, less so in the case of the female with broad hips and narrow shoulders where a mild downward slope towards the head already exists (Fig. 8.4). The angle to which the table should be tilted varies, therefore, from

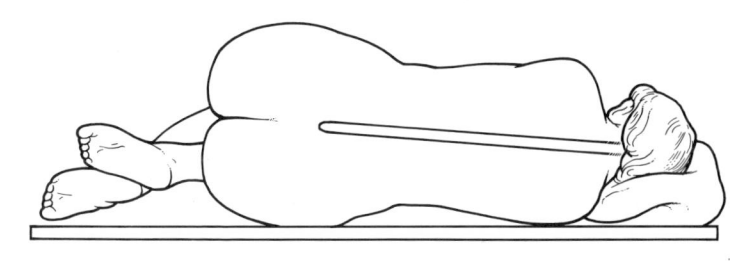

Fig. 8.4 In women, however, the column may incline downwards towards the head.

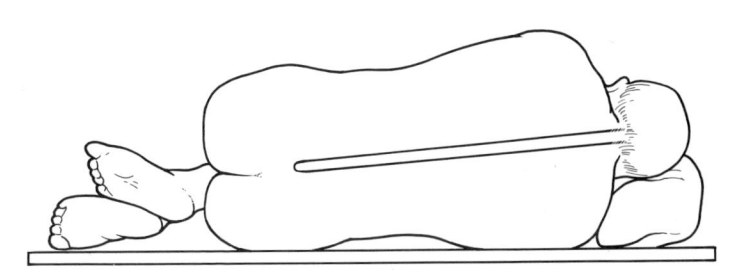

Fig. 8.5 In men the inclination may be downwards towards the coccyx. (After Mushin, 1943.)

194 LUMBAR PUNCTURE AND SPINAL ANALGESIA

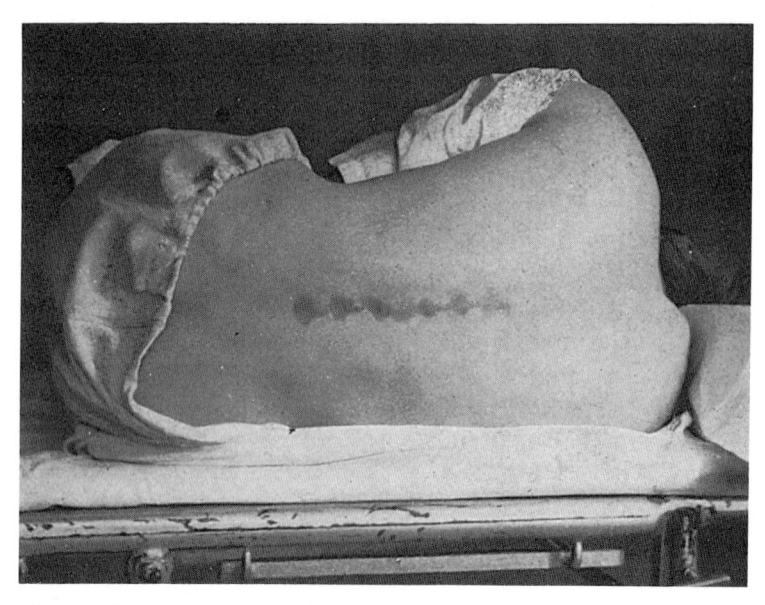

Fig. 8.6 The vertebral column is horizontal.

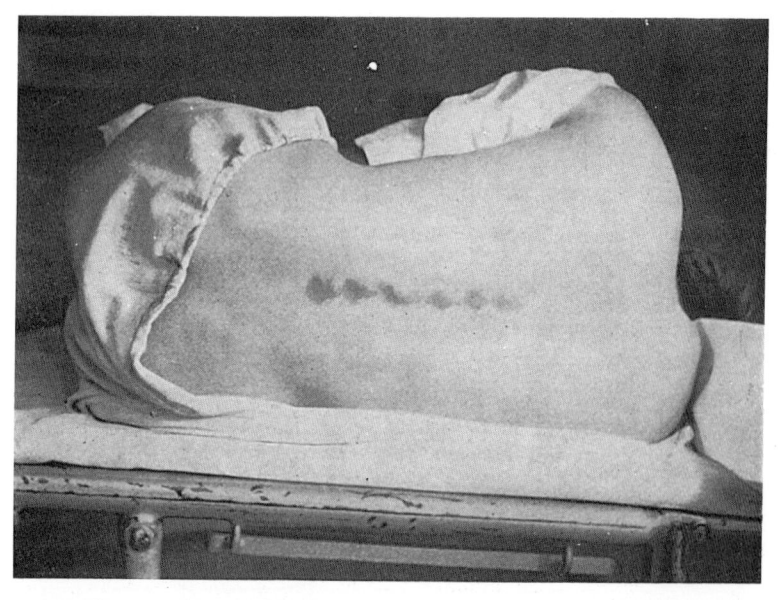

Fig. 8.7 If a heavy spinal analgesic solution is to be used for abdominal surgery, the table must be tilted until, as in this illustration, it is obvious that a line joining the spinous processes slopes downwards towards the head.

patient to patient. Precision is unnecessary, but the angle must be sufficient for it to be quite clear that the slope of the line joining the tips of the spinous processes is downwards towards the head. Not till then is the back flexed and lumbar puncture performed. The heavy analgesic solution injected will at once start to travel cephalwards (Fig. 8.13).

The inclination of the vertebral column is a factor of great importance in determining the spread of a heavy spinal analgesic solution.

As soon as the injection is finished, the needle is withdrawn and the patient rolled on to his back. The heavy analgesic solution continues its downward course into the thoracic hollow. On its journey some of the drug is adsorbed or 'fixed' by the nerve roots, and some absorbed by the venous plexuses which abound there (Jones, 1930). These two processes are fairly constant, so that in practice the vertebral level reached by the drug depends on the amount injected. If the amount is small, the downward flow soon peters out, automatically limiting the level of analgesia. If the volume of injected solution is large, any which remains unabsorbed or unadsorbed will continue its downward trek to the most dependent part of the thoracic curve which, because of the slope of the table, will now be about T.4–5. Here any remaining local analgesic solution will pool. Just as surely as the heavy solution flows *down* one side of the thoracic curve, so it will not flow *up* the other and over the cervical vertebrae towards the 3rd, 4th and 5th cervical roots which supply the diaphragm, and the vital centres. Such a reversal of the natural forces is out of the question, so that it is entirely unnecessary to give the patient an extra pillow to guard against a fanciful upward spread of heavy fluid.

Barbotage

Barbotage (from the French *barboteur*, tame duck, and used in the sense of puddling, dabbling or stirring up).

The term is applied to the technique by which a local analgesic solution is injected into the spinal canal, after which the movement of the piston is reversed and fluid is withdrawn into the syringe. This to-and-fro action of the piston which simulates that of a mechanical pump sets up currents which carry the drug far afield. The extent of the distribution, which is not accurately predictable, is determined by the mass of local analgesic drug, the speed with which the injection is made and the number of times it is repeated. The method was described in 1907 (Bier, 1908), given a name by Le Filliatre (Le

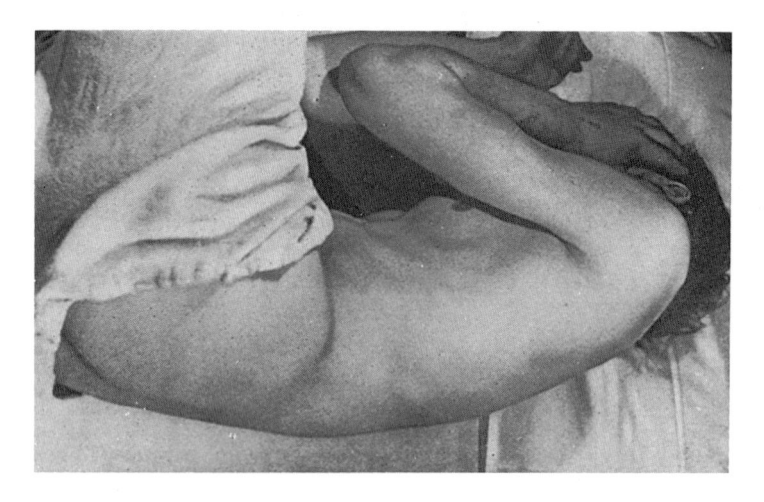

Fig. 8.8 The patient in position for lumbar puncture — viewed from above.

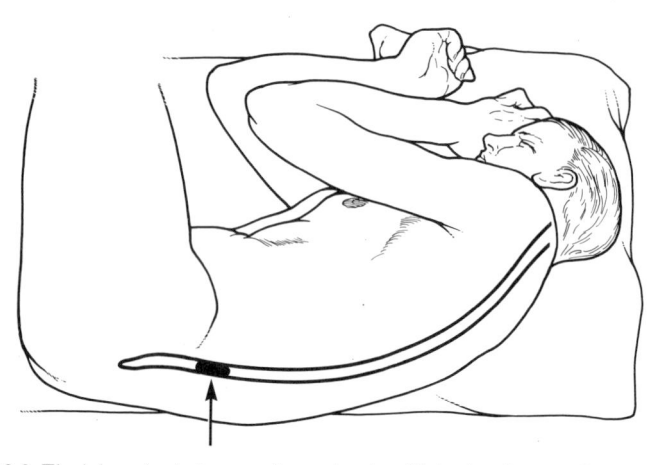

Fig. 8.9 The injected solution remains at the site of injection, between L. 2–3.

Filliatre, 1921) and popularised by Labat (Labat, 1930). It has been suggested that if the patient coughs immediately after the analgesic has been injected the spread of effect will be increased, but recent work has not supported this (Dubelman and Forbes, 1979).

Turbulent currents are set up if an injection is made rapidly enough into the dural canal, and these influence the extent of the spread of the injected solution beyond the site of puncture. Rapid injection is facilitated by a needle of large bore, and a syringe of small diameter (Macintosh, 1957). With the fine needles now in vogue it is difficult

INTRADURAL ANALGESIA (SUBARACHNOID BLOCK) 197

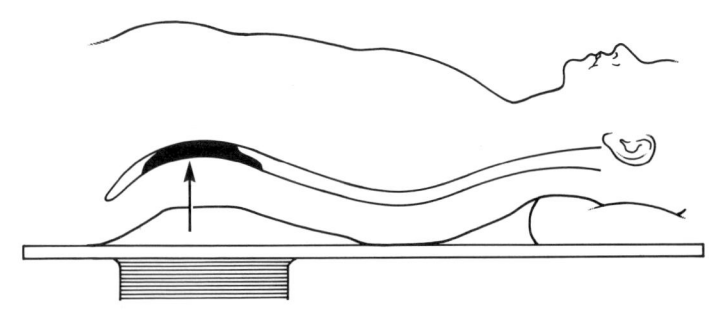

Fig. 8.10 When the patient rolls over on to his back the height of the lumbar convexity corresponds to the level L.2–3. The heavy solution now runs down both slopes. The part running into the sacral concavity is completely wasted as far as providing analgesia for abdominal surgery is concerned.

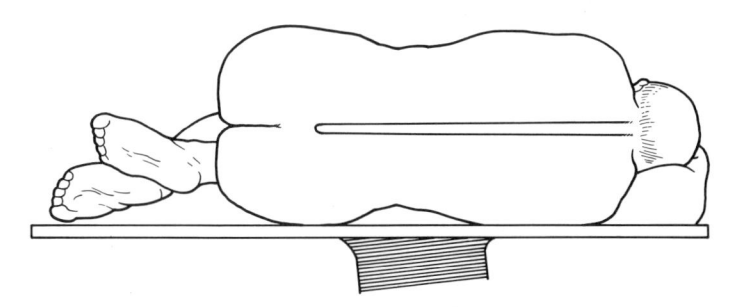

Fig. 8.11 The table is tilted until it is quite obvious that the vertebral column inclines downwards towards the head.

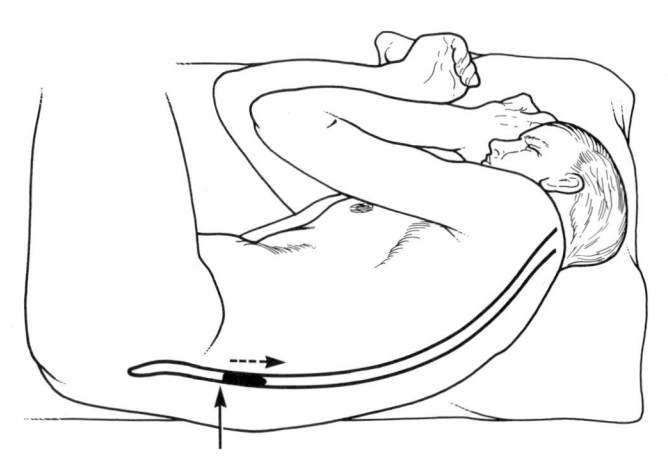

Fig. 8.12 The precise site of injection is immaterial. The solution at once runs down the incline. Contrast with Fig. 8.9.

to inject sufficiently rapidly to affect distribution. However, even with the slow currents resulting from the use of fine needles, the spread can be increased by repeating the injection several times.

Workers of experience (Nolte and Farrar, 1983) report that, using the sitting position, minimal barbotage (0.5 ml × 2) through a 25 gauge needle increases the height of the block by an average of two segments and greater barbotage (1 ml × 2) via a 22 gauge needle increases height of block by an average of three to four segments. Others (Chambers, 1982) have found barbotage to be unreliable in increasing the cephalad spread of plain solutions. Conversely, slowing the rate of injection is likely to prevent unduly wide spread from taking place (McClure et al, 1982).

Volume

Recent studies relating the volume of analgesic solution injected intradurally to the degree of spread have been conflicting. Using plain solution of bupivacaine, 0.5 per cent, many workers have reported that volume influenced spread (Cameron et al, 1981; Nightingale and Marstrand, 1981; Farrar and Nolte, 1982) whereas others have found that volume bore little relationship to spread (Wildsmith et al, 1981a). Workers using hyperbaric solutions also differ. One group (Löfström et al, 1982) found that 15 mg of bupivacaine produced the same segmental level of block whether given in a 2 or 3 ml volume, while others (Sundres et al, 1982) showed that doubling the volume from 1.5 to 3 ml did result in higher levels of analgesia. Workers in Edinburgh (Chambers et al, 1982b) found that varying the volume between 2 and 4 ml when 0.5 per cent bupivacaine was used did not affect spread, though when the concentration was increased to 0.75 per cent, different volumes did result in different segmental levels. They found that the major effect of increasing the dose of bupivacaine was to increase duration of action rather than height of block.

Hyperbaric solutions

These solutions have been used for many years and have stood the test of time. The authors have obtained reliable results using them for surgical procedures below the diaphragm, but appreciate that afferent impulses can still ascend via the vagus nerve. These can be blocked at the cardia by local infiltration on the part of the surgeon or by light general anesthesia in order to reduce the incidence of 'bucking' when the upper abdomen is explored.

Glucose can be added to local analgesic solutions by the operator, or he may elect to use one of the commercially available hyperbaric solutions. Hyperbaric cinchocaine is supplied in 3 ml ampoules containing 0.5 per cent of the drug and 6 per cent glucose. This solution does not stand repeated autoclaving without deterioration but it produces excellent analgesia, usually for several hours. Amethocaine is not as stable in glucose solution as other analgesic agents and it is usual to mix it with glucose from another sterile ampoule immediately before use. Whereas a 1 per cent aqueous solution is isobaric for practical purposes and remains so if mixed with an equal volume of normal saline, a mixture with an equal volume of 10 per cent glucose gives a resulting solution of 0.5 per cent amethocaine in 5 per cent glucose with a specific gravity of 1021 at 25°C (Wildsmith et al, 1981b).

Mepivacaine has been used as a 4 per cent solution in 10 per cent glucose and is satisfactory for intradural block for operations lasting less than one hour (Dunn et al, 1963; Siker et al, 1966). Other agents which have proved more popular overseas than in the UK include lignocaine 5 per cent in glucose up to 7.5 per cent (Adams, 1956) and prilocaine 5 per cent in 5 per cent glucose (Fisher and Bryce-Smith, 1971). Procaine has lost favour due to its short duration of action.

Bupivacaine solutions can be rendered hyperbaric if 4 ml 0.5 per cent plain solution are mixed with 1 ml 20 per cent glucose; this results in a solution containing 0.4 per cent bupivacaine and 5 per cent glucose with a specific gravity of 1014 (Goodison and Joysala, 1979).

Plain solutions

Analgesic solutions without addition of glucose were known for many years as iso- or hypobaric solutions. The 1:1500 solution of cinchocaine in 0.5 per cent saline had popularity following its introduction by Howard Jones in 1930 (Jones, 1930) and was used by Jones and others (Wilson, 1934; Lake, 1938; Macintosh, 1957). In the US, 0.1 per cent amethocaine hydrochloride in distilled water also enjoyed popularity (Lund and Cameron, 1945). These solutions have not been commercially available in Britain for many years, though interest in plain solutions has recently been revived owing to the ready availability of bupivacaine 0.5 per cent.

Although bupivacaine was synthesised in 1957 and was used clinically by Telivuo in 1963, some time elapsed before anaesthetists realised that it was a safe agent for intradural injection (Ekblom and Widman, 1966), but in recent years there have been many reports of its successful use (Nolte et al, 1977; Lanz et al, 1979; Moore, 1979; Cameron et al, 1981; Chambers et al, 1981a; Farrar and Nolte, 1982; Ryan et al, 1983), an average of 0.22 ml 0.5 per cent bupivacaine being required to block each segment (Nolte and Stark, 1979). Nolte (1982) reported experience with over 13 000 intradural blocks using 3 ml 0.5 and 0.75 per cent bupivacaine plain injected with minimal barbotage over an average time of 15 seconds with the patient sitting. A resultant level of sensory block between T.7 and T.9 was found, though occasionally above T.5, after a latent period of up to eight minutes. Other workers (Chambers et al, 1981a) found the plain bupivacaine solution satisfactory for operations on the perineum, legs and groin, but not for lower abdominal surgery.

The 0.5 per cent solution in distilled water is slightly hypobaric, which may be advantageous in that the patient can lie on the painless side in conditions such as fractured neck of femur and a unilateral block may result (Casale, 1982). The commercially available 0.5 per cent bupivacaine plain (Marcain) has a specific gravity of 1004 at room temperature (Chambers et al, 1981a), falling to 0997 at body temperature.

Procaine has been used in 5 per cent solution, often by dissolving crystals in cerebrospinal fluid (Labat, 1930), but has lost favour due to its short duration of action.

Choice of analgesic drug, dose and concentration

The choice of analgesic drug for intradural block has often been dependent upon availability. This is indeed one of the factors which has aroused interest in bupivacaine which has for many years been available for extradural block in 0.5 per cent solution. For most major surgical procedures, a duration of action in excess of one hour is desirable and this will rule out consideration of agents such as procaine and mepivacaine. In the UK this is likely to mean that the choice lies between heavy cinchocaine and plain bupivacaine. There is now good evidence that the last is satisfactory for surgical operations on the perineum, legs, hip joint and groin, but that spread is unreliable for intra-abdominal surgery for which on present evidence heavy solutions are more dependable. Plain bupivacaine can of course be made hyperbaric by addition of glucose by the anaesthetist to aid cephalad spread (see p. 199).

Whereas cinchocaine has been used for intradural block in concentrations varying from 1:1500 to 1:200 (0.067 to 0.5 per cent), bupivacaine has usually been employed in concentrations of at least 0.5 per cent. Solutions of bupivacaine stronger than 0.75 per cent are unsatisfactory for intradural block as a precipitate is then likely to form when the solution mixes with cerebrospinal fluid (Moore, 1982). When 0.75 per cent is used, however, a higher level of spread may occur even if the patient is in the sitting position during injection (Tuominen et al, 1982).

Experienced workers have suggested a level of segmental block appropriate for various surgical procedures (Cousins and Bridenbaugh, 1980). The authors, however, are well aware of the dangers of dogmatism and recognise that the height of analgesia required may vary according to the severity and type of the surgical lesion as well as by the physical build of the patient and the gentle technique (or otherwise) of the surgeon. Table 8.1 gives some recommended doses which it is hoped may form a helpful general guide.

Table 8.1 Some recommended doses (ml)

	Standard Heavy Solution (ml)	Plain Bupivacaine 0.5%
Haemorrhoidectomy	0.8–1.0	
Cystoscopy + cystodiathermy	1.0–1.2	
Adult circumcision	1.0–1.2	
Transurethral resection of the prostate gland	1.0–1.2	
Pelvic floor repair	1.4–1.8	3 ml or 4 ml
Posterior colpo-perineorrhaphy	1.0–1.2	
Vaginal hysterectomy	1.6–1.8	
Surgery of the lower limb	1.0–1.2	
Operation for fractured hip	1.0–1.2	
Total hip replacement	1.2–1.4	
Herniorrhaphy	1.2–1.8	
Retropubic prostatectomy	1.4–1.6	
Interval appendicectomy	1.4–1.8	3 to 4 ml
Abdominal hysterectomy	1.4–1.8	with added
Lower segment Caesarean section	1.4–1.8	glucose
Colono-rectal surgery	2.0–2.2	
Upper abdominal surgery	2.0–2.2	

Note: Experience shows that these are average doses but that the extent of spread is variable and capricious in clinical practice.

Addition of vasoconstrictor agents

The use of adrenaline and phenylephrine to prolong the effects of intradural block is well documented, a dose as high as 0.5 mg (0.5 ml of 1:1000 solution) of adrenaline being mixed with the local analgesic drug before injection (Egbert and Deas, 1960; Moore, 1965). One of the authors (R. S. A.) has personal experience of this technique in association with hyperbaric amethocaine and can testify to its effectiveness. Recent studies, however, suggest that whereas adrenaline may increase the duration of effect when amethocaine is used, its addition to hyperbaric solutions of bupivacaine (Chambers et al, 1982a) or lignocaine (Chambers et al, 1981b) does not result in clinically significant prolongation of analgesia.

Adrenaline added to local analgesic solutions for intradural injection will reduce the already very low concentrations of analgesic drug in the systemic circulation found when plain solutions are used. Adrenaline added to local analgesic solutions lowers the pH. This effect is less if adrenaline is freshly added by the anaesthetist since commercial mixtures are deliberately made more acid in order to prevent deterioration of the adrenaline.

The advantages of the addition of adrenaline to analgesic solutions for intradural injection are doubtful. There is also the supposition that adrenaline may compromise the blood supply to the spinal cord in some patients, especially in those suffering from atheroma, hypovolaemia or hypotension.

All things considered, the authors have a lack of enthusiasm for the continued use of vasoconstrictor drugs in this context, although use in the extradural space is often recommended.

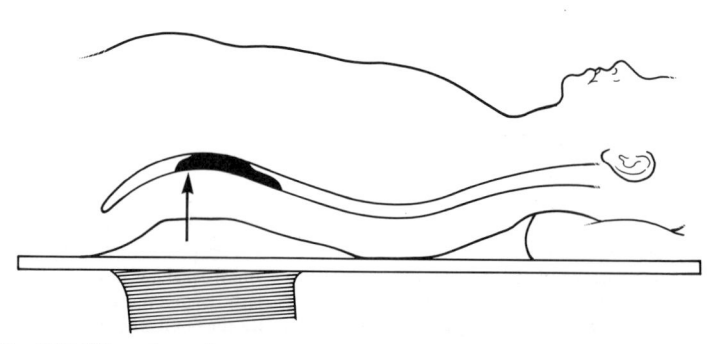

Fig. 8.13 When the patient turns on to his back the solution flows on towards the thoracic concavity.

INTRADURAL ANALGESIA (SUBARACHNOID BLOCK) 203

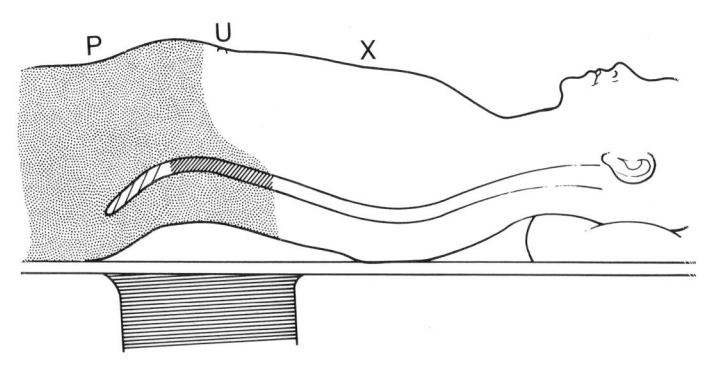

Fig. 8.14 1.4 ml of a standard heavy solution has just reached the 11th thoracic nerve roots anaesthetising the abdominal wall to just below the umbilicus.

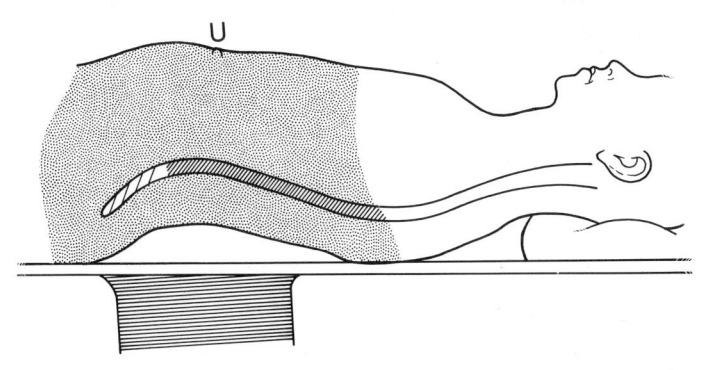

Fig. 8.15 If 2 ml of solution is injected some of it will reach the thoracic concavity which, because of the slope of the table, is at the level of about T.5: any excess of solution will pool here, and cause no harm. Analgesia high enough for any abdominal operation is assured.

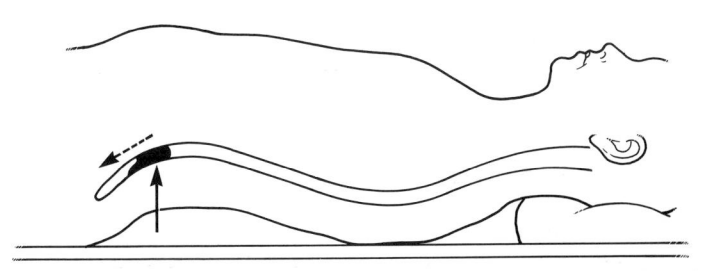

Fig. 8.16 A heavy analgesic solution injected into the dural canal low down (L.4–5) when the vertebral column is horizontal, gives particularly disappointing results for abdominal surgery. When the patient rolls on to his back the point where the dura has been pierced is on the sacral slope of the lumbar convexity. The solution runs into the sacrum: little, if any, runs cephalwards to reach even the lowest intercostal nerves.

Intradural spinal analgesia for the surgeon

Occasionally, a doctor may have to undertake surgery on a patient, far from modern facilities and inadequately assisted. In such circumstances intradural spinal analgesia forms a reasonably safe and efficient form of pain relief for many operations on the lower abdomen, legs and perineum.

The patient, not too heavily premedicated, should have his blood-pressure recorded and should have a cannula inserted into a suitable vein on the arm which will be uppermost during the lumbar puncture (if this is performed in the lateral position). He will probably be benefited by the intravenous infusion of 500 ml or more of isotonic fluid. The surgeon should then scrub up, tap the theca and inject the analgesic solution; 2–4 ml of 0.5 per cent plain bupivacaine, 1.5 to 2 ml of heavy lignocaine 5 per cent, or heavy cinchocaine 0.5 per cent, might well be suitable. The patient should then be turned into the supine position and carefully observed for fifteen minutes with blood-pressure estimations at five minute intervals. There must be positive evidence of a successful block such as inability to move the legs and complete relaxation of the lower abdomen. If at the end of this time the general condition of the patient is satisfactory and the blood-pressure is 80 mmHg or over, the surgeon should scrub again and commence the operation. It is important that there should be someone of intelligence and humanity seated at the head of the table, not only to keep a record of the blood-pressure and the adequacy of the respiration, but also to give comfort and encouragement to the patient during this time of inevitable strain.

Mental distress or apprehension on the part of the patient can be ameliorated by the intermittent injection into the intravenous line of a suitable sedative such as Thalamonal, 0.5 ml, diamorphine, 1 mg, midazolam 5 mg, or diazepam, 5 mg, but no analgesic can compensate for an inadequate block; nor can intravenous thiopentone. If thought necessary, the attendant can hold an anaesthetic face mask in position through which oxygen is given.

A falling or persistently low blood-pressure can be corrected by elevating the legs on two pillows, by increasing the volume and speed of the intravenous infusion, or by the intravenous injection of a pressor drug such as ephedrine, 10 mg.

The occasional anaesthetist is advised against attempting lumbar extradural block.

REFERENCES

Adams, B. W. (1956) Lignocaine spinal analgesia in transurethral prostatectomy. *Anaesthesia*, 2, 297.
Barker, A. E. (1907) Clinical experiences with spinal anaesthesia in 100 cases. *British Medical Journal*, 1, 665.
Barker, A. E. (1908a) A second report on clinical experiences with spinal analgesia, with a second series of 100 cases. *British Medical Journal*, 1, 264.
Barker, A. E. (1908b) A third report on clinical experiences with spinal analgesia. *British Medical Journal*, 2, 453.
Bier, A. (1908) *Deutsche Zeitschrift für Chirurgie*, 95, 373.
Brown, D. T., Wildsmith, J. A. W., Covino, B. G. & Scott, D. B. (1980) Effects of baricity on spinal anaesthesia with amethocaine. *British Journal of Anaesthesia*, 52, 589.
Cameron, A. E., Arnold, R. W. & Ghoris, M. W. (1981) Spinal analgesia using bupivacaine plain. *Anaesthesia*, 36, 318.
Casale, F. F. (1982) Correspondence. *Anaesthesia*, 37, 602.
Chambers, W. A., Edstrom, H. H. & Scott, D. B. (1981a) Effect of baricity on spinal anaesthesia with bupivacaine. *British Journal of Anaesthesia*, 53, 279.
Chambers, W. A. (1982) Editorial. Intrathecal bupivacaine. *British Journal of Anaesthesia*, 54, 799.
Chambers, W. A., Littlewood, D. G., Logan, M. R. & Scott, D. B. (1981b) The effect of added epinephrine on spinal anesthesia with lidocaine. *Anesthesia and Analgesia*, 60, 417.
Chambers, W. A., Littlewood, D. G. & Scott, D. B. (1982a) Effect of added vasoconstrictors on spinal anaesthesia with hyperbaric bupivacaine. *British Journal of Anaesthesia*, 54, 230P.
Chambers, W. A., Littlewood, D. G., Edstrom, H. H. & Scott, D. B. (1982b) Spinal anaesthesia with hyperbaric bupivacaine: effect of concentration and volume administered. *British Journal of Anaesthesia*, 54. 75.
Cousins, M. J. & Bridenbaugh, P. O. (1980) *Neural Blockade*. Philadelphia: Lippincott.
Crawford, J. S. (1979) Experiences with spinal analgesia in a British obstetric unit. *British Journal of Anaesthesia*, 51, 531.
Dubelman, A. M. & Forbes, A. R. (1979) Does cough increase the spread of spinal anesthesia? *Anesthesia and Analgesia*, 58, 306.
Dunn, R. E., Gee, H. L., Carnes, M. A. & Fabian, L. W. (1963) Spinal anesthesia with mepivacaine hydrochloride. *Anesthesia and Analgesia*, 42, 49.
Egbert, L. D. & Deas, T. C. (1960) Effect of epinephrine on the duration of spinal anesthesia. *Anesthesiology*, 21, 345.
Ekblom, L. & Widman, B. (1966) L. A. C. 43 and tetracaine in spinal anaesthesia. *Acta Anaesthesiologica Scandinavica* Suppl., 23, 419.
Farrar, M. D. & Nolte, H. (1982) Spinal analgesia using bupivacaine 0.5 per cent. Correspondence. *Anaesthesia*, 37, 91.
Fisher, A. & Bryce-Smith, R. (1971) Spinal analgesic agents. A comparison of cinchocaine, lignocaine and prilocaine. *Anaesthesia*, 26, 324.
Goodison, R. R. & Joysala, A. (1979) Agents for spinal analgesia: hyperbaric bupivacaine. *Anaesthesia*, 34, 375.
Jones, H. W. (1930) Spinal anaesthesia. A new method and a new drug: Percaine. *British Journal of Anaesthesia*, 7. 146.
Labat, G. (1930) *Regional Anesthesia*, p. 522, 2nd edn. Philadelphia: Saunders.
Lake, N. C. (1938) Precision in spinal anaesthesia. *Lancet*, 2, 241; ibid. (1958), 1, 387.
Lanz, E., Schellenberg, B. & Theiss, D. (1979) Lokale Spinalanaesthesie mit Bupivacaine und Tetracaine. *Regional Anesthesia*, 2, 25.

Le Filliatre, G. (1921) *Précis de Rachianaesthésie Générale*. Paris: Libraire le François.

Löfström, J. B., Bengtsson, M. & Edström, H. H. (1982) Bupivacaine in spinal anaesthesia. *Proceedings of the European Society of Regional Anaesthesia* (Edinburgh), p. 32.

Lund, P. C. & Cameron, J. D. (1945) Hypobaric Pontocaine: a new technique in spinal anesthesia. *Anesthesiology*, 6, 565.

McClure, J. H., Brown, D. T. & Wildsmith, J. A. W. (1982) Effects of injected volume and speed of injecton on the spread of spinal anaesthesia with isobaric amethocaine. *British Journal of Anaesthesia*, 54, 917.

Macintosh, R. R. (1957) *Lumbar Puncture and Spinal Analgesia*, p. 116, 2nd edn. Edinburgh: Livingstone.

Moore, D. C. (1965) *Regional Block*. Springfield: Thomas.

Moore, D. C. (1979) Comparison of bupivacaine (Marcaine) with tetracaine (Pontocaine) for spinal block for intra-abdominal pelvic surgery. *Anesthesiology*, 51, S211.

Moore, D. C. (1982) Precipitation of local anesthetic drug in cerebrospinal fluid. *Anesthesiology*, 57, 134.

Mushin, W. W. (1943) Concerning spinal analgesia. *Postgraduate Medical Journal*, 19, 175.

Nightingale, P. J. & Marstrand, T. (1981) Subarachnoid anaesthesia with bupivacaine for orthopaedic procedures in the elderly. *British Journal of Anaesthesia*, 53, 369.

Nolte, H. (1982) Bupivacaine in spinal anaesthesia. *Proceedings of the European Society of Regional Anaesthesia* (Edinburgh), p. 30.

Nolte, H. & Farrar, M. D. (1983) Correspondence. *Anaesthesia*, 38, 811.

Nolte, H. & Stark, P. (1979) Die Dosis-Wirkungsrelation des isobaren Bupivacain zur Spinalanaesthesie. *Der Anaesthesist*, special section, 1.

Nolte, H., Schiker, K., Gergs, P., Meyer, J. & Stark, P. (1977) Zur Frage der Spinalanaesthesie mit isobaren Bupivacain, 0.5%. *Der Anaesthesist*, 26, 33.

Pflug, A. E., Aasheim, G. M. & Beck, H. A. (1976) Spinal anesthesia: bupivacaine versus tetracaine. *Anesthesia and Analgesia*, 55, 489.

Robertson, D. H., Sewerentz, H. & Holmes, F. (1978) Subarachnoid spinal analgesia: a comparative survey of current practice in Scotland and Scandinavia. *Anaesthesia*, 33, 913.

Ryan, D. W., Pridie, A. K. & Copeland, P. F. (1983) Plain bupivacaine 0.5%: a preliminary evaluation as a spinal anaesthetic agent. *Annals of the Royal College of Surgeons*, 65, 40.

Siker, E. S., Wolfson, B., Stewart, W. D., Pavilack, P. & Pappas, M. T. (1966) Mepivacaine for spinal anaesthesia: effects of changes in concentration and baricity. *Anesthesia and Analgesia*, 45, 191.

Sinclair, C. J., Scott, D. B. & Edström, H. H. (1982) Effect of Trendelenburg position on spinal anaesthesia with hyperbaric bupivacaine. *British Journal of Anaesthesia*, 54, 497.

Sundres, K. O., Vaagenes, P., Skretting, P., Lind, P. & Edström, H. H. (1982) Spinal analgesia with hyperbaric bupivacaine: effects of volume of solution. *British Journal of Anaesthesia*, 54, 69.

Tattersall, M. P. (1983) Isobaric bupivacaine and hyperbaric amethocaine for spinal anaesthesia. A clinical comparison. *Anaesthesia*, 38, 115.

Telivuo, L. (1963) A new long-acting local anaesthetic solution for pain relief after thoracotomy. *Annales chirurgiae et gynaecologiae Fenniae*, 52, 513.

Tuominen, M., Kalso, E. & Rosenberg, P. H. (1982) Effects of posture on the spread of spinal anaesthesia with isobaric 0.75% or 0.5% bupivacaine. *British Journal of Anaesthesia*, 54, 313.

Wildsmith, J. A. W., McClure, J. H. & Brown, D. T. (1981a) Effect of injected volume on the spread of spinal anaesthesia. *British Journal of Anaesthesia*, 53, 1103.

Wildsmith, J. A. W., McClure, J. H., Brown, D. T. & Scott, D. B. (1981b) Effects of posture on the spread of isobaric and hyperbaric amethocaine. *British Journal of Anaesthesia*, **53**, 273.

Wilson, W. E. (1934) Intrathecal nerve root block: some contributions and a new technique. *Proceedings of the Royal Society of Medicine*, **27**, 323.

9

Extradural analgesia

Extradural block may be used for the relief of pain during and, if desired, following surgical operations, for the relief of chronic pain, for the relief of pain in labour, for the reduction of bleeding by producing hypotension during surgery, or to supplement light general anaesthesia, thereby suppressing the transmission of afferent impulses and autonomic and hormonal responses to surgery (Germann et al, 1979).

Extradural spinal block requires precision and adequate time must be allowed by the anaesthetist so that proper positioning of the patient, careful identification of the space and observation of the effects of the injection are made before surgical procedures are allowed to commence. In the opinion of the authors, the patient should arrive in the anaesthetic room at least half an hour before the proposed time of surgery.

It is not every anaesthetist, patient or surgeon who has a temperament suitable for surgery under regional analgesia. The anaesthetist must have confidence in the technique and in his own expertise. The anxious or uncooperative patient should seldom be subjected to spinal injection or to awareness of the operation, even if it does not involve physical discomfort, unless other considerations are overwhelming. The surgeon must appreciate that gentleness is required especially in the patient who is awake. When, however, the surgeon and anaesthetist work as a team and both have faith in the technique and, when the procedure has been properly explained to the patient, we are of the opinion that the method is an excellent one for operations on the lower abdomen, pelvis, perineum and for laminectomy, as well as in obstetric patients both for pain relief and for operative delivery. In this book we do not describe extradural analgesia for operations on the thorax, for a consideration of which we refer our readers to the textbook by Bromage (Bromage, 1978a). We advise the anaesthetist, unless he is very expert, not to insert the needle higher than the L.2/L.3 interspace, to avoid damage to the cord. The expert may consider a level between T.6 and T.8 as a logical site for injection for upper abdominal surgery. Injection between T.12 and L.1 has little to recommend it as it does not necessarily avoid the cord or allow deposition of the analgesic solution in the most advantageous site, which is between T.6/7 and T.7/8. During surgical operations the good analgesia and muscle relaxation, accompanied by a relatively ischaemic field and contracted bowels, compares very favourably with general anaesthesia, while the absence of post-spinal headache, when the dura is not punctured, is a clear advantage over intradural block.

Before an anaesthetist embarks on central neural blockade he should make a superficial physical examination of the central nervous system, looking out for abnormal or absent tendon reflexes and gross disorders of sensation of the limbs, including paraesthesiae. He should enquire as to the history of previous neurological abnormalities and he should chart his findings on the patient's notes if they are negative or if abnormalities are found. Whether these, if present, should contraindicate spinal block will depend on many factors (Crawford et al, 1981) and in cases of doubt a neurological opinion should be obtained. These enquiries should be conducted before the day of operation, ideally in a pre-anaesthetic clinic.

We prefer to introduce the lumbar puncture needle and observe the effects of intradural or extradural block with the patient conscious, although suitably sedated. This allows easy positioning in which the patient can co-operate. The insertion of a needle through a weal of local analgesic seldom causes real discomfort unless many attempts are made or unless the needle makes frequent contact with bone in the difficult case. The periosteum is sensitive. It also enables the anaesthetist to satisfy himself as to the success (or failure) of the injection by checking for skin analgesia and the disappearance of reflexes such as the knee and ankle jerks and the tone of the muscles of the anterior abdominal wall, and sometimes of the anal sphincter. Injection with the patient awake is certainly safer and simpler when the anaesthetist wishes to make his injection with the patient sitting.

If, alternatively, the choice is to establish anaesthesia first, the possibility of airway obstruction with the patient breathing spontaneously in the lateral position while the block is being put in, must always be borne in mind. Doses of intravenous or inhalation agents necessary to produce a quiet, still and relaxed patient during the insertion of the needle are much greater than those necessary to keep a patient peacefully asleep, once the block has been established.

In a minority of our patients, in order to guarantee a free airway with spontaneous respiration during the injection of the analgesic solution or during the operation, we resort to tracheal intubation using a muscle relaxant or topical laryngeal analgesia, aided by a small dose of intravenous barbiturate (Bromage, 1978b). This might apply when there are anatomical peculiarities about the upper airway, when the position on the operating table is steeply head-down or lateral or when the duration of the surgical procedure is likely to be prolonged. Obesity often makes intubation desirable. When intubation is planned it can be done conveniently in the anaesthetic room either before or after the block is established. There is a risk that the intravenous barbiturate injected with a relaxant to facilitate the intubation may cause a low blood-pressure which may summate with the developing hypotension of the block. We have seen severe cardiovascular depression result from this and so we usually prefer to intubate before the block, should a tube be thought necessary, so that hypotension due to the barbiturate has worn off before that due to the block makes itself felt.

Approach to the extradural space

Extradural block is most commonly performed in the lumbar region, the approach being identical with that for lumbar puncture (see Ch. 7). The needle may be inserted in the mid-line, i.e. the sagittal plane of the body, or 1 cm laterally. (White 1982). There is evidence that in the mid-line the space is wider and less vascular (Usubiaga et al, 1967). In each case the tough ligamentum flavum must be identified and advancement of the needle discontinued when the needle point leaves that structure before it pierces the dura.

Extradural injection can also be carried out at other points along the spinal column. In the mid-thoracic region, the needle must be angled more acutely (40 degrees) with the skin (Simpson et al., 1961; Dawkins and Steel, 1971). Fortunately, this very angulation renders accidental dural puncture unlikely as the Tuohy needle will probably 'toboggan' along the dura. Entry in the mid-thoracic region presents problems owing to the overlapping of the spines of these vertebrae but can be approached by the lateral or paramedial route (see Ch. 7).

Block in the cervical region has been undertaken for the relief of intractable pain and for operations on the thyroid, arm, hand and breast. This route should not be embarked on lightly as such important structures as the cervical cord and phrenic nerve roots are in the vicinity of the needle point. The authors have no personal experience of this approach.

Extradural sacral or caudal block, by injection through the sacrococcygeal membrane, is the subject of a separate section (p. 227).

Identification of the extradural space

It has already been described how the lumbar puncture needle on its way to the intradural space pierces the tough ligamentum flavum and then crosses the extradural space to reach the dura mater itself. If the operator can arrest the progress of the needle while the point is in the extradural space, injections can be made so that local analgesic solution spreads to affect the nerve roots as they cross that space. In one method of doing this, the anaesthetist takes advantage of the change in resistance as the needle point leaves the tough ligament to enter the space filled with loose areolar tissue and vessels (Fig. 7.16). As a majority of patients have a negative pressure in the extradural space, this fact is also made use of when a number of other methods of locating the space are used.

The skilled worker can usually determine the point when this occurs by sensing the change in resistance to advancement of the needle, but in order to magnify such loss of resistance it is usual to employ some visual or tactile aid. A number of devices have been recommended but most experienced anaesthetists prefer to attach a syringe to the hub of the needle. The syringe may be of any convenient size, though a 10 ml syringe is often preferred, and may be filled with air or fluid or even a combination of the two. Steady pressure on the plunger of a syringe filled with saline, local analgesic solution or distilled water, as the needle point traverses the ligamentum flavum will result in injection of a small amount as soon as the needle point enters the extradural space. The needle may be advanced continuously or in 1 mm steps. Others prefer the syringe to be filled with air. The plunger of the syringe can then be 'bounced' on the cushion of air as the needle progresses and some air will be injected as the needle point enters the space. Loss of resistance means that air no longer 'bounces' the plunger back. The authors prefer to use this 'loss of resistance to the injection of fluid or air' test. Some workers have reported hearing a bubbling sound when the extradural space is entered (Mirakhur and Bandopadhyay, 1973; Rauscher, 1975).

When extradural injection is contemplated the dura should not be punctured. In rare cases when the needle is advanced too far, this mistake may be made. An occasional reason may be the presence of a median dorsal fold in the dura in the mid-line in the lumbar region which decreases the size of the extradural space (Husemeyer et al, 1978). The advantage of a lumbar puncture needle of small diameter to minimise the incidence of spinal headache is no longer significant, because a larger bore needle magnifies the pressure changes which are important in identification. Flow of fluid through a tube is proportional to the fourth power of the diameter (Poiseuille). A wide bore needle is necessary if a catheter is to be introduced (16 to 18 gauge) while a 20 gauge thin walled needle is satisfactory for the single injection. The fine needle, up to 25 gauge, recommended for intradural puncture is not necessary and may make identification of the extradural space less easy. There is a good reason for always using a Tuohy needle for extradural injection, both 'one-shot' and when a catheter is to be used; technique is thereby standardised. Markings at 1 cm intervals on the shaft of the needle, the first being 4 cm from the point (Lee, 1960), assist the anaesthetist by making the depth of the needle point known throughout the injection. A special syringe may be used for the same purpose (Williams, 1975). The space may be encountered 3 to 3.5 cm from the skin in thin subjects, but is more commonly found between 4 and 5 cm. Some prediction of depth can be made from an examination of a lateral radiograph of the spine (Sloss et al, 1970).

A few words should be written about some of the other methods used to identify the extradural space. The sign of the hanging drop (Gutiérrez, 1932) is popular in some quarters: a drop of saline or analgesic fluid is placed on the hub of the needle, with its tip in the ligamentum flavum; it is sucked in as the point enters the extradural space. The disappearance of the drop into the lumen of the needle is caused by the negative pressure in the extradural space, though it is now appreciated that this negative pressure is not present in every patient. The method, however, has its advocates, who find the technique reliable in their hands, especially in the thoracic or cervico-thoracic regions. In the dog, radiographs have shown dimpling of the dura by the needle point as it advances, together with a progressive and measurable decrease in extradural pressure (Aitkenhead et al, 1979).

The Macintosh spring-loaded needle (Macintosh, 1953; Salt, 1963) contains a spring-loaded stylet which is propelled forwards when the space is reached. The hub of the needle is provided with wings to facilitate control of the advancement of the needle (Macintosh, 1948). The Iklè syringe is also spring-loaded to work on a similar principle (Iklè, 1950).

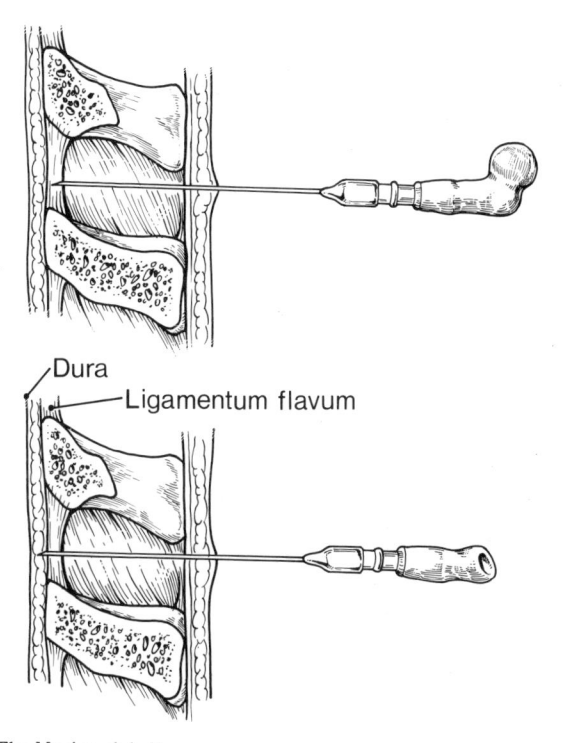

Fig. 9.1 The Macintosh balloon.

Macintosh also described the Oxford balloon (Macintosh, 1950). This probably provides the most obvious end-point of any indicator. The balloon is attached to the hub of the needle already placed in the ligaments and is then inflated with air, using a 2 ml syringe and a very fine needle. The balloon remains distended, about the size of a cherry stone, until the needle point enters the extradural space when it suddenly deflates (Fig. 9.1). For success it is important to ensure an airtight junction between needle and balloon and for the needle point to be already placed among tough ligaments. Repeated sterilisation, however, shortens the working life of these balloons and stocks must be replaced regularly.

Odom's indicator (Odom, 1936) is a classic piece of apparatus for identification of the extradural space. It is a fine bore glass tube which contains a bubble of air in saline and is attached to the hub of the spinal needle. The air bubble moves towards the hub of the needle as the space is entered, due to the negative pressure usually present there. Brooks has modified this indicator by the addition of a small glass bulb to the operator's end of the tube (Brooks, 1957). If the air in this bulb is warmed slightly it provides a head of pressure to accentuate movement of the air bubble inwards as resistance is lost. Massey Dawkins described how such an apparatus can be fashioned from an ordinary household thermometer with the mercury removed and the end ground down to fit the needle hub (Dawkins, 1972). Recently, another simple derivative of Odom's indicator has been described (Mustafa and Milliken, 1982). A segment of clear plastic extension drip-tubing, 10 cm in length, to which is attached a male Luer connection is filled with local analgesic solution, then shaken so that an air bubble can enter its lumen. It is attached to the lumbar puncture needle which is carefully advanced. When the extradural space is entered there will be a sudden movement of the bubble and oscillations synchronous with the heartbeat.

There are other designs based on this basic principle, such as the drip indicator (Dawkins, 1961; Baraka, 1972) which starts to drip as the space is entered. In this case the weight of a column of fluid provides the pressure head.

The Oxford Epidural Space Detector (Evans, 1982) consists of a lightweight polypropylene syringe with a very low friction piston which is held under tension by a rubber strap and an arrangement whereby it is made to contain 4 ml of air at a pressure of 80 mm of mercury. The syringe is connected securely to a winged Macintosh spinal needle the point of which has been accurately placed in either the interspinous or the yellow ligament. The needle is further advanced and when its point reaches the extradural space the piston moves rapidly inwards.

It is clear from the above discussion that the loss of resistance while quite definite is nevertheless of small magnitude. It follows that the apparatus used must be of the highest quality. Syringes must not stick, needles must remain patent, and the needle hub must make an airtight fit with any indicator. Difficulties can be avoided when equipment is well maintained and due care is taken. The anaesthetist is particularly advised to avoid contamination of syringes and needles with glove powder, and to check their patency and free movement immediately prior to use. While some anaesthetists use plastic disposable syringes when identifying the extradural space, the authors prefer the glass syringe with either a ceramic or metal piston, which gives the best results in their hands, especially when loss of resistance to the injection of air is used to determine the end-point. All-glass syringes properly lubricated with silicone oil, which withstands autoclaving, are preferred by other workers. Very occasionally this resistance to injection cannot be demonstrated and the important landmark is lost. It may be because of the spongy nature of the yellow ligament, because the needle point has entered a small cyst in the interspinous ligament which sometimes occurs in old people (Sharrock, 1979), or because the point has wandered too laterally into the yielding tissue of the erector spinae. Whatever the cause the anaesthetist is perplexed; injection of solution may fail to produce analgesia and advancement may result in dural puncture. It is in such circumstances that the marked needle (Lee, 1960; Doughty, 1974) can be so helpful as it enables the anaesthetist to know to what distance from the skin the point has advanced. If it is (on average) about 4 cm deep it is in 'tiger country' and great care and experience will be required if dural puncture is to be avoided. The rate of injection has little effect on the spread of the block although the dependent side usually sustains a higher block when the injection is given in the lateral position (Husemeyer and White, 1980). A rate of dural puncture of 1 per cent should be aimed at and may be bettered (MacDonald, 1983).

Once the extradural space has been positively identified, the injection of analgesic solution should be performed slowly, occupying a period of one to two minutes. Care must be taken not to inject too much air during identification of the space as a bubble may prevent the analgesic solution making contact with one or more nerve roots, thus causing a patchy block. Large volumes of air may also result in surgical emphysema, for example in the supraclavicular area (Laman and McLeskey, 1978), or venous air embolism (Naulty et al, 1982). Some workers inject a test dose of analgesic solution to make sure that none has been deposited in the intradural space with the risk of total spinal block. 2 ml of 0.5 per cent bupivacaine solution can be used (Peters, 1983); larger doses than this may cause high levels of block if injected intradurally, particularly in the obstetric patient. Others inject 1 ml of hyperbaric lignocaine 5 per cent with 1: 200 000 adrenaline and wait for five minutes. They then test for motor loss in the legs and feet which would suggest an intradural injection, as would tachycardia due to adrenaline, should the needle point have inadvertently entered a blood vessel (Moore and Batra, 1982). We would not object to this precaution. *The final test of the correct location of the needle point in the extradural space is the ease of injection of the local analgesic solution, no force being required for this.* Once the space is identified negative pressure from a 2 ml syringe should be applied to the needle; the absence of cerebrospinal fluid or blood is a reassuring sign. If the anaesthetist is still in doubt as to the exact position of the needle point the injection of 2 ml of distilled water may help him to decide as it will produce a stab of discomfort in the conscious patient or slight movement if he is lightly anaesthetised, if the point is in the extradural space (Lund, 1966). Rapid injection of 2 ml of air causes no discomfort if the needle point is in the extradural space; otherwise the patient will experience discomfort (Ducrow, 1980). The direction of the needle bevel and the rate of injection have little effect on the spread of solution or the extent of the block (Boskowski and Levinski, 1982; Burn and Langdon, 1982; Park et al, 1982b) although the dependent side usually sustains a higher block when the injection is given in the lateral position (Husemeyer et al, 1980; Seow et al, 1983). Many papers have been written on the identification of the extradural space (Dawkins, 1963; Dawkins and Steel, 1971).

Following the injection of local analgesic solution, the anaesthetist must monitor most carefully the patient's vital signs in case hypotension, respiratory depression or signs of drug toxicity arise. The most critical time is the 20 minutes following extradural (or intradural) injection.

A technique employing both continuous extradural and 'one-shot' intradural block has been described (Coates, 1982; Mumtaz et al, 1982) in which the extradural space is identified using a 16 to 18 g Tuohy needle. Through this a longer (by 1 cm) (Forster, 1983) 25 g needle is inserted into the theca and solution suitable for an intradural block is injected. The inner needle is then removed and replaced by a catheter carefully guided into the extradural space. The patient thus receives a rapidly acting intradural block and can have the advantage of postoperative pain relief following the injection of either local analgesic solution or of a narcotic analgesic. Only one lumbar injection is required. Another method requires two lumbar injections, one for the intradural drug and the second, perhaps at a different level, for the extradural catheter (Brownridge, 1981). Thus, during the operation profound muscular relaxation of rapid onset is provided without the danger of the absorption of toxic amounts of drug into the systemic circulation, while postoperative analgesia can be easily arranged.

Complications

Accidental dural puncture will occasionally occur even when the anaesthetist is experienced. That the solution which flows from the needle is cerebrospinal in origin, and not a backflow of the fluid used for the test injection, can be confirmed because it feels warm to the bare skin of the anaesthetist's wrist, and it has the ability to turn the colour of a test strip containing glucose oxidase (Dextrostix) by virtue of the glucose it contains. Cerebrospinal fluid will also affect a protein sensitive test strip because of the albumen it contains (Berry, 1958). Local analgesic solution causes cloudiness if dropped into 2.5 per cent solution of thiopentone solution (Clatterberg, 1977). The anaesthetist faced with this annoying complication has three choices. He can abandon the block and give a general anaesthetic; he can proceed to intradural block with an appropriate solution; he can leave the needle in situ to occlude temporarily the hole in the dura and give an extradural block, using an adjacent space and withdrawing both needles after a short interval. Of the three, we incline to adopt the last, provided that no technical difficulty is anticipated and the anaesthetist has time to carry out the procedure without the necessity for undue haste. Using these precautions we do not believe that a significant amount of analgesic fluid will pass directly into the intradural space, but if the needle is merely withdrawn and the extradural space identified a second time in the same intervertebral space, there is a risk of inadvertent intradural leakage which may cause spread to a higher segmental level than is desired (Hodgkinson, 1981).

Massive spread

Total spinal block is likely to occur when the large volume of solution intended for extradural blockade is inadvertently given into the intradural compartment. The analgesic drug is then likely to spread up to the cervical region of the cord to involve the entire sympathetic outflow and the phrenic nerves (C. 3, 4 and 5). The blood-pressure falls to low or unrecordable levels and apnoea ensues. The patient loses consciousness, in part due to the extensive deafferentation which occurs, but also because of cerebral hypoxia.

We believe that total central neural blockade may very occasionally follow genuine extradural injection (Woerth et al, 1977; Findley and Shandro, 1982) though the onset of block in the cervical region is likely to be slower than when the solution is injected intradurally. Hypotension is usually less severe as there is time for compensatory mechanisms to develop and frank apnoea may not occur. It is unlikely that the concentration of local analgesic drug in the cervical region will be great enough to paralyse the phrenic motor roots (C. 3, 4, 5) while medullary ischaemia, secondary to hypotension, is unlikely to be severe enough to cause respiratory paralysis. If the patient stops breathing it may be as a result of toxicity following systemic absorption of the local analgesic drug (Scott, 1981). Another possibility is the accidental *subdural* extra-arachnoid injection of local analgesic solution. The subdural space is potential only, lying between the dura mater and arachnoid membranes which are normally in close apposition. Radiological studies (Boyes and Norman, 1975; Mehta and Maher, 1977) show that it is possible for the tip of the needle to be in this space and for injected fluid to spread in a rostral direction. A high level of block may occur over a period of 15 to 20 minutes; the clinical picture is then one of progressive depression of respiration leading to apnoea, but with time for the cardiovascular system to adjust to the increasing vasomotor block, so that the sudden hypotension seen after intradural injection does not occur. Systolic arterial pressure often levels at about 80 mmHg. The subject is well discussed by Collier (1982a).

Toxic effects due to absorption of local analgesic drug are not often seen in clinical practice, but muscle twitching or frank convulsions can occur as a result of inadvertent intravascular injection or due to rapid absorption from the extradural space. This complication may be more frequent following sacral rather than lumbar injection (Prentiss, 1979). Aspiration tests should always be carried out prior to injection and the needle reinserted, usually in an adjacent intervertebral space, should blood flow freely from the needle. The relatively large doses of local analgesic drug used in extradural block for surgical operations sometimes approach the maximum permitted amount and there is an advantage in adding adrenaline to the solution to retard the rate of absorption. A satisfactory concentration is 1: 200 000 (5 µg/ml).

Convulsions, should they occur, may be treated by the intravenous injection of small and, if necessary, repeated doses of 25 to 50 mg of thiopentone, or a rapidly acting muscle relaxant, e.g. suxamethonium 25 mg or diazepam 1 to 5 mg (Moore et al, 1979). Oxygen should be administered by IPPV as hypoxia and hypercapnia accompany generalised fits. The high blood level of local analgesic drug responsible for the cerebral hyperexcitability soon falls due to metabolism, and the emergency is then past. Convulsions may be associated with metabolic acidosis (Scott, 1981). They may be localised, possibly due to transitory ischaemia of the cord caused by adrenaline (Nadkarni and Tondare, 1981). The causation and treatment of convulsions are discussed at length by Moore and his colleagues (1979).

Cardiovascular collapse

This may follow extradural injection as a result of toxic effects due to inadvertent leakage into veins, or to rapid local absorption. It has been suggested that signs of cardiovascular toxicity may appear earlier following high blood levels of the longer-acting drugs bupivacaine and etidocaine than with lignocaine (Albright, 1979) where there is a wide margin between central nervous system toxicity and cardiovascular depression (Scott, 1981). Cardiovascular collapse may of course also arise as a result of extensive vasomotor blockade with resultant dilatation of the vascular bed, especially in the hypovolaemic subject. A contributory cause may be unopposed vagal action causing severe bradycardia. The hypotensive patient should be treated along the usual lines including intravenous infusion, tilting the table head down, raising the legs, drugs, oxygen and, if necessary, cardiac compression. Elevation of the legs, however, in a patient in advanced pregnancy may do more harm than good as aorto-caval compression may be increased thereby (Collier, 1982a).

When local analgesic solutions are used in clinically appropriate doses and concentrations, a true irritative effect on the cauda equina or spinal cord following either intra- or extradural injection is very rare (Steen and Michenfelder, 1979). Prolonged spinal nerve involvement has followed extradural injection of etidocaine (Ramanathan et al, 1978).

A successful extradural puncture may be difficult in patients with spina bifida occulta, where there may be a patch of hair and a deep mid-line cleft, and after previous laminectomy involving the area where the puncture is proposed.

We cannot stress too strongly that the anaesthetist should never undertake extradural block unless he has the means to treat these potentially lethal complications and of course the same remarks apply to intradural block. A bag and mask must be available to ventilate the lungs, preferably with oxygen. *An indwelling needle or drip must always be in situ before commencement of the extradural injection so that intravenous fluids may be infused rapidly and restorative drugs administered.*

Patchy analgesia

Sometimes one or more dermatomes remain unblocked (Roberts, 1972) but the incidence of this unsatisfactory complication, especially if it occurs in the woman in labour (Bray and Carrie, 1978), is seen less frequently if the carbonated salts of lignocaine and prilocaine are substituted for the hydrochloride (Bromage, 1972). The 1st and 5th lumbar and the 1st sacral roots appear to be affected more frequently than other roots. Unilateral block, unplanned, can also be a complication. The incidence of patchy analgesia is not increased in patients who have had previous extradural injections (Bray and Carrie, 1978).

Catheters

The insertion of a catheter into the extradural space is nowadays commonplace, as the advantages of extended periods of analgesia in obstetric practice and for postoperative pain relief are appreciated (see Ch. 13). Tuohy designed a special needle with a curved Huber point to facilitate the introduction of a catheter (Tuohy, 1945). It was originally used for continuous, or serial, intradural block and found a particular indication when the short-acting drug procaine was popular in spinal analgesia and the length of the operation was uncertain. It also enabled the anaesthetist to titrate the dose in unfit or emergency patients. Today, however, catheters are almost always confined to the extradural space (Curbelo, 1949), thus avoiding the possible dangers of intradural infection and the high incidence of spinal headache consequent on the large rent made in the dura. The catheter may break and it is arguable that a remnant of plastic material is better left alone, after telling the patient or his friends. Other fragments of plastic material left in the body, e.g. joints, ears, eyes, seldom cause harm.

Modern catheters are made of plastic polyvinyl chloride, polytetra-fluoro-ethylene (Teflon) or nylon, and are non-toxic, non-irritant, flexible and individually packed and sterilised by gamma radiation. They are designed to be passed through a 18 gauge thin walled needle and should have an internal diameter of 0.6 mm and an external diameter of 0.9 mm. They may be fitted with a standard Luer mount (Lee, 1962) and may be used with a bacterial filter. Marks can be placed on the catheter to allow accurate estimation of the length remaining in the extradural space (Lee, 1962; Doughty, 1974). The tip should be blunt to minimise trauma to the dura or to vessels (Fig. 6.4).

The 16/18 gauge Tuohy needles are wider than the usual spinal needle and the Huber point is designed to guide the catheter as it passes from the needle into the extradural space and to prevent its impingement on the dura. It is important therefore that the point should be aligned towards the head of the patient as the needle is inserted. The Huber point is relatively blunt and this means that some force is required to push the needle through the tough ligaments, so that care is necessary if control is not to be lost, with the risk of accidental dural puncture. The bluntness is in some degree a safety factor, since it may result in 'tenting' of the dura without perforation. If, however, dural puncture does take place then the chances of the patient developing a headache subsequently are high, and in addition, 6th nerve palsy has been described (Macintosh and Bryce Smith, 1951). The dura may also be punctured by the catheter itself either during insertion or later (Philip and Brown, 1976) with the risk of intradural injection and the possibility of total spinal analgesia (Youngman, 1956; Moir and Hesson, 1965; Quader and Waldron, 1976). A catheter, like a needle, may be wrongly sited so that the injection of a test dose of either 1 ml of hyperbaric lignocaine with adrenaline or 2 ml of 0.5 per cent bupivacaine with adrenaline will soon cause motor loss in the feet and legs, if it is in the intradural space, or tachycardia from the adrenaline if its tip lies within a vessel (Moore and Batra, 1982).

Technical difficulties sometimes arise as attempts are made to pass the catheter through the Tuohy needle. There is often a little resistance when the tip of the catheter passes the point of the needle to enter the extradural space, as a change in direction occurs. Slight alteration of the position of needle and catheter, together with that modicum of good fortune without which work of this kind becomes impossible, will often ensure success. The wise anaesthetist will always check that the catheter runs freely within the needle before commencing the block. If necessary the catheter can be lubricated with local analgesic solution before it is inserted into the needle. The dead-space in the hub of the spinal needle allows the catheter, during insertion, to move laterally and even to kink. To enable direct force to be applied to the catheter when it is in precisely straight alignment, the cut-off nozzle of the syringe used for local analgesic skin infiltration can be inserted into the hub of the needle, so removing the dead-space. This keeps the catheter in a straight line and allows maximum insertion pressure (Keane, 1983). On rare occasions it is impossible to proceed at this stage and the needle and catheter should be withdrawn together. There is the danger of slicing off the catheter tip if it is withdrawn with the needle left in position (Macmurdo and McKenzie, 1979). If the catheter contains a stylet, it must be withdrawn so that 1 to 2 cm of the distal end of the catheter is free of it and is relatively soft and atraumatic.

It is a mistake to advance the catheter in the extradural space in the hope of reaching segmental levels at a distance from the point of entry. Several studies (Sanchez et al, 1967; Bridenbaugh et al, 1968; Usubiaga et al, 1970) have shown that it may move in a bizarre direction and even pass out through an intervertebral foramen or become knotted; resulting analgesia is then likely to be inadequate. The catheter should always be matched for length against the extradural needle (Lee, 1962; Doughty, 1974) and not more than 3 to 4 cm should be inserted into the extradural space. Occasionally, a fresh approach may be necessary. The subdural space may be entered accidentally (Boyes and Norman, 1975; Mehta and Maher, 1977).

Care is required in fixation with adhesive strapping to prevent both kinking and dislodgement. A transparent surgical dressing makes a good fixative as it enables the anaesthetist to see if blood has entered the catheter (Duffy, 1982), and of course safeguards must be taken to prevent bacterial contamination. Full aseptic technique must be maintained throughout the whole procedure and a bacterial filter with a pore size of 2 microns used when the catheter is left in place for an extended period. It has been suggested too that even the initial injection should be made through a filter, as this will prevent entrance not only of organisms but also of foreign particles such as glass or plastic (Crawford et al, 1975). This does, however, increase resistance to injection so that the anaesthetist loses one of the valuable confirmatory signs that the injection is into the correct space. On the other hand, Bromage has experience of over 30 000 cases of continuous block without a filter and with no infection (Bromage, 1978c).

The advantage of the catheter technique in the operating theatre is that the duration of analgesia can be extended when the operative procedure is of long duration. It is also useful when the extent of the surgery is not known at the start or when the fitness of the patient is suspect, so that small incremental doses can be used. Early positioning of a catheter also saves delay when the exact time of the commencement of the operation cannot be forecast.

Catheters are suitable also for postoperative analgesia (Utting and Smith, 1979) and in obstetrics. If necessary, a catheter can be left in position for 72 hours or even for up to a week, provided proper aseptic precautions are taken. When repeated injections are required for the control of chronic pain, acute tolerance or tachyphylaxis may account for poor results. Doses injected within 20 minutes of each other are cumulative while doses given at longer intervals are not (Albright, 1978). Substitution of a different agent may improve matters. A continuous drip of 0.125 per cent bupivacaine solution into the extradural space, driven by an infusion pump at a rate of 5 drops a minute (20 ml/h), has given good results (Ross et al, 1980).

Difficulty in withdrawing a catheter has been reported due to nipping but this can sometimes be overcome by asking the patient to extend the back (Ballance, 1981). The unfortunate complication of a knotted catheter has occurred, in the reports, with the method of management (Brown and Politi, 1979; Blass et al, 1981; Riegler and Pernetzky, 1983).

The anaesthetist can satisfy himself that the catheter is correctly placed in the extradural space if he flushes it out with analgesic solution until he gets a fluid level. With the patient lying on his side, the open end of the catheter is raised to the upper iliac crest and is then lowered to the vertebral column, when the fluid level should be seen to rise. This free rise and fall is important and in its absence the position of the catheter should be altered. If the catheter has entered the intradural space the fluid level continues to rise on movement of the free end (Daykin, 1982; Shah, 1982).

Once in position, aspiration tests should be performed to ensure that accidental intravascular cannulation or thecal puncture has not occurred (Carr and Hehre, 1962; Moir and Hesson, 1965; Kalas and Hehre, 1972). Blockage of the catheter by blood clot can be prevented by filling its lumen with analgesic solution before it is inserted.

Teflon catheters marked 'opaque' may not be visible to X-rays in the extradural space. If the anaesthetist is unfortunate enough to cause a small piece of catheter to be retained in the body of the patient he is not necessarily guilty of malpractice, whereas the vain pursuit of a small piece of plastic material into the recesses of the body may be considered so. It is of course important if this occurs that the patient or his friends should be told about it. Teflon is the least reactive type of catheter. A double catheter technique for major surgery has been described (Myint, 1976). Patterns of pain after operation vary with the sex of the patient, the site of the operation and the time of day. Study of the individual patient will often enable his needs for relief of pain to be met successfully by altering the rate and contents of the solution injected (Gjessing and Tomlin, 1979).

Spread of solution in the extradural space

The extent of the extradural space has been described in Chapter 2. Theoretically, injected analgesic solution may spread along the length of the spinal cord to block segmental roots anywhere from the upper cervical to the lower sacral roots, and may also pass laterally into the paravertebral spaces. This, however, would require a larger volume of solution than is customarily used for extradural block. Spread of any solution will depend on the volume injected as well as on a number of other factors.

The site of injection is important. In the thoracic region the extradural space is relatively narrow and a small volume (3 to 5 ml) may block several segments. In the lumbar region larger volumes are needed as the space is wider here, while in caudal blocks still greater amounts are required as the extradural space fills the cavity of the sacral canal below the level of S. 1 or 2 where the dura ends. The extradural space also narrows in the lumbo-sacral region and this fact, combined with the extra thickness of the nerve roots here, has been alleged to be the cause of the occasional failure to block the S. 1 and S. 2 roots (Galindo et al, 1975).

The speed of injection also affects the extent of the block. Too rapid injection may result in spread to higher levels but with patchy analgesia (Erdemir et al, 1965). There is therefore no advantage to be gained by such a manoeuvre which is moreover uncomfortable for the patient. The spread of solution is not much influenced by the direction of the catheter tip or the needle bevel point (Burn and Langdon, 1982).

Gravity has a part to play in the spread of solutions in the extradural space, though it has nothing like the same importance as in intradural block. Although studies with radio-opaque solutions and radioisotope tracers have failed to show any effect of posture on spread (Nishimura et al, 1959; Burn et al, 1973), clinical experience with the smaller volumes used in obstetric analgesia has shown that the adoption of appropriate posture is helpful (see Ch. 12) (Grundy et al, 1978a). Keeping the patient on the side for 10 minutes results in a higher block on the dependent side than on the upper side, by an average of three segments (Husemeyer and White 1980). When chloroprocaine is given in 5 per cent dextrose solution instead of an equal volume of saline, to a patient in the sitting position, the height of the block is reduced (Park & Eastwood, 1980).

Full term pregnancy is a condition which has a well established effect on dose requirements. This is thought to be due to increased intra-abdominal pressure and caval compression with resultant distension of veins in the extradural space. The engorged veins have the effect of diminishing the volume of the extradural space so that the amount of fluid injected will spread further. These effects are not peculiar to the pregnant uterus and the anaesthetist should beware lest any sizeable abdominal tumour has a similar action. The volume of solution injected must thus be smaller in these cases.

The presence of arteriosclerosis leads to diminished dose requirement and therefore the volume injected into the extradural space may spread to a higher level than in normal patients. The decrease in dose per segment observed may be due to decreased rate of absorption by arteriosclerotic vessels, leaving more drug available to block nerve fibres (Bromage, 1969). Other workers suggest that degenerative vascular disease, height of the patient (other than extreme variations) and age have only small effects on the spread of the solution (Grundy et al, 1978b). Most anaesthetists of experience will, however, have seen unexpectedly high spread follow injection of a reasonable dose of analgesic solution (Mesry, 1976; Soni and Holland, 1981). One explanation for this is spread up the subdural space (Mehta and Maher, 1977). Arteriosclerotic patients may also have narrowed intervertebral foramina so that less loss of fluid occurs laterally.

Radiological studies (Burn et al, 1973) have, however, failed to show a relationship between patient height, rate of injection, posture and age on the one hand, with spread in the extradural space on the other. They led to the conclusion that the volume of solution used and the site of injection were the most important factors. However it is possible that radio-opaque material and analgesic drugs do not spread in an identical manner. The authors remain convinced that with advancing age, that is greater than 20 or 30 years, dosage should be reduced so that a patient aged 70 for suprapubic prostatectomy might well require 15 to 20 ml of 1.5 per cent lignocaine injected in the lumbar region. Estimation of dosage for any particular individual requires, from the experienced anaesthetist, a good deal of intelligent guesswork. We would prefer to give rather too much than too little as a general rule. supporting the blood-pressure as necessary, because the results of inadequate block can be very inconvenient to all concerned. We have sometimes seen a patient in whom the height of block has not been adequate for the proposed operation. For example, after the abdomen is opened, stimuli arising during exploration of the upper abdomen can result in tightening of the abdominal muscles, extrusion of the gut, nausea, vomiting and hypotension. Para-oesophageal infiltration of local analgesic solution by the surgeon is thought by some workers to prevent stimuli passing up the vagi and to make the conduct of anaesthesia for upper abdominal surgery smoother. Both in general anaesthesia and in regional block, a gentle surgeon will obtain better results than his more heavy handed colleagues.

Dosage

It is not possible to recommend specific doses for every surgical procedure as so many factors are involved in the spread of the local analgesic solution. The following suggestions apply to fit young patients only, who are to remain awake during the operation, or when the proposed sedative or light general anaesthetic used to provide comfort for the patient do not add significantly to analgesic requirements.

For injection in the lumbar region, using 1.5 per cent lignocaine solution with 1:200 000 adrenaline: 35 to 40 ml for upper abdominal procedures, 30 to 35 ml for operations confined to the lower abdomen and 25 to 30 ml for perineal operations such as the repair of prolapse where some fall in arterial pressure to provide a relatively ischaemic surgical field is desired. A block to a lower level (T.10) is needed for analgesia only, while an operation on the posterior vagina and perineum for a posterior repair can be painlessly performed if the sacral nerves alone are blocked, requiring 20 to 25 ml of solution.

It cannot be stressed too forcibly that these doses must be reduced with advancing age, the presence of arteriosclerosis and abdominal tumours of sufficient size to cause compression of the vena cava, and when the patient has cardiovascular disease or hypovolaemia or appears to be in poor general condition (Bromage, 1962). A given volume of 1.5 per cent lignocaine solution gives a higher block in patients over 40 to 50 than in younger ones, but doubling the dose does not double the number of segments blocked (Park et al, 1982a). The dose response curve differs in the old from the young. For example it has been shown that using bupivacaine 0.75 per cent solution for an upper thoracic block 20 to 25 ml is required in the 20 to 40 age group, 15 to 20 ml in the 40 to 60 group and 6 to 10 ml in those over 60, catheter inserted at L.2–3 interspace (Sharrock, 1978).

It has been suggested (Moore and Bridenbaugh, 1977) that safe amounts for injection into the extradural space, regardless of age, sex, weight, height and underlying disease and strength of solution are bupivacaine 225 mg with adrenaline, etidocaine 450 mg with adrenaline, or mepivacaine 500 mg with adrenaline. Patients who have received 0.75 per cent solution of bupivacaine need close supervision after injection as complete absorption and the onset of toxic signs may be delayed for up to 100 minutes. They will occur much more rapidly of course if the injection is intravascular (Bhate, 1983).

We recommend that when the agent used is bupivacaine 0.5 or 0.75 per cent with adrenaline, the dosage in millilitres required should be about two-thirds or rather less, than with 1.5 per cent lignocaine solution. Increasing the concentration of bupivacaine and etidocaine from 0.5 and 1 per cent respectively to 0.75 and 1.5 per cent, produces a more rapid onset of both motor and sensory blockade, with an extended duration and fewer unsatisfactory blocks. Increasing the concentration of prilocaine from 2 to 3 per cent has no advantages; it is probably the least toxic of the commonly used drugs and results in satisfactory blockade (Scott et al, 1980). Dosage is as for lignocaine. Etidocaine may be used in 1 per cent solution, with or without the addition of adrenaline. It has about half the potency of bupivacaine but about twice that of lignocaine (Bromage et al, 1974). Chloroprocaine is weaker, about 3 per cent being required for operative surgery and half this for analgesia in labour (Foldes and McNall, 1952; Foldes and Davis, 1954; Allen and Johnson, 1979). Mixtures of chloroprocaine with a long-acting agent offer the combined advantages of a short latent period with a long duration of effect (Cunningham and Kaplan, 1976). Mixtures of lignocaine and bupivacaine for extradural block, both of them amide-linked drugs with similar routes of excretion, are not recommended (Seow et al, 1982) although other workers (Magee et al, 1983) see a clinical advantage in that latency is reduced without shortening duration.

Sacral injection

The sacrococcygeal membrane can be pierced by a short sharp needle to enter the sacral canal. A 21 gauge, 40 mm needle is ideal for this purpose. The procedure is relatively simple if the landmarks are easily palpable but variations in anatomy do occur and occasionally difficulties arise, particularly in obese subjects.

The authors find it advantageous to have the patient in the prone position with two pillows placed under the pelvis, the legs fairly

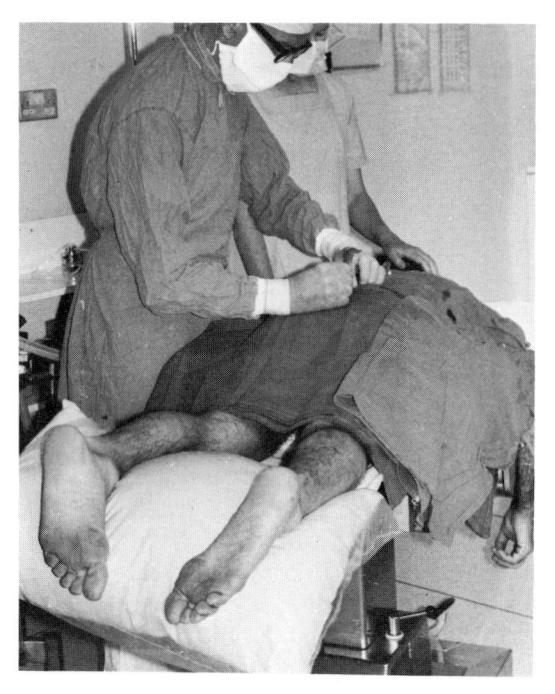

Fig. 9.2 Note the position of the legs.

widely separated and the toes turned inwards (Fig. 9.2). This last position is to take the tone out of the gluteal muscles and so to reduce the depth of the intergluteal cleft. Other workers prefer the lateral position which is especially indicated in obstetric practice, unless the patient adopts the knee-elbow attitude.

The usual skin preparation must be carried out and strict aseptic precautions taken. Antiseptic solutions containing spirit must be kept away from the perianal and scrotal regions as this will cause stinging pain.

The sacral hiatus is palpated and will be found to resemble the space between the knuckles of the hand when the fingers are flexed. A weal of local analgesic solution is raised in the skin with a fine intradermal needle and then the 21 gauge needle is inserted through it at an angle of 20 degrees with the perpendicular, to pierce the skin and membrane. A slight 'snap' can often be felt as the needle point pierces the membrane. The direction of the needle must now be changed by some 45 degrees towards the intergluteal cleft so that the needle can be advanced into the canal of the sacrum (Figs. 9.3 and 9.4). The needle should be kept in the mid-line at all times: it

EXTRADURAL ANALGESIA 229

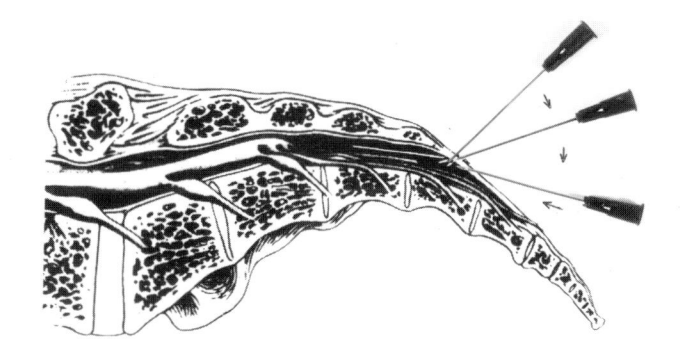

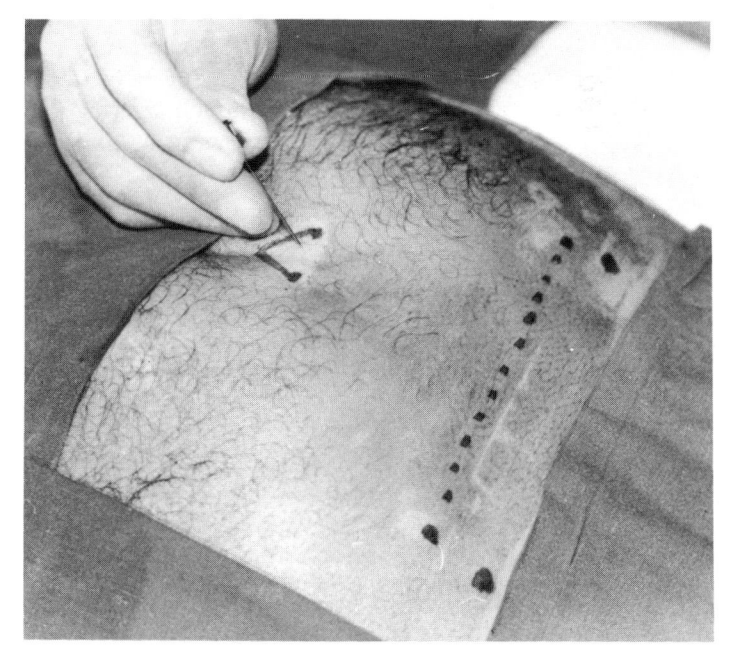

Figs 9.3 and 9.4 Insertion of needle into sacral canal (see text). The authors advise the use of a short needle (e.g. 40 mm, 21 gauge) to reduce the risk of dural puncture.

should not advance more than 2 cm from the sacrococcygeal membrane. The needle point may now be in any one of six positions. It may lie between the skin and the sacrum in which case the injection of 2 ml of air will produce crepitation to the touch. It may be lying between the sacral bone and its periosteum and injection then will require great force. It may be in the theca so that cerebrospinal fluid can be aspirated: this in spite of the fact that in the average patient the dural sac ends at the level of the posterior superior iliac spines or the second piece of the sacrum. It may have entered an extradural vein so that blood can be aspirated. It may have passed through the anterior wall of the sacrum, possibly injuring the rectum or in the obstetric patient, the fetal head (Dawkins, 1972). Lastly, and hopefully, it lies snugly and correctly in the extradural space, in which case the injection of a little air or solution requires no force, nor does this cause any swelling superficial to the sacrum. The appearance of blood on aspiration requires a slight alteration in the position of the needle point until no further blood appears, as intravascular injection of any sizeable volume of analgesic solution with adrenaline can lead to signs of toxicity, or the needle can be moved laterally if its point is in the canal. If cerebrospinal fluid is aspirated into the syringe the procedure must be either converted into an intradural block using a small volume of an appropriate solution, or it must be abandoned.

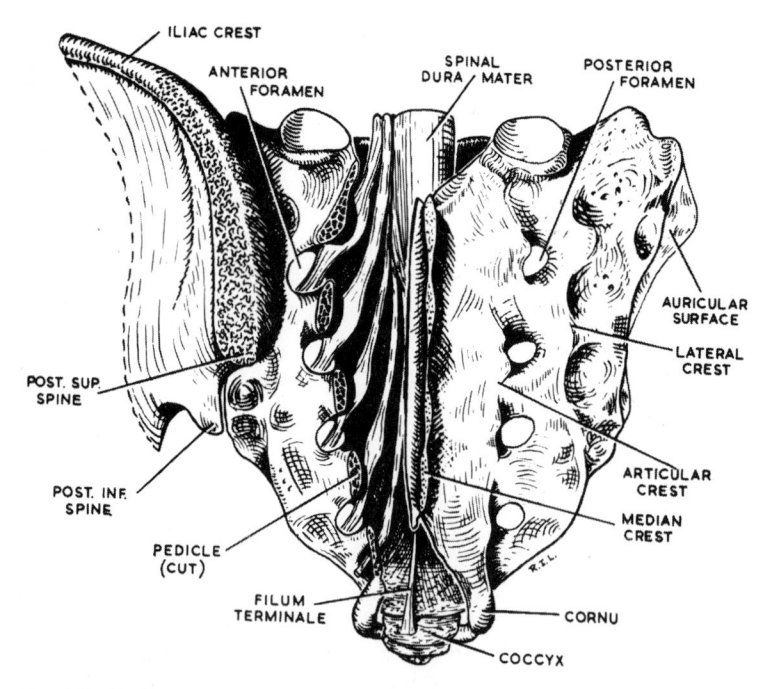

Fig. 9.5 The sacrum from behind. The five pedicles and the laminae have been cut through on the left side to show the sheaths of dura mater around the nerve roots. (Reproduced by kind permission of Professor R. J. Last, *Regional Anatomy*, Churchill Livingstone.)

Sacral injection is often easier in negroes than in white patients (Norenberg et al, 1979). Injection into the sacral canal should not be undertaken unless palpation of the area suggests that success will be likely. A failure of between 5 and 10 per cent can be expected depending on the experience of the anaesthetist.

A catheter may be inserted into the sacral extradural space via a suitable wide bore needle (Hingson and Southworth, 1942). The use of a 16 gauge Teflon intravenous cannula with needle stylet has also been recommended (Owens et al, 1973). In this way, serial injections can be given to provide prolonged pain relief in obstetrics, and after haemorrhoidectomy and similar operations.

Solutions injected into the sacral canal can pass throughout the length of the extradural space to reach the cervical area, but such a high block requires a near toxic amount of analgesic solution. Sacral injection is most satisfactory for operations on those structures supplied by the sacral and lumbar nerve roots. Larger amounts of local analgesic drug are required to block a segment in the sacral than in the lumbar area, while the onset of analgesia is slower. Hypotension and convulsions are always a possibility and careful and frequent observations of the level of the blood-pressure must be made. Large volumes of solution injected into the sacral canal increase the risks of toxicity without achieving increased height of block, partly due to leakage of solution through the anterior and posterior sacral foramina, and partly due to the difficulty in forcing solution round the lumbo-sacral angle. One method of achieving block of the lumbar nerves is to insert a catheter above this angle. Injected solution is then more likely to remain within the extradural space (Bryce-Smith, 1954).

Sacral or caudal block is particularly useful when the sacral segments alone are required to be blocked. It is therefore useful in such operations as haemorrhoidectomy, though when the surgeon requires maintenance of sphincter tone, general anaesthesia is to be preferred. Other operations which can be carried out satisfactorily under sacral block include cystoscopy, transurethral resection of the prostrate, pelvic floor repair, especially posterior colporrhaphy and perineorrhaphy, and operations on the lower extremity, e.g. Keller's operation.

There is no need to detain a patient in hospital overnight following a sacral block, provided that full muscular power has returned to the legs and that the cardiovascular system is stable.

Sepsis is a greater hazard in sacral than in lumbar block owing to the proximity of the anus, an infection rate of 0.2 per cent being quoted (Dawkins, 1972). Breakage of the needle or catheter is also commoner in sacral than in lumbar block.

In the authors' experience, toxic manifestations as a result of absorption of the local analgesic agent into the systemic circulation are commoner after sacral than after lumbar injection. This may be partly due to the use of larger doses in an attempt to ensure satisfactory levels of analgesia, but also may be associated with greater ease of administering an accidental injection directly into a vessel in this site. *It is our firm conviction that no sacral or lumbar block should be conducted without there being a patent needle in a vein, as the treatment of the signs of toxicity such as cardiovascular depression or convulsions requires instant intravenous injection of a suitable restorative.*

Caudal analgesia in infants and children

This is a useful technique (Fortuna, 1967), especially when combined with light general anaesthesia, for surgery below the umbilicus and for relief of postoperative pain, e.g. after circumcision (Lunn, 1979). Any associated sympathetic blockade is generally well tolerated by young children. It is usually necessary to give ketamine 2 mg/kg, i.m., thiopentone or light general anaesthesia to prevent movement during the injection and to keep the child asleep during the operation. Location of the sacral canal is usually easy, but once the sacrococcygeal membrane has been pierced, the needle should not be advanced further because in young children the dural sac may extend below the second piece of the sacrum and dural puncture is always possible.

There is discussion as to the nature of the drug and the dosage which should be injected. The volume of solution is important in calculating the correct dose, and correlating the dose with body weight has given satisfactory results in many hundreds of patients (Schulte-Steinberg and Rahlf, 1970, 1977; Takasaki et al, 1977; Soliman et al, 1978; Lunn 1979; Jensen, 1981; McGown, 1982). There are other workers of experience who prefer to correlate dosage with age (Kay, 1974; Davenport, 1981).

Lignocaine works well because of its relative lack of toxicity, its central sedative effect and its rapid onset (McGown, 1982) and the 1 per cent solution to which adrenaline 1: 200 000 has been added is satisfactory. Examples of dosages used for circumcision include:
1. Schulte-Steinberg and Rahlf, 1970. Bupivacaine 0.25 per cent with adrenaline, or lignocaine 1 per cent with adrenaline; 0.1 ml/year per dermatome to be blocked.

2. Kay, 1974. Bupivacaine plain 0.5 per cent solution with adrenaline, 0.5 ml/year of age.
3. Davenport, 1981. Bupivacaine 0.5 per cent solution, 0.5 ml/year.
4. Soliman et al, 1978. Plain bupivacaine 0.25 per cent or lignocaine 1 per cent with adrenaline, 1 ml/year.
5. Lunn. 1979. Plain bupivacaine 0.5 per cent, 1.5 mg/kg body weight.
6. Armitage, 1979. Plain bupivacaine 0.25 per cent, 0.5 to 1.25 mg/kg.
7. McGown, 1982. Lignocaine 1 per cent solution with adrenaline, 1: 200 000 (0.55 ml/kg).

For block to T.11 (testicular and inguinal surgery), 1.7 mg/kg body weight.

For block to L.2 (surgery of lower limb with tourniquet), 1.1 mg/kg.

For block to S.3 (operations on the penis and vulva), 0.55 mg/kg.

It is wise to limit the dosage of 1 per cent lignocaine to 10 mg/kg and of 0.25 per cent bupivacaine to 2.5 mg/kg.

Like all other techniques of pain relief problems can occur, and among complications reported have been dural puncture, hypotension, cardiac arrest, respiratory arrest, regurgitation of gastric contents and total central neural blockade. If the anaesthetist is alert he should be able to spot such abnormalities early on, treat them and prevent harm coming to the child (McGown, 1982).

Signs of successful lumbar extradural block

On completion of the extradural injection the anaesthetist must look for signs that successful block has been achieved. Some 10 minutes should be allowed for these to become manifest, although latency — the time between the completion of the injection and the onset of the effects — will vary somewhat according to the analgesic drug used. The signs are usually quicker in onset with intradural than with extradural block and with lignocaine than with bupivacaine

The conscious patient may exhibit facial pallor as a result of reflex vasoconstriction in an effort to maintain arterial pressure. He may also admit that his legs feel heavy or numb, or have 'pins and needles'. An objective test is to elicit the tendon reflexes, the ankle and the knee jerks. If these were previously brisk but are now absent, this is good evidence of block in the appropriate segments, S.1 and 2 in the case of the ankle jerks and L.2–4 for the knee jerks (Westphal's sign), named the 'knee-jerk' by Sir William

Gowers (1845–1915) in 1879 (Gowers, 1879). Relaxation of the anal sphincter, tested by rectal examination with the finger, also suggests the presence of sacral block. Some voluntary movement of the legs is usually possible following extradural block but this is perfectly compatible with good clinical relaxation. The lower limbs are usually paralysed after intradural analgesia, this being the basis of the test dose of analgesic solution to recognise inadvertent intradural injection.

A fall in arterial pressure is a good confirmatory sign although it is not always present and can have other causes. Additional positive signs which may be observed are legs warm to palpation with dilated veins as a result of sympathetic block, and a scaphoid abdomen due to the relaxation of the muscles of the abdominal wall and diminished intra-abdominal pressure due to contraction of the intestines. The patient with a high segmental block is not able to cough forcefully while his attempts to do so do not stiffen the abdominal wall.

Pinprick sensitivity is a useful method of eliciting segmental levels of block in the conscious and co-operative patient, although in the experience of the authors, this degree of definition is unnecessary in the majority of clinical situations. Testing sensation by stroking the skin with an ether soaked swab, or an ethyl chloride spray is more elegant but gives poor information in the heavily sedated patient or where communication is difficult. The level of sensory blockade in both intra- and extradural analgesia can be tested by applying bursts of electric current at tetanic frequencies using a nerve stimulator (Andrade and Wilinski, 1980). Muscle weakness or paralysis in relation to joint movement will also give useful information. Plantar flexion of the ankle is controlled by S.1 and S.2, while dorsiflexion is controlled by L.4 and 5; flexion of the knee joint by L.5 and S.1; extension of the knee by L.3 and 4; extension of the hip by L.4 and 5; flexion of the hip by L.2 and 3 (see Fig. 9.6).

The final test of a successful spinal block is the absence of response to surgical stimulation. There should be no reaction when the skin is incised and on opening the peritoneal cavity the abdominal wall should be relaxed, and the bowel contracted and unobtrusive.

The choice between intradural and extradural block

The physiological effects of both types of block are mainly the result of paralysis of spinal nerves emerging from the cord, sensory, motor

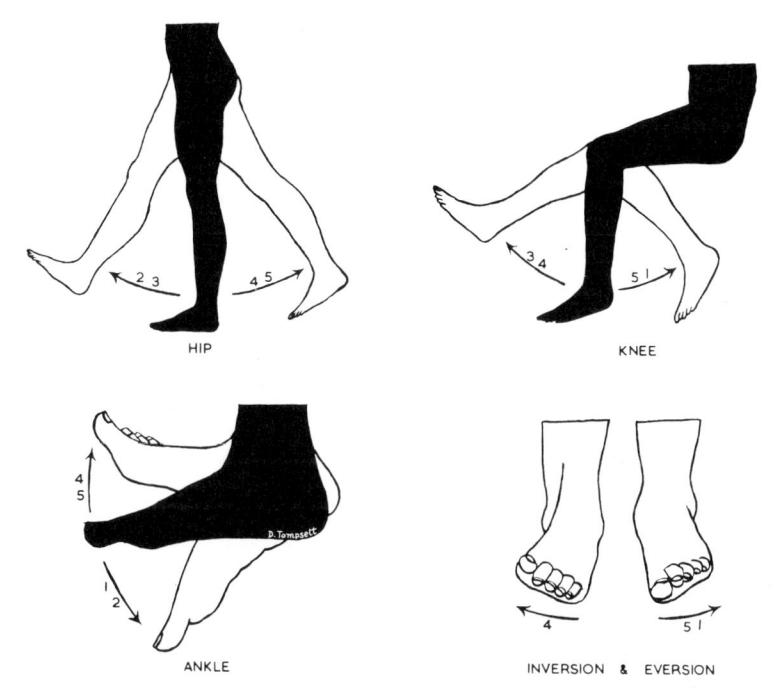

Fig. 9.6 The segmental innervation of the movements of the lower limb. (Reproduced by kind permission of Professor R. J. Last, *Regional Anatomy*, Churchill Livingstone.)

and autonomic. There are however a few significant differences which may sway the clinical anaesthetist in his choice between the two methods.

Intradural block is easier to teach, quicker to perform, and its effects usually come on more rapidly. The total dose of analgesic drug to be injected is so small that for practical purposes the risks of toxic absorption into the systemic circulation can be ignored: this is certainly not always so following extradural injection. The height of block can be more readily controlled when a suitable amount of a hyperbaric solution is injected into the intradural space and gravity used to limit spread or when plain 0.5 per cent bupivacaine is used.

While extradural injection of a suitable amount of local analgesic solution of adequate strength gives very good muscular relaxation of the anterior abdominal wall, suitable for an extensive intra-abdominal exploration, most experienced workers would agree that the relaxation produced by intradural block is slightly more profound. This may be an advantage when working with a surgeon who demands an almost corpse-like flaccidity, and also in the occasional patient who combines obesity with stiff, tough and unyielding anterior abdominal wall muscles.

Why then do so many anaesthetists prefer extradural injection? The idea that by keeping the needle point and analgesic solution outside the dura, neurological complications can be avoided is not valid in the light of recent reports (p. 291). Undoubtedly, the major advantage of avoiding dural puncture is the absence of the complication of post-lumbar puncture headache, which may be severe and distressing and may, in addition, delay the patient's discharge from hospital. Its incidence is low if a 25 g lumbar puncture needle is used. It cannot be denied that the slight technical difficulties of performing a satisfactory extradural puncture add to the attraction of the method to the anaesthetist, if it is applied in suitable circumstances.

There are also differences in the extent of the zones of differential blockade, sensory, sympathetic and motor between the two sites of injection. For a given level of sensory blockade intradural injection of local analgesic solution causes interruption of more sympathetic fibres and hence, theoretically, more fall in blood-pressure than extradural block. On the other hand, intradural injection results in motor block being two segments lower than sensory block, but this does not hold for extradural injection (Greene, 1969). In our opinion, the differences are of little practical importance when a choice has to be made between intra- and extradural block for surgical operations. The relative absence of motor paresis during extradural blockade is however advantageous when analgesia is required but preservation of motor function is desirable, as when it is proposed to extend analgesia into the postoperative period, and in obstetric analgesia for vaginal delivery. The use of indwelling catheters has become more popular in recent years, and although they have been used for intradural block (Lemmon, 1940; Lee, 1943) most anaesthetists would now consider the hazards of infection to be much greater than when the extradural site is chosen. Moreover, the large bore needle necessary for the introduction of a catheter makes a relatively big hole in the dura mater when this is penetrated, with a consequent high incidence of postoperative headache.

REFERENCES

Aitkenhead, A. R. Hothersall, A. P., Gilmour, D. G. & Ledingham, I. M. (1979) Dural dimpling in the dog. *Anaesthesia*, **34**, 14.

Albright, G. A. (1978) *Anaesthesia in Obstetrics*, p. 239. London: Addison-Wesley.
Albright, G. A. (1979) Cardiac arrest following regional anesthesia with etidocaine and bupivacaine. *Anesthesiology*, **51**, 285.
Allen, P. R. & Johnson, R. N. (1979) Subarachnoid injection during extradural analgesia for labour using 2-chloroprocaine. *Anaesthesia*, **34**, 874.
Andrade, R. A. & Wilinski, J. A. (1980) Monitor of sensory level during epidural spinal anesthesia. *Anesthesiology*, **52**, 189.
Armitage, E. N. (1979) Caudal block in children. *Anaesthesia*, **34**, 396.
Ballance, J. H. W. (1981) Difficulty in the removal of an epidural catheter. *Anaesthesia*, **36**, 71.
Baraka, A. (1972) Correspondence. *British Journal of Anaesthesia*, **44**, 122.
Berry, A (1958) A test for cerebrospinal fluid. *Anaesthesia*, **13**, 100.
Bhate, H. (1983) Correspondence. Systemic reaction caused by epidural bupivacaine 0.75 per cent. *Anaesthesia*, **38**, 71
Blass, N. H., Roberts, R. B. & Wiley, J. K. (1981) The case of the errant epidural catheter. *Anesthesiology*, **54**, 419.
Boskowski, N. & Levinski, A. (1982) The effect of the direction of the needle bevel on lumbar epidural analgesia. **37**, 216.
Boyes, J. E. & Norman, P. F. (1975) Accidental subdural analgesia. *British Journal of Anaesthesia*, **47**, 1111.
Bray, M. C. & Carrie, L. E. S. (1978) Unblocked segments in obstetric epidural block. *Anaesthesia*, **33**, 232.
Bridenbaugh, L. D., Moore, D. C., Bagdi, P. & Bridenbaugh, P. O. (1968) The position of plastic tubing in continuous block techniques — an X-ray study of 552 patients. *Anesthesiology*, **29**, 1047.
Bromage, P. R. (1962) Spread of analgesic solutions in the extradural space and their site of action. *British Journal of Anaesthesia*, **34**, 161.
Bromage, P. R. (1969) Ageing and epidural dose requirements. *British Journal of Anaesthesia*, **41**, 1016.
Bromage, P. R. (1972) Unblocked segments in epidural analgesia for relief of pain in labour. *British Journal of Anaesthesia*, **44**, 676.
Bromage, P. R. (1978a) *Epidural Anesthesia*, p. 486. Philadelphia: Saunders.
Bromage, P. R. (1978b) *Epidural Anesthesia*, p. 476. Philadelphia: Saunders.
Bromage, P. R. (1978c) *Epidural Anesthesia*, p. 226. Philadelphia: Saunders.
Bromage, P. R., O'Biern, P. & Dunford, L. A. (1974) Etidocaine: an evaluation for regional analgesia in surgery. *Canadian Anaesthetists' Society Journal*, **21**, 523.
Brooks, W. (1957) An epidural indicator. *Anaesthesia*, **12**, 227.
Brown, R. A. & Politi, V. L. (1979) A knotted epidural catheter. *Canadian Anaesthetists' Society Journal*, **26**, 142.
Brownridge, P. (1981) Correspondence, Epidural and subarachnoid analgesia for elective Caesarean section. *Anaesthesia*, **36**, 70.
Bryce-Smith, R. (1954) The spread of solutions within the extradural space. *Anaesthesia*, **9**, 201.
Burn, J. M. & Langdon, L. (1982) Correspondence. The effect of the direction of the needle bevel in lumbar epidural analgesia. *Anaesthesia*, **37**, 698.
Burn, J. M., Guyer, P. B. & Langdon, L. (1973) The spread of solutions injected into the epidural space. A study using epidurograms in patients with the lumbo-sciatic syndrome. *British Journal of Anaesthesia*, **45**, 338.
Carr, M. F. & Hehre, F. W. (1962) Complications of continuous lumbar peridural anesthesia. 1. Inadvertent dural puncture. *Anesthesia and Analgesia*, **41**, 349.
Clatterberg, J. (1977) Local anesthetic versus spinal fluid. *Anesthesiology*, **46**, 309.
Coates, M. B. (1982) Correspondence. Combined subarachnoid and epidural techniques. *Anaesthesia*, **37**, 89.
Collier, C. (1982a) Collapse after epidural injection following inadvertent dural puncture. *Anesthesiology*, **57**, 427.
Collier, C. (1982b) Correspondence. *Anaesthesia and Intensive Care*, **10**, 92.

Crawford, J. S., Willams, M. E. & Veales, S. (1975) Correspondence. Particulate matter in the extradural space. *British Journal of Anaesthesia*, **47**, 807.

Crawford, J. S., James, F. M., Nolte, H., Van Steenberge, A. & Shah, J. L. (1981) Regional analgesia for patients with chronic neurological disease and similar conditions. *Anaesthesia*, **36**, 82.

Cunningham, N. L. & Kaplan, J. A. (1976) A rapid onset, long acting regional anesthetic technique. *Anesthesiology*, **41**, 509.

Curbelo, M. M. (1949) Continuous peridural segmental anesthesia by means of a ureteral catheter. *Anesthesia and Analgesia, Current Researches*, **28**, 13.

Davenport, H. T. (1981) *Paediatric Anaesthesia*, 3rd edn. London: Macmillan.

Dawkins, C. J. M. (1961) A drip epidural indicator. *Anaesthesia*, **16**, 102.

Dawkins, C. J. M. (1963) The identification of the epidural space: a critical analysis of various methods employed. *Anaesthesia*, **18**, 66.

Dawkins, C. J. M. (1972) In Doughty, A. (ed.) *Proceedings of the Symposium on Epidural Analgesia in Obstetrics*, London: Lewis.

Dawkins, C. J. M. & Steel, G. C. (1971) Thoracic extradural (epidural) block for upper abdominal surgery. *Anaesthesia*, **26**, 41.

Daykin, A. P. (1982) A test to show correct placement of epidural catheter. *Anaesthesia*, **37**, 863.

Doughty, A. (1974) A precise method of cannulating the lumbar epidural space. *Anaesthesia*, **29**, 63.

Ducrow, M. (1980) The extradural space. *British Journal of Anaesthesia*, **52**, 241.

Duffy, B. L. (1982) Securing the epidural catheter. *Canadian Anaesthetists' Society Journal*, **29**, 636.

Erdemir, H. A., Soper, L. E. & Sweet, R. B. (1965) Studies of factors affecting peridural anesthesia. *Anesthesia and Analgesia*, **44**, 400.

Evans, J. M. (1982) The Oxford Epidural Space Detector. *Lancet*, **2**, 1432.

Findley, I. & Shandro, J. (1982) Delayed onset spinal after epidural analgesia. *Anaesthesia*, **37**, 602.

Foldes, F. F. & Davis, D. L. (1954) The spinal fluid concentrations of 2-chloroprocaine following its epidural administration in man. *Journal of Pharmacology and Experimental Therapeutics*, **110**, 18.

Foldes, F. F. & McNall, P. G. (1952) 2-chloroprocaine: a new anesthetic agent. *Anesthesiology*, **13**, 287.

Forster, S. J. (1983) Correspondence. Combined subarachnoid and epidural techniques. *Anaesthesia*, **38**, 72.

Fortuna, A. (1967) Caudal analgesia: a simple and safe technique in paediatric surgery. *British Journal of Anaesthesia*, **39**, 165..

Galindo, A., Hernandez, J., Benarides, O., Ortegon de Munoz, S. & Bonica, J. J. (1975) Quality of spinal extradural anaesthesia: the influence of spinal nerve root diameter. *British Journal of Anaesthesia*, **47**, 41.

Germann, P. A. S., Roberts, J. G. & Prys-Roberts, C. (1979) The combination of general anaesthesia with epidural block; I. The effects of sequence of induction on haemodynamic variables and blood gas measurements in healthy patients. *Anaesthesia and Intensive Care*, **7**, 229.

Gjessing, J. & Tomlin, P. J. (1979) Patterns of postoperative pain: a study of the use of continuous epidural analgesia in the postoperative period. *Anaesthesia*, **34**, 624.

Gowers, W. (1879) The knee-jerk. *Medical Times and Gazette*, **2**, 524.

Greene, N. M. (1969) *Physiology of Spinal Anaesthesia*, p. 227, 2nd edn. Baltimore: Williams & Wilkins.

Grundy, E. M., Rao, L. N. & Winnie, A. P. (1978a) Epidural anesthesia and the lateral position. *Anesthesia and Analgesia*, **57**, 95.

Grundy, E. M., Ramamurthy, S., Patel, K. P., Mani, M. & Winnie, A. P. (1978b) Extradural analgesia revisited. *British Journal of Anaesthesia*, **50**, 805.

Gutiérrez, A. (1932) Anesthesia metamerica peridural. *Revista de Cirugia* (Buenos Aires), **12**, 665.

Hingson, R. A. & Southworth, J. L. (1942) Continuous caudal anesthesia. *American Journal of Surgery*, **58**, 665.

Hodgkinson, R. (1981) Total spinal block after epidural injection into an interspace adjacent to an inadvertent dural puncture. *Anesthesiology*, **55**, 593.

Husemeyer, R. P. & White, D. C. (1980) Lumbar extradural injection and pressures in pregnant women. *British Journal of Anaesthesia*, **52**, 55.

Husemeyer, R. P., White, D. C. & Smolenski, T. (1978) The shape of the lumbar extradural space with reference to accidental dural puncture. *British Journal of Anaesthesia*, **50**, 631P.

Husemeyer, R. P., White, D. C., Park, Y. R. & Eastwood, D. W. (1980) Dextrose affects gravitational spread of epidural anesthesia. *Anesthesiology*, **52**, 439.

Iklè, A. (1950) Preliminary report on a new techn... for epidural anaesthesia. *British Journal of Anaesthesia*, **22**, 150.

Jensen, B. H. (1981) Caudal block for postoperative pain relief in children with genital operations: a comparison. *Acta Anaesthesiologica Scandinavica*, **25**, 373.

Kalas, D. B. & Hehre, F. W. (1972) Continuous lumbar peridural anesthesia in obstetrics. VIII. Further observations on inadvertent lumbar puncture. *Anesthesia and Analgesia*, **51**, 192.

Kay, B. (1974) Caudal block for postoperative pain relief in children. *Anaesthesia*, **29**, 610.

Keane, P. W. (1983) Correspondence. Insertion of epidural catheters. *Anaesthesia*, **38**, 701.

Laman, N. & McLeskey, C. H. (1978) Supraclavicular subcutaneous surgical emphysema following lumbar epidural anesthesia. *Anesthesiology*, **48**, 219.

Lee, J. A. (1943) Serial spinal analgesia. *Lancet* **2**, 156.

Lee, J. A. (1960) Specially marked needle to facilitate extradural block. *Anaesthesia*, **15**, 186.

Lee, J. A. (1962) A new catheter for continuous extradural analgesia. *Anaesthesia*, **17**, 248.

Lemmon, W. T. (1940) A method of continuous spinal anesthesia. A preliminary report. *Annals of Surgery*, **111**, 141.

Lund, P. C. (1966) *Peridural Analgesia and Anesthesia*, p. 70. Springfield: Thomas.

Lunn, J. N. (1979) Postoperative analgesia after circumcision. *Anaesthesia*, **34**, 552.

MacDonald, R. (1983) Correspondence. *Anaesthesia*, **38**, 71.

Macintosh, R. R. (1948) A new needle for spinal analgesia. *Lancet*, **2**, 612.

Macintosh, R. R. (1950) Extradural space indicator. *Anaesthesia*, **5**, 98.

Macintosh, R. R. (1953) Extradural space indicator. *British Medical Journal*, **1**, 398.

Macintosh, R. R. & Bryce-Smith, R. (1951) Sixth nerve palsy after lumbar puncture and spinal analgesia. *British Medical Journal*, **1**, 275.

Macmurdo, S. D. & McKenzie, R. (1979) Mishap with an epidural catheter. *Anesthesiology*, **50**, 260.

Magee, D. A., Sweet, P. T. & Holland, A. J. C. (1983) Epidural anaesthesia with mixtures of bupivacaine and lidocaine. *Canadian Anaesthetists' Society Journal*, **30**, 174.

McGown, R. G. (1982) Extradural analgesia in children. *Anaesthesia*, **37**, 806.

Mehta, M. & Maher, R. (1977) Injection into the extra-arachnoid subdural space. *Anaesthesia*, **1931**, 760.

Mesry, S. (1976) Massive epidural spread of local analgesics. *Anaesthesia*, **31**, 576.

Mirakhur, R. K. & Bandopadhyay, A. (1973) An auditory guide to the extradural space. *Anaesthesia*, **28**, 707.

Moir, D. D. & Hesson, W. R. (1965) Dural puncture by an epidural catheter. *Anaesthesia*, **20**, 373.

Moore, D. C. & Batra, M. S. (1982) Further consideration concerning the compounds of an effective test dose prior to epidural block. *Anesthesiology*, **57**, 141.

Moore, D. C. & Bridenbaugh, L. D. (1977) Factors determining dosages of amide type local anesthetic drugs. *Anesthesiology*, **47**, 263.

Moore, D. C., Balfour, R. I. & Fitzgibbon, D. (1979) Convulsive arterial plasma levels of bupivacaine and response to diazepam therapy. *Anesthesiology*, **50**, 454.

Mumtaz, M. H., Daz, M. & Kuz, M. (1982) Correspondence. Combined subarachnoid and epidural techniques. *Anaesthesia*, **37**, 90.

Mustafa, K. & Milliken, R. A. (1982) A simple device for the identification of the epidural space. *Anesthesiology*, **57**, 330.

Myint, 0. (1976) A double catheter technique for major surgery. *Anaesthesia*, **31**, 575.

Nadkarni, A. V. & Tondare, A. S. (1981) Localised clonic convulsions after spinal anesthesia with lidocaine and epinephrine. *Anesthesia and Analgesia*, **60**, 945.

Naulty, J. S., Ostheimer, G. W., Datta, S., Knapp, R. & Weiss, J. B. (1982) Incidence of venous air embolism during epidural catheter insertion. *Anesthesiology*, **57**, 410.

Nishimura, N., Kitahara, T. & Kusakabe, T. (1959) The spread of lidocaine and 1-131 solution in the epidural space. *Anesthesiology*, **20**, 785.

Norenberg, A. J., Johanson, D. C. & Gravenstein, J. S. (1979) Racial differences in sacral structure. *Anesthesiology*, **50**, 549.

Odom, C. B. (1936) Epidural anesthesia. *American Journal of Surgery*, **34**, 547.

Owens, W. D., Slater, E. E. & Battit, G. E. (1973) A new technique of caudal anesthesia. *Anesthesiology*, **39**, 451.

Park, W. Y., Hagins, F. M., Rivat, E. L. & Macnamara, T. E. (1982a) Age and epidural dose responses in adult men. *Anesthesiology*, **56**, 318.

Park, W. Y., Poon, K. C., Massengale, M. D. & Macnamara, T. E. (1982b) Direction of needle bevel and epidural anesthetic spread. *Anesthesiology*, **57**, 327.

Park, Y. R. & Eastwood, D. W. (1980) Dextrose affects gravitational spread of epidural anesthetic. *Anesthesiology*, **52**, 439.

Peters, G. C. (1983) Correspondence. *Anaesthesia*, **38**, 72.

Philip, N. H. & Brown, W. V. (1976) Total spinal anesthesia late in the course of obstetric epidural block. *Anesthesiology*, **34**, 340.

Prentiss, J. E. (1979) Cardiac arrest following caudal anesthesia. *Anesthesiology*, **50**, 51.

Quader, M. A. & Waldron, B. A. (1976) Multiple epidural taps by epidural catheter. *Anaesthesia*, **31**.793.

Ramanathan, S., Chalon, J., Richards, M., Patel, C. & Turndorf, H. (1978) Prolonged spinal nerve involvement after epidural anesthesia with etidocaine. *Anesthesia and Analgesia*, **57**, 361.

Rauscher, L. A. (1975) An auditory guide to the location of the extradural space. *Anaesthesia*, **30**, 98.

Riegler, R. & Pernetzky, A. (1983) Irremovable epidural catheter due to a sling and a knot. *Regional Anesthesia*, **6**, 19.

Roberts, R. B. (1972) Occurrence of unblocked segments during continuous lumbar epidural analgesia for pain relief in labour. *British Journal of Anaesthesia*, **44**, 628.

Ross, R. A., Clarke, J. E. & Armitage, E. N. (1980) Postoperative pain prevention by continuous epidural infusion. *Anaesthesia*, **35**, 663.

Salt, R. H. (1963) Correspondence. Identification of extradural space. *Anaesthesia*, **18**, 404.

Sanchez, R., Acuna, L. & Rocha, F. (1967) An analysis of the radiological visualization of the catheters placed in the epidural space. *British Journal of Anaesthesia*, **39**, 485.

Schulte-Steinberg, O. & Rahlf, V. W. (1970) Caudal anaesthesia in children. *British Journal of Anaesthesia*, **42**, 1093.

Schulte-Steinberg, O. & Rahlf, V. W. (1977) Spread of extradural analgesia in children; a statistical study. *British Journal of Anaesthesia*, **49**, 1027.

Scott, D. B. (1981) Editorial. Toxicity caused by local anaesthetic drugs. *British Journal of Anaesthesia*, **53**, 553.

Scott, D. B., McClure, J. H., Giasi, R. N., Seao, J. & Covino B. G. (1980) The

effect of the concentration of local anaesthetic drugs in extradural block. *Anaesthesia and Intensive Care*, **9**, 150.
Seow, L. T., Lips, F. J. & Cousins, M. J. (1983) Effect of lateral posture on epidural blockade for surgery. *Anaesthesia and Intensive Care*, **11**, 97.
Seow, L. T., Lips, F. J., Cousins, M. J. & Mather L. E. (1982) Lidocaine, bupivacaine mixture for epidural blockade. *Anesthesiology*, **56**, 177.
Shah, J. L. (1982) A test to show correct placement of epidural catheter. *Anaesthesia*, **37**, 426.
Sharrock, N. E. (1978) Epidural anesthetic dose responses in patients 20–80 years old. *Anesthesiology*, **49**, 425.
Sharrock, N. E. (1979) Recordings of and anatomical explanations for false positive loss of resistance during lumbar extradural analgesia. *British Journal of Anaesthesia*, **51**, 253.
Simpson, B. R., Parkhouse, J., Marshall, R. & Lambrechts, W. (1961) Extradural analgesia and the prevention of postoperative respiratory complications. *British Journal of Anaesthesia*, **33**, 628.
Sloss, M. T., Forbes, A. M., Moreley, T. R. & Plumpton, F. S. (1970) Applied anatomy of the epidural space prediction of the distance between the skin and lumbar epidural space. *Proceedings of the III Asian Australasian Congress of Anaesthesiology*, p. 305 Chatswood (Australia) Butterworths.
Soliman, M. G., Ansara, S. & Laberge, R. (1978) Caudal anaesthesia in children. *Canadian Anaesthetists' Society Journal*, **25**, 226.
Soni, N. & Holland, R. (1981) Extensive lumbar epidural block. *Anaesthesia and Intensive Care*, **9**, 150.
Steen, P. A. & Michenfelder, J. R. (1979) Neurotoxicity and local anesthetics. *Anesthesiology*, **50**, 437.
Takasaki, M., Dohi, S., Kawabata, Y. & Takahashi, T. (1977) Dosage of lidocaine for caudal anesthesia in infants and children. *Anesthesiology*, **47**, 307.
Telivuo, L. (1963) A new long-acting local anaesthetic solution for pain relief after thoracotomy. *Annales chirurgiae et gynaecologiae Fenniae*, **52**, 513.
Tuohy, E. B. (1945) The use of continuous spinal anesthesia — utilizing the ureteral catheter technique. *Journal of the American Medical Association*, **128**, 262.
Usubiaga, J. E., Dos Reis, A. & Usubiaga, L. E. (1970) Epidural misplacement of catheters and mechanisms of unilateral blockade. *Anesthesiology*, **32**, 158.
Usubiaga, J. E., Wilinski, J. A. & Usubiaga, L. E. (1967) Epidural pressure and its relation to spread of anesthetic solutions in the epidural space. *Anesthesia and Analgesia*, **46**, 440.
Utting, J. E. & Smith, J. M. (1979) Postoperative analgesia. *Anaesthesia*, **34**, 320.
White, D. C. (1982) In Kaufman, L. (ed.) *Anaesthesia Review*, ch. 10. Edinburgh: Churchill Livingstone.
Williams, R. A. J. (1975) A syringe for extradural analgesia. *Anaesthesia*, **30**, 288.
Woerth, S. D. Bullard, J. R. & Alpert, C. C. (1977) Total spinal anesthesia: a late complication of epidural anesthesia. *Anesthesiology*, **47**, 380.
Youngman, H. R. (1956) Toxic reactions to epidural anesthesia. *Anesthesiology*, **17**, 632.

10

Management of the patient during the operation

The successful and safe supervision of the patient during the operation requires just as much skill and experience as the actual injection of the local analgesic drug. It is not every surgeon, nor indeed every patient who readily accepts this form of analgesia, however perfect the anaesthetist's technique may be.

Before the patient is moved from the anaesthetic room into the operating theatre the anaesthetist should make up his mind whether the patient is to remain awake during the operation or is to be made unconscious. This will depend on the preferences and customs of the anaesthetist, on the wishes of the patient and on the temperament of the surgeon. There are some patients who should never be operated on in the conscious state just as there are some surgeons who should never be allowed to operate unless the patient is quietly asleep. We have found that there are few patients who prefer to be awake during surgery, but in certain countries in Asia this is not so and the avoidance of the loss of consciousness is one of the great attractions of spinal analgesia (Nabi, 1966).

If the spinal block is to be accompanied by general anaesthesia to what depths should this be carried and which agents and techniques should be employed? The choice of both is wide and each worker will have his favourites. Methods and techniques range from nitrous oxide and oxygen, with or without an intravenous supplement of analgesic or barbiturate; nitrous oxide and oxygen with the addition of a volatile supplement such as halothane, trichloroethylene or enflurane. Ether and air also has its advocates. If the surgical procedure is expected to be lengthy, especially if the steep head-down or lateral position is required, e.g. in operations on the colon, rectum or kidney, tracheal intubation makes for safety and smoothness. In such patients spinal analgesia provides excellent muscular relaxation, contraction of the bowel, and relative wound ischaemia, together with spontaneous respiration which may from time to time require manual assistance.

We have found intermittent intravenous injections of thiopentone very serviceable for maintaining a light level of unconsciousness during operations under spinal block. Restlessness can frequently be quelled by the intravenous injection of small (0.5 mg) doses of diamorphine (heroin). Using this method the amount of thiopentone needed seldom exceeds 300 mg and that of diamorphine 2.5 mg even for lengthy procedures. Other sedative drugs which have been recommended during the operation include 0.8 per cent solution of chlormethiazole (Heminevrin; Hemineurin) at a commencing drip rate of 20 ml min (Wilson et al, 1969; Schweitzer, 1978; Seow and Ryall, 1982), diazepam 2.5 to 5 mg (Gjessing and Tomlin, 1977), Thalamonal and low dose ketamine and diazepam (Austin, 1980). Etomidate as a sedative agent in patients undergoing hip surgery under extradural block has given good results (as has midazolam). An initial dose of 60 μ/kg/min for the first minute, followed by a stepwise reduction over 10 minutes to a maintenance level of 5 to 7 μg/kg/min, gives a uniform level of sedation (Birks et al, 1983).

We cannot stress too strongly that general anaesthesia should be provided whenever the block is demonstrably inadequate. The fact of partial or complete failure should be honestly faced and full general anaesthesia instituted. Repeated doses of an intravenous barbiturate should not be used to try to disguise a failed regional technique. General anaesthesia is also necessary when the scope of surgery extends outside the zone of analgesia or when the passage of time results in recovery, partial or complete, from the block.

Spinal analgesia should not be undertaken unless there is access to a vein (e.g. an intravenous infusion or indwelling needle such as a 'butterfly' and an anaesthetic machine with all reasonable ancillary aids, or a device for IPPV with air or oxygen such as an Ambu resuscitator is to hand. Solutions for intravenous infusion, pressor agents, atropine, suction, etc. should all be available. Nothing but good can follow the administration of oxygen during the operation and this can be given via a nasal catheter, an oxygen mask or an anaesthetic face mask, with or without nitrous oxide. Atropine can be administered in the event of bradycardia accompanied by hypotension. Quite small intravenous doses of 0.1 mg are often sufficient to restore cardiac output.

Respiration must be carefully watched the whole time, and should tidal exchange become abnormally shallow, intermittent positive pressure ventilation must be commenced without delay in the form of assisted or controlled respiration, with added oxygen. We have on a number of occasions seen a patient under extradural block and with a stable cardiovascular system, stop breathing. This may be due to the toxic effect of lignocaine. More rarely, if the apnoea is accompanied by hypotension it may be due to the so-called total spinal, from inadvertent intradural injection. It may also result from spread of solution in the extradural or in the subdural space. Respiratory depression must never pass unnoticed.

Throughout the operation, the blood-pressure must be monitored and, if necessary, steps must be taken to maintain it at a suitable level. An intravenous infusion is valuable here and when the cardiovascular system is healthy, the first 500 ml of fluid may be administered quickly. The authors have found Hartmann's solution (compound sodium lactate solution) useful, otherwise isotonic saline or 5 per cent glucose may be used. We have often found that the infusion of 200 to 1000 ml of plasma volume expander, as the block is taking effect, will prevent a serious fall in blood-pressure. Pressor drugs are seldom indicated: they may certainly produce a rise in arterial pressure but only at the expense of peripheral vasoconstriction with the risk of hypoxia at tissue level. Nevertheless, in rare instances when the pressure has dropped suddenly they provide the most rapid means of restoring the situation when combined with intravenous fluids. It should be understood, however, that central neural blockade interferes with the normal homeostatic response to haemorrhage, and blood transfusion should be given when hypotension is associated with blood loss.

The patient with an established block may not withstand movement readily. For this reason the authors prefer to give the spinal injection with the patient already on the operating table. Subsequently, all movements of the patient should be made with care and smoothness. Whenever the legs are lowered from the lithotomy position, the table should be inclined head downwards to compensate for the change in haemodynamics. Likewise, blood-pressure should be checked as soon as the patient arrives in the postoperative room.

The preoperative management of the patient before spinal analgesia does not differ greatly from management before general anaesthesia. Nervous and apprehensive patients will require relatively heavy sedation, and for this every anaesthetist will have his favourite drugs: opiates (e.g. papaveretum 10 to 20 mg or morphine 5 to 10 mg), pethidine (50 to 100 mg), neurolept agents (e.g. Thalamonal 1 to 2 ml), barbiturates (e.g. pentobarbitone 100 to

200 mg) or a benzodiazepine derivative (e.g. Diazemuls 10 to 20 mg). Other techniques include the administration of Althesin in a continuous drip or midazolam (Hypnovel), which has been recently introduced. Midazolam is gaining popularity because its duration of action is shorter than that of diazepam. It has a half life of two hours and its use is associated with amnesia. The dose required intravenously is of the order of 0.07 mg/kg, the total dose used being in the range of 2.5 to 10.0 mg. It is our preference to introduce the spinal needle and observe the effects of intradural or extradural injection with the patient conscious, though suitably sedated. This allows easy positioning of the patient and avoids the possibility of airway obstruction which can so easily occur in the anaesthetised subject. Moreover the doses of intravenous or inhalation agents necessary to produce light general anaesthesia, once the block is established, are much less than those required to ensure a relaxe l patient with absence of movement during insertion of a spina needle.

The maintenance of a free airway in a patient lightly asleep from intravenous agents during a successful block may require judgement and experience. Unobstructed respiration especially if the head is fully rotated to one side may require nothing other than careful observation. The insertion of a Guedel pharyngeal airway of suitable size may be quite satisfactory, although sometimes it will cause the patient to cough. The insertion of a soft nasopharyngeal airway, size 6 to 8, preceded by spraying of the naris with 4 per cent cocaine solution to cause both analgesia and decreased vascularity of the nasal mucosa often works well, although we have seen it cause epistaxis which is both inconvenient and unsightly. Both the oropharyngeal and the nasopharyngeal tube should be inserted following a small dose of intravenous barbiturate. Lastly, it is the custom of some anaesthetists to support the patient's jaw throughout the operation while administering a gaseous anaesthetic mixture.

We do, however, recommend tracheal intubation once general anaesthesia has been induced whenever the patient's position on the operating table or his anatomical peculiarities make it difficult to ensure a free airway throughout the operation. If it is decided to intubate after the local analgesic drug has been injected, care is necessary that the barbiturate and relaxant used for intubation do not further lower the blood-pressure, which is already being affected by the inactivation of the vasoconstrictor fibres. Most careful observation is necessary at this stage so that severe hypotension can be detected early and steps taken to control it. Another method of inserting a tracheal tube is following transtracheal analgesia (Bromage, 1978).

Drugs such as hyoscine and atropine which block the action of acetylcholine may have disadvantages. Quite apart from causing dryness of the mouth, they will prevent maximum contraction of the intestine by inhibiting the activity of the vagus.

REFERENCES

Austin, T. R. (1980) Low dose ketamine and diazepam during spinal analgesia. *Anaesthesia*, **35**, 391.
Birks, R. J. S., Edbrook, D. L. & Mundy, J. V. B. (1983) Correspondence. *Anaesthesia*, **38**, 295.
Bromage, P. R. (1978) *Epidural Anesthesia*, p. 476. Philadephia: Saunders.
Gjessing, J. & Tomlin, P. J. (1977) Intravenous sedation and regional analgesia. *Anaesthesia*, **32**, 63.
Nabi, R. A. (1966) Anaesthesia in the tropics. *British Medical Journal*, **2**, 1525.
Schweitzer, S. A. (1978) Chlormethiazole (Hemineurin) infusion as a supplemental sedation during epidural block. *Anaesthesia and Intensive Care*, **6**, 248.
Seow, L. T. & Ryall, R. G. (1982) Minimal haemolytic effects from 0.8 per cent chlormethiazole infusion in volunteer subjects. *Anaesthesia*, **37**, 646.
Wilson, J., Stephen, G. W. & Scott, D. B. (1969) A study of the cardiovascular effects of chlormethiazole. *British Journal of Anaesthesia*, **41**, 840.

11

Indications and contraindications

Indications

In the day-to-day practice of many anaesthetists there are none. Other workers of experience employ spinal intradural or extradural analgesia very frequently for abdominal operations and for interventions on the perineum and lower extremities. Many surgeons in Britain are unfamiliar with the technique while others are never so happy as when their anaesthetists employ spinal analgesia on their patients.

The method is most useful in robust young adults who are to be operated on for hernia repair or for lesions in the lower abdomen. It is widely used in obstetrics for normal delivery, for forceps extraction and for Caesarean section. While the introduction of muscle relaxants 40 years ago reduced the need for spinal analgesia, it is still a fact that the effects of this form of pain relief on body chemistry and metabolism are minimal. It allows spontaneous respiration to take place, usually avoiding the use of a tracheal tube, without the disadvantages of underventilation, avoids deep general anaesthesia and makes muscle relaxants unnecessary, thus avoiding the occasional harmful side-effects of this group of drugs. It can of course be used with light general anaesthesia to produce muscle relaxation and ischaemia.

For many years we have used spinal block, usually extradural, sometimes intradural, for the great majority of our patients requiring abdominal and perineal gynaecological operations. Coming fresh to the hospital, our gynaecological colleagues first tolerated our methods, soon accepted them, and then warmly appreciated the form of pain relief for the conditions produced, including relative lack of bleeding, freedom from reflex response to surgical stimuli and satisfactory post-operative recovery. They are now inclined to raise an eyebrow if general anaesthesia is suggested! We have personal experience of some hundreds of operations on the vertebral column, laminectomies etc. where the method of analgesia with its associated ischaemia adds significantly to the success of the procedure. For such operations extradural block is strongly requested by the surgeons in the great majority of cases (Thorne, personal communication) although intradural analgesia is preferred by some workers (Abouleish, 1981). Operations on the anal and perianal regions are well conducted under block analgesia, sacral extradural or low intradural. It must be pointed out, however, that we have worked with some surgeons who prefer the anaesthetist not to provide the complete relaxation of the anal sphincter associated with these forms of regional block.

It is not our aim to popularise either form of spinal analgesia; in fact, we think its use should be more restricted than it formerly was. For example, it would now be difficult to justify its choice for thoracic or for high abdominal surgery in the very ill patient, for here the physiological trespass would be great and the patient would need the most careful supervision, so that the anaesthetist capable of dealing with this delicate situation is likely to achieve, with general anaesthesia, equally good operating conditions with less anxiety. Central neural blockade has been used more and more frequently in recent years for surgery of the hip, both for total replacement and for fixation of fractures. Good results have been reported in spite of the fact that many patients are elderly. For example, there is a report (Thorburn et al, 1980) of two groups of patients, one receiving general anaesthesia, the other intradural block; in the spinal group there was a significantly reduced incidence of deep vein thrombosis after operation, and also in the need for and frequency of blood transfusion because of a 50 per cent decrease in the amount of blood lost. The resulting hypotension in the spinal group of patients gave rise to no increase in cardiac, cerebral or renal complications. There is evidence that deep vein thrombosis after operation is related to the amount of blood lost, so this very worrying sequel is not so often seen after spinal block (Sculco and Ranawat, 1975; Keith, 1977; McLaren et al, 1978; Davis et al, 1980; Thorburn et al, 1980; Davis and Lawrenson, 1981; Chin et al, 1982).

No doubt spinal analgesia could be dispensed with, but much would be lost. Like Nabi (Nabi, 1966), we have found it a boon in the occasional patient who dreads being made unconscious. On the physical side the procedure provides excellent operating conditions, with minimal metabolic upset, for lesions below the umbilicus. Few will deny the attractions for prostatectomy, both suprapubic and endoscopic, though the possible increased fibrinolytic effects of extradural block may cause concern for an operation where fibrinolysis is already pathologically increased due to urokinase release (Simpson et al, 1982). Amputation of the leg in elderly and atherosclerotic and diabetic patients can also be carried out conveniently under central neural blockade. Our experience of spinal analgesia, intradural or extradural for Caesarean section, has been entirely favourable and we believe that the patient is likely to benefit, on balance, from its use in such major interventions as resections of the colon, Wertheim's hysterectomy, total cystectomy (Ryan, 1982) and abdomino-perineal resection of the rectum. It is said to reduce the incidence of breakdown of the anastomosis of the colon (Aitkenhead et al, 1978; Pither, 1983). This fact has been confirmed in the dog where intradural block increased colon blood flow and so, presumably, aided healing after intestinal incision and suture (Aitkenhead et al, 1980). Nor should the needs of developing countries be overlooked. Here, shortage of staff, and economics play their parts in determining choice of method of pain relief. In mission hospitals, single-handed doctors may be faced with lists of minor operations such as hernia repairs, hydrocoeles and circumcisions; we are convinced of the value of spinal analgesia in such circumstances. The technique of lumbar puncture is usually simple in these flexible young patients, and since analgesia need not extend much above the umbilicus, little skill is needed in supervising the patient throughout the operation, and in the postoperative period the menaces of obstructed airway and inhalation of vomitus are eliminated (see p. 256). Spinal analgesia is an economical way of achieving pain relief (Farman, 1962; Nabi, 1966), a factor easily overlooked in our relatively affluent society. The cost is a fraction of that involved in the administration of general anaesthesia. It has been suggested that better X-ray pictures following femoral aortography can be obtained when pain is abolished by extradural block instead of by general anaesthesia (Miller et al, 1980). Certain types of neurological disease are not regarded as absolute contraindications to central neural blockade by some workers of experience in the UK, in Europe and in the US (Crawford et al, 1981). The authors of this book would, however, urge caution and prudence before contemplating block in patients suffering from such abnormalities. Many workers tend to avoid block in elderly patients, largely because of their fear of the hypotension almost invariably accompanying this form of pain relief. There are others who report good results in old people (Nightingale and Marstrand, 1981) especially when undergoing lower limb surgery (McKenzie et al, 1980). Phaeochromocytoma surgery is always a difficult problem for the anaesthetist so that various methods of management have been advocated over the years, extradural analgesia being one of them (Cousins and Rubin, 1973; Bromage, 1978; Stonham and Wakefield, 1983). A morbidly obese patient who is about to undergo an operation on the lower abdomen or the lower limbs is seldom welcomed by the anaesthetist. Such patients can be managed satisfactorily by extradural analgesia together with light general anaesthesia and, if necessary, IPPV (Buckley et al, 1983). If the catheter is left in place, injections given as necessary in the postoperative period will provide excellent pain relief without unduly depressing respiration (Fox et al, 1981). The patient with chronic respiratory disease, with irritable bronchial tree, active cough reflexes and a tendency to wheeze, may well be a candidate for central neural blockade, certainly for operations on the lower abdomen, perineum and legs. In these individuals the avoidance of the use of potentially irritant vapours and, in particular, the absence of any need for tracheal intubation may be expected to result in a smooth operative and immediate postoperative course without laryngospasm, bronchospasm, coughing and the changes in blood gases which may then follow.

Since the Polish surgeon, Johan von Mickulicz-Radecki (1850–1905), Professor of Surgery in Breslau showed over a four-year period, 1896–1900, that the incidence of postoperative chest complications was very similar after regional and general anaesthesia, surgeons and anaesthetists have been debating the best form of pain relief in patients with chronic lung disease. The skilled anaesthetist today can usually manage both techniques with safety and relative absence of harmful after-effects with either method. We do not regard either intradural or extradural analgesia as noticeably safer in these patients than general anaesthesia. Each patient and each operation must be assessed individually (Raven, 1971).

Continuous extradural block

Outside the operating room, extradural block has been employed in a variety of circumstances (Atkinson et al, 1982). An indwelling catheter with its tip in the extradural space allows serial injections of analgesic solution to be made to maintain block over a period of hours or days.

Postoperative pain relief can be provided by this technique, the method being specially useful in those individuals who have difficulty in expectoration and in whom postoperative atelectasis is particularly likely to occur; serial injections or continuous infusion can be employed (Griffiths, 1981). The analgesia produced enables vigorous coughing and physiotherapy to take place, since the quality of pain relief is superior to that provided by the narcotic analgesics.

The catheter can be introduced in the thoracic region, either between T.1 and T.4, or between T.8 and T.9 a procedure which need be no more difficult than when performed in the more usual lumbar area, if the acute angle of the thoracic spines is borne in mind. Indeed the direction which a needle must take if inserted between T.4 and T.7. (see Fig. 2.5a) is so oblique that injection at this level is not advised. There are workers who, at this level, prefer to use the hanging drop method for identification of the space with the patient in the sitting position, as the ligamentum flavum is less robust here than it is lower down (Dawkins and Steel, 1971). Small doses of local analgesic drug, e.g. between 7 and 10 ml of 0.25 or 0.5 per cent bupivacaine, can be injected as required, with good relief of pain following operations on the abdomen. The patient must lie down for some 20 minutes after each injection, but following this brief period of recumbency there is usually no reason why he should not walk about his room, as falls in blood-pressure are uncommon (Simpson et al., 1961). Prolonged dilatation of the bladder by fluid has been used as distension therapy for both the unstable bladder and for the amelioration of carcinoma (Ramsden et al, 1976). For the latter very unpleasant disease, extradural block by means of a catheter must go to a sensory level of T.8 but must also provide a low blood-pressure in the region of 80 mmHg (Helmstein, 1972).

Opinions differ on the effect of this method of pain relief after operation, on respiratory function. The usual fall in functional residual capacity with accompanying hypoxaemia, seen after upper abdominal surgery, is less than when narcotic analgesics are used (Spence and Smith, 1971), but extradural block after lower abdominal surgery (Drummond and Littlewood, 1977) or major hip surgery (Modig, 1976) may confer no special advantages in terms of respiratory function, as indicated by blood gas analysis.

Relief of pain in obstetrics by continuous extradural block is considered in Chapter 12.

A catheter or plastic cannula placed in the sacral canal can also be the route through which local analgesic solution is injected. There may be an indication here for the relief of pain following operations such as haemorrhoidectomy or posterior colpoperineorrhaphy or operations on the lower limb. Single shot injections of bupivacaine 0.5 per cent may produce a worthwhile period of analgesia in these cases. Similarly, following circumcision in children, a dose of 0.5 ml of 0.5 per cent bupivacaine with adrenaline per year of age has been recommended (Kay, 1974) or 0.55 ml of 1 per cent lignocaine with adrenaline 1:200 000 per kg of body weight (McGown, 1982). Sacral block has found a place in the management of patients suffering from ankylosing spondylitis in whom both tracheal intubation and lumbar injection may well prove to be difficult (De Board et al, 1981). Sacral block through an indwelling catheter will often provide satisfactory postoperative pain relief after orthopaedic operations on the lower limb. Injections through a catheter placed in the sacral extradural space are also of value in the relief of pain in labour (see Ch. 12, and Atkinson et al, 1982).

Contraindications

We seldom use either form of central neural blockade for operations in the upper abdomen. The level of blockade must be high and must reach T.5; hypotension may be profound; general anaesthesia is usually required and we do not find that even infiltration of the vagus near the oesophageal hiatus by the surgeon will always block vagal reflexes. We do not use the method for operations on the thorax, but the subject is well discussed by Bromage (1978). Lumbar puncture is unwise in patients who have had a subarachnoid haemorrhage, unless preceded by a C.A.T. scan (Duffy, 1982) although this opinion is disputed by some neurologists (Teddy et al, 1983). Spina bifida occulta is a relative contraindication and the condition may be suspected in a patient with a tuft of hair, deep dimpling or a port wine stain in the lumbar area (Farmer, 1975). Constrictive pericarditis, where both preload and afterload are compromised, is a disease requiring careful consideration as is any patient with obstruction of the vena cava which cannot be controlled. All would agree that the patient who has bled profusely and in whom blood replacement is inadequate is likely to do better under general anaesthesia than under any form of central neural blockade.

Spinal analgesia should not be attempted on an unwilling patient; and the surgeon too must be co-operative, for heavy handling of the tissues can make the procedure miserable for all concerned. The more ill the patient, the more inclined is the experienced anaesthetist to choose general anaesthesia in preference to spinal analgesia. Over the latter he has less immediate control, and it is seldom indicated in patients with hypovolaemia, dehydration, bleeding diseases, those on anticoagulants or with severe anaemia; and a recent episode of cerebrovascular insufficiency is a relative contraindication. The risk of surgery in a patient with a recent history of myocardial infarction is increased whatever the method of pain relief (Tarhan and Moffitt, 1972) and spinal analgesia should not be considered here unless the blood-pressure can be maintained, tachycardia avoided and the patient can be kept in a position which favours venous return to the heart. Indeed the anaesthetist is advised to consider carefully the indication for central neural blockade in any patient with a history of severe myocardial disease, particularly when the mechanical pump action of the heart may not be able to respond to the physiological changes induced by the block. Those with tight mitral stenosis, for example, and patients on treatment with negative inotropic or chronotropic drugs may not be able to compensate for changes in cardiac preload so that reduction of the cardiac output is likely to occur, resulting in diminished supply of oxygenated blood to the myocardium itself. It cannot be denied that experience of the management of patients in intensive therapy units which may involve mechanical ventilation, sedation and intensive monitoring, has made the administration of light general anaesthesia safe for many critically ill patients. For medico-legal reasons, it would appear advisable to consider, most carefully, spinal analgesia in a patient with any abnormality of the central nervous system whether it be degenerative or infective, acute, inactive or healed. Marked deformity of the back or chronic backache are relative contraindications and skin sepsis, at the site of puncture, an absolute one.

REFERENCES

Abouleish, E. (1981) Spinal anesthesia for laminectomy. *Anesthesia and Analgesia*, **60**, 169.

Aitkenhead, A. R., Wishart, H. Y. & Peebles Brown, D. A. (1978) High spinal nerve block for large bowel anastomosis. *British Journal of Anaesthesia*, **50**, 177.

Aitkenhead, A. R., Gilmore, D. G., Hothersall, A. P. & Ledingham, M. (1980) Effects of subarachnoid nerve block on arterial PCO_2 and on colon blood flow in dogs. *British Journal of Anaesthesia*, **52**, 1071.

Atkinson, R. S., Rushman, G. B. & Lee, J. Alfred (1982) *A Synopsis of Anaesthesia*, p. 448, 9th edn. Bristol: Wright.

Bromage, P. R. (1978) *Epidural Anesthesia*. Philadelphia: Saunders. p. 501.

Buckley, F. P., Robinson, N. B., Simonowitz, D. A. & Dellinger, E. P. (1983) Anaesthesia in the morbidly obese. A comparison of anaesthetic and analgesic regimens for upper abdominal surgery. *Anaesthesia*, **38**, 840.

Chin, S. P., Abou Madi, M. N. et al (1982) Blood loss in total hip replacement: extradural versus phenoperidine anaesthesia. *British Journal of Anaesthesia*, **54**, 491.

Cousins, M. J. & Rubin, R. B. (1973) The intraoperative management of phaeochromocytoma with total epidural sympathetic blockade. *British Journal of Anaesthesia*, **46**, 78.

Crawford, J. S., James, F. M., Nolte, H., Van Steenberge, A. & Shah, J. L. (1981) Regional analgesia for patients with chronic neurological disease and similar conditions. *Anaesthesia*, **36**, 821.

Davis, F. M. & Lawrenson, V. G. (1981) Spinal anaesthesia or general anaesthesia for emergency surgery in elderly patients. *Anaesthesia and Intensive Care*, **9**, 352.

Davis, F. M., Quince, M. & Lawrenson, V. G. (1980) Deep vein thrombosis and anaesthetic technique in emergency hip surgery. *British Medical Journal*, **281**, 1528.

Dawkins, C. J. Massey & Steel, G. C. (1971) Thoracic extradural (epidural) block for upper abdominal surgery. *Anaesthesia*, **26**, 41.

De Board, J. W., Ghia, J. N. & Guilford, W. B. (1981) Caudal anesthesia in a patient with ankylosing spondylitis. *Anesthesiology*, **54**, 104.

Drummond, G. B. & Littlewood, D. G. (1977) Respiratory effects of extradural analgesia after lower abdominal surgery. *British Journal of Anaesthesia*, **49**, 999.

Duffy, G. P. (1982) Lumbar puncture in spontaneous subarachnoid haemorrhage. *British Medical Journal*, **285**, 1163.

Farman, J. V. (1962) Two problems of anaesthesia in the underdeveloped countries. *British Journal of Anaesthesia*, **34**, 897

Farmer, T. W. (1975) *Pediatric Neurology*, p. 428, 2nd edn. Hagerstown: Harper & Rowe.

Fox, G. S., Whalley, D. G. & Bevan, D. R. (1981) Anaesthesia for the morbidly obese. *British Journal of Anaesthesia*, **53**, 811.

Griffiths, D. P. G. (1981) Postoperative pain prevention by continuous epidural infusions. *Anaesthesia*, **36**, 214.

Helmstein, K. (1972) The treatment of bladder carcinoma by hydrostatic pressure technique. *British Journal of Urology*, **44**, 434.

Kay, B. (1974) Caudal block for postoperative pain relief in children. *Anaesthesia*, **29**, 610.

Keith, I. (1977) Anaesthesia and blood-loss in total hip replacement. *Anaesthesia*, **32**, 444.

McGown, R. G. (1982) Caudal analgesia in children. *Anaesthesia*, **37**, 806.

McKenzie, P. J., Wishart, H. Y., Dewes, K. M. S., Gray, I. & Smith, G. (1980) Comparison of effects of spinal anaesthesia on postoperative oxygenation and perioperative mortality. *British Journal of Anaesthesia*, **52**, 49.

McLaren, A. D., Stockwell, M. C. & Reid, V. T. (1978) Anaesthetic techniques for surgical correction of fractured neck of femur. *Anaesthesia*, **33**, 10.

Miller, P. A., Fagraeus, L., Johnsrude, I. S. Jackson, D. C. & Mills, S. R. (1980) Epidural anesthesia in aortofemoral arteriography. *Annals of Surgery*, **192**, 227.

Modig, J. (1976) Respiration and circulation after total hip replacement surgery. A comparison between parenteral analgesics and continuous lumbar epidural block. *Acta Anaesthesiologica Scandinavica*, **20**, 225.

Nabi, R. A. (1966) Anaesthesia in the tropics. *British Medical Journal*, **2**, 1525.

Nightingale, P. J. & Marstrand, T. (1981) Subarachnoid anaesthesia for orthopaedic procedures in the elderly. *British Journal of Anaesthesia*, **53**, 369.

Pither, C. E. (1983) Correspondence. *British Medical Journal*, **286**, 1352.

Ramsden, P. D., Smith, J. C. & Dunn, M. (1976) Distension therapy for unstable bladder. *British Journal of Urology*, **48**, 623.

Raven, M. B. (1971) Comparison of spinal with general anesthesia in patients with chronic lung disease. *Anesthesiology*, **35**, 319.

Ryan, D. W. (1982) Anaesthesia for cystectomy: a comparison of two anaesthetic techniques. *Anaesthesia*, **37**, 554.

Sculco, T. P. & Ranawat, C. (1975) The use of spinal anesthesia for total hip replacement arthroplasty. *Journal of Bone and Joint Surgery*, **57A**, 173.

Simpson, B. R., Parkhouse, J. & Marshall, R. (1961) Extradural analgesia and the prevention of postoperative respiratory complications. *British Journal of Anaesthesia*, **33**, 628.

Simpson, P. J., Radford, S. G., Forster, S. J., Cooper, G. M. & Hughes, A. O. (1982) Fibrinolytic effects of anaesthesia. *Anaesthesia*, **37**, 3.

Spence, A. A. & Smith, G. (1971) Postoperative analgesia and lung function: a comparison of morphine with extradural block. *British Journal of Anaesthesia*, **43**, 144.

Stonham, J. & Wakefield, C. (1983) Phaeochromocytoma in pregnancy: Caesarean section under epidural analgesia. *Anaesthesia*, **38**, 654.

Tarhan, S. & Moffitt, E. A. (1972) Myocardial infarction after general anesthesia. *Journal of the American Medical Association*, **220**, 1451.

Teddy, P. J., Briggs, M. & Adams, C. B. T. (1983) Correspondence. *British Medical Journal*, **286**, 143.

Thorburn, J., Louden, J. R. & Vallance, R. (1980) Spinal and general anaesthesia in total hip replacement. *British Journal of Anaesthesia*, **52**, 1117.

Thorne, T. C. (1978) Personal communication.

12

Intradural and extradural spinal analgesia in obstetrics

Every anaesthetist is well aware of the unhappy combination of 'the full stomach' and general anaesthesia. It is not so generally realised, however, that a woman in labour must be regarded as having a 'full' stomach even though she has not taken anything by mouth for some hours. This applies with particular emphasis if labour has been prolonged and stressful. Should vomiting occur under general anaesthesia, the situation is all the more dangerous because the increased bulk of the patient makes more difficult any change of posture which may be required to maintain a clear airway. Statistics of pain relief in obstetrics show that inhalation of vomitus is the most common cause of mortality and morbidity. Any anaesthetist who has seen a woman under general anaesthesia, in the lithotomy position for the application of forceps, vomiting fluids imbibed hours previously, or at a Caesarean section, has seen copious vomiting before it was possible to intubate the unconscious patient, will not soon forget the spectacle.

Spinal analgesia offers certain clear advantages. Inhalation of vomitus is eliminated. The firm tone of the uterine muscle ensures prompt contraction after delivery, reduces blood loss, and if the use of forceps is intended, delivery is facilitated and trauma to the fetal head is minimised because of the profound relaxation of the pelvic floor.

History

There can be little doubt that when in 50 years time the intelligent mothers-to-be look back on the methods of pain relief in normal labour we employ today on their grandmothers, they will regard our practice as derisory. Although we ourselves know that they are better than open drop chloroform or Minnitt's nitrous oxide and air, they leave very much to be desired. Techniques of regional block were seldom employed 50 years ago whereas today they are gaining in popularity and increasing in safety with lessons to be learned from tracing their development. However, there is still a very long way to go before we are in sight of a satisfactory solution to the problem.

Intradural analgesia

Soon after the introduction of spinal analgesia by August Bier and Tuffier in 1899 (see Ch. 1) the new method was employed for operations on many parts of the body, and it is not surprising that it was used, or possibly misused, in obstetrics as early as 1900 (Kreis, 1900). Labat was clearly not an enthusiast for the n ethod in labour, a view also held by those who benefited from his teaching at the Mayo Clinic. Nor was the method much used in Europe until the visit of George P. Pitkin of New Jersey who was a competent anaesthetist and a superb salesman for what he called 'controllable spinal anaesthesia'. This took place in 1929 and, as a result of it, spinal analgesia underwent a revival of interest if not of popularity and its employment in obstetrics shared in this (Pitkin, 1927). When Pitkin returned to his own hospitals, interest in spinal analgesia waned although it was practised by a few enthusiasts, among whom was R. C. Thomas of Croydon (Thomas, 1944). Saddle-block was described by Adriani in 1946 (Adriani and Roma-Vega, 1946).

Extradural sacral (caudal) block

Single injection of procaine into the sacral extradural canal was described by Stoeckel of Marburg in 1909 (Stoeckel, 1909) for normal delivery and soon afterwards by Schlimpert and Schneider (Schlimpert and Schneider, 1910; Schlimpert, 1911) who used 50 ml of 1 per cent procaine solution. This pioneering work owed something to Arthur Laewen of Konigsberg, a general surgeon who found that the activity of procaine injected into the canal was potentiated by the addition of sodium bicarbonate (Laewen, 1910a, 1910b) In the US sacral analgesia was used in the Mayo Clinic in obstetrics in 1923 (Meeker and Bonar, 1923) and also by Rucker (1930) and Baptisti (1939).

A pioneer, almost completely unknown to English-speaking anaesthetists until recently, was Eugen Bogdan Aburel (Curelaru and Sandu, 1982). Aburel was born in Rumania in 1899, graduated in his native country and did postgraduate work in Paris. He wrote many of his scientific papers in French. In 1936 he became Professor of Obstetrics and Gynaecology in Iassy in Rumania and nine years later moved to the capital city, Bucharest. In 1930 he worked out the afferent nerve pathways of labour pains (Aburel, 1930) and in addition devised a satisfactory method of controlling them by the injection into the sacral canal through a fine malleable tube similar to a ureteric catheter, of 30 ml of 0.5 per cent cinchocaine solution, which could be repeated as required (Aburel, 1931). This valuable original work did not receive the worldwide notice that it deserved, due to political and linguistic reasons, and so had scant influence.

One of the most important advances, important not only because of its scientific value but because it also led directly to a large number of women throughout the world receiving relief from the distressing pains of labour, was the discovery by J. G. P. Cleland of the University of Oregon of the anatomy of the afferent course of the pains associated with labour (Cleland, 1933). Like Aburel before him, but unaware of the articles in the French literature, Cleland devised a practical technique for analgesia in labour. He advocated bilateral paravertebral somatic block of T.10 and T.11, together with sacral analgesia by means of 20 ml of 1 per cent procaine or 1:1500 cinchocaine injected into the sacral canal. Cleland worked in the department of physiology, first at McGill University, Montreal, then in the University of Oregon, using animals, mainly dogs for his investigations. This work set in motion the energies and enthusiasm of Robert Hingson and his colleagues who by their skill and persistence led to the technique soon to be called continuous caudal anesthesia being very widely practised in the US and to a lesser extent in Britain (Edwards and Hingson, 1942; Hingson and Edwards, 1942; Hingson and Southworth, 1942; Galley, 1949). At first Hingson and his followers used a malleable metal needle for continuous blocks, following the work on continuous spinal analgesia by Lemmon (Lemmon, 1940) but this very soon gave way to a plastic catheter (Adams et al, 1943). Today a plastic intravenous cannula attached to a length of plastic tubing is often used.

Extradural lumbar block

An early report describing injection of a single dose of local analgesic solution into the extradural space came in 1938 (Graffagnino and Seyler, 1938) from New Orleans. The continuous method, employing first a malleable needle and later a catheter, was pioneered by Flowers and his colleagues in 1949 (Flowers et al, 1949). Later developments included the substitution of the long-acting bupivacaine for lignocaine following the work of

Duthrie et al (1968), its use in continuous extradural block and the improvement in the quality of plastic catheters. The Huber pointed needle, which was devised by Tuohy for continuous intradural analgesia (Tuohy, 1945), was adapted by the Cuban anaesthetist Curbelo for continuous extradural block and simplified the performance of this type of pain control (Curbelo, 1949).

There was sporadic enthusiasm for continuous extradural analgesia in labour during the 1950s and 1960s but it was not until the advent of the long-acting bupivacaine together with the publicity following a press report at the 4th World Congress of Societies of Anaesthesiologists held in London in 1968 that the knowledge of the possibilities of the technique became known to the general public in the UK. Once that knowledge became widespread, potential patients were naturally not only willing but in many cases insistent on having this method of pain control during their own labour. Since then it has been used with increasing frequency in the hospitals of the world (Bromage, 1961; Brandstater, 1966). Only history will be able to tell us if this method of providing painless labour is a wise one.

Nerve supply of the uterus

The motor innervation of the uterus is not known for certain, although it is often stated that efferent impulses leave the cord between the 5th and the 10th thoracic segments, while contractions can continue normally in a uterus which has been deprived of nervous impulses. Motor activity seems to depend on humoral factors (Vasicka and Hutchison, 1963). Provided the blood-pressure is kept within normal limits, high spinal analgesia does not affect uterine tone or contractions (Bromage, 1961). Successful spontaneous vaginal delivery has been reported after inadvertent total spinal analgesia (Lund, 1971) and after paraplegia due to trauma and to poliomyelitis, which is not without pain, as the sensory innervation is not affected (Robertson, 1963).

Afferent impulses from the uterus pass to the spinal cord via the posterior roots of T.11, 12, L.1, 2 and even L.3 (Mair, 1939). The efferent nerve supply to the cervix and perineum, and the afferent supply from the same structures, travel in S.2–4.

Extradural block in obstetrics

Extradural analgesia is now accepted as a most effective method of pain relief during childbirth. The quality of relief obtained is superior to that provided by other techniques. While the dangers associated with general anaesthesia are normally avoided, the usual precautions should be taken in case general anaesthesia is required later. Nothing should be taken by mouth apart from routine antacids or H_2 antagonists. Analgesia can be obtained by a single injection, while the insertion of a catheter ensures a prolonged period of freedom from pain. Possible toxic effects are minimised because small doses can be used and repeated as necessary. At the same time, extradural block gives complete analgesia which will allow the performance of obstetric operations without the mother or the fetus being subjected to the risks of general anaesthesia.

There are, however, difficulties. Successful placement of a catheter into the extradural space requires a degree of expertise not possessed by all hospital doctors. There is a shortage of anaesthetists in many countries, especially those possessing the necessary skills for this type of work, and this results in many hospitals not being able to provide a regular extradural service. It is, however, quite possible for an extradural pain relief service to be provided by junior and senior obstetricians provided that they have been properly trained in the use of the technique and in the management of its complications (Taylor et al, 1977; Ghosh-Ray et al, 1980). The absence of a resident anaesthetist is not necessarily a contraindication to this type of organisation provided the medical personnel in the labour suite have been adequately trained (Adamson, 1973; Brown and Vass, 1977). In a series of over 300 reported consecutive cases of extradural analgesia provided by obstetricians (Taylor et al, 1977) there was a successful block with pain relief in 98 per cent of patients and a dural puncture rate of 2 per cent. The importance of fetal monitoring during the conduct of the labour was emphasised. Midwives also have to be trained in the supervision of patients undergoing this form of analgesia. The remote, but nevertheless haunting, possibility of serious neurological sequelae following spinal block (see Ch. 13) which is catastrophic when it occurs in a young woman with small children to look after must also be considered. That such misfortunes have taken place after extradural analgesia is without doubt. The fact remains that extradural block is a reasonably safe form of pain relief in obstetric practice in the vast majority of patients. Few will deny them the clear advantages which this method provides in spite of the small risk involved.

Extradural block gives very good analgesia, while the patient remains alert and co-operative. This is very advantageous during the second stage of labour, and the concentration of the drug used for the block should ideally be such as to provide analgesia but avoid motor impairment. A criticism of this method in labour is that the incidence of operative delivery is increased (Moir and Willocks, 1967), a finding which has been disputed (Doughty, 1969; Noble and de Vere, 1970; Bailey, 1983), but another study (Hoult et al., 1977) found that instrumental delivery was five times more common and malposition of the fetal head three times more common when extradural analgesia was employed than in mothers not receiving regional block.

The cardiovascular system in the obstetric patient

As pregnancy proceeds the heart enlarges, with an increase in both the thickness of the muscle and the volume of its chambers. Cardiac output increases from about 4.5 l/min to 6 l/min by the 10th week of pregnancy and the increase is maintained until term unless factors such as caval compression operate. There is a rise in both stroke volume and heart rate. Peripheral resistance is considerably reduced in pregnancy and systolic and diastolic arterial pressures usually fall in mid-pregnancy (the latter, more than the former) but return to non-pregnant levels as term approaches.

From the 32nd week of pregnancy the size of the gravid uterus has become sufficient to cause compression of the inferior vena cava in most subjects when the supine position is assumed (Kerr et al, 1964; Lees et al, 1967; Lees et al, 1970). Usually compensatory mechanisms come into play with diversion of venous blood via the paravertebral and azygos veins, a condition sometimes described as *latent* caval compression syndrome. In a minority of women such compensatory mechanisms are inadequate, venous return to the heart is seriously impeded and a gross fall in cardiac output results in a severe fall in arterial pressure. This is a situation of *overt* caval compression which results in the *supine hypotensive syndrome of pregnancy*. The significance of this condition to the anaesthetist (Scott, 1968) should not need emphasising. Whether caval compression is latent or overt, placental blood flow is reduced, but by interrupting the compensatory mechanisms which maintain arterial pressure the anaesthetist may convert the latent to the overt syndrome with resultant acute danger to mother and fetus. Reduction of placental blood flow may lead to a fall of arterial oxygen tension in fetal blood, together with acidosis.

When the patient goes into labour and the fetus descends the birth canal, caval compression may become less significant. However, uterine contractions may partly occlude the uterine arteries and reduce placental blood flow temporarily. Uterine contractions are thought to result in diminished pelvic perfusion and a fall of pulse pressure in the legs in one-third of normal labours if the patient maintains the supine position — the Posiero effect (Posiero, 1967).

Fortunately, these harmful actions can be largely overcome by turning the patient into the lateral position (Crawford et al, 1972; Downing et al, 1974; Drummond et al, 1974; Eckstein and Marx, 1974; Crawford, 1975b) or, where this is not possible, by tilting the patient to one side either by manipulation of the operating table controls or by inserting a wedge under the buttock. Tilt to the left is preferred (Buley et al, 1977) but tilt to the right can be tried if the former is not effective.

It is important to prevent hypotension which may result from extradural block. Not only should due attention be paid to posture but fluids should be infused intravenously to prevent hypovolaemia (Wollman and Marx, 1968); up to 2000 ml of Hartmann's solution may be administered (Lewis et al, 1983) while other workers advocate a proportion of polygelatine (Hallworth et al, 1982). Pressor agents should also be available. Prophylactic intramuscular ephedrine (Gutsche et al, 1982) cannot be relied upon to prevent hypotension (Rolbin et al, 1982). Ephedrine may be administered intravenously in doses of 10 to 30 mg to control blood-pressure falls associated with extradural block. It is the pressor drug of choice as it maintains both maternal arterial blood-pressure and placental blood flow better than other pressor agents (Schnider et al, 1968; Ralston et al, 1974). Alpha adrenergic drugs cause a substantial reduction in uterine artery blood flow and are to be avoided. Ephedrine does cross the placenta and may give rise to an increase in fetal heart rate.

Spinal block, whether intradural or extradural, is likely to cause a fall in arterial pressure which may become profound in the presence of caval compression. Even with the most careful management the incidence of hypotension has been reported to be as high as 80 per cent (Clark et al, 1976). Examination of fetal blood from the umbilical artery shows an association between maternal hypotension and fetal acidosis (Marx et al, 1969; Datta and Brown, 1977; Corke et al, 1982), though not between maternal hypotension and differences in Apgar scores (Marx et al, 1969; Ralston and Schnider, 1978). It is likely that duration of hypotension is more important than its degree in its effect on fetal well-being (Ebner et al, 1960). Short periods of hypotension, less than two minutes, are unlikely to give rise to fetal depression (Corke et al, 1982).

In some hospitals, extradural block is offered to all obstetric patients in whom no contraindication exists (Romine et al., 1970; Crawford, 1972a; Crawford, 1972b; Moore et al., 1974). Where resources and medical policy do not allow this, priority may be given to those patients with pre-eclampsia, slow painful labour, or cardiac or respiratory distress. The technique is also useful when the fetus is considered at risk or when operative intervention is likely, as in a trial of labour.

Extradural analgesia is clearly undesirable when the patient objects to it, when a skilled anaesthetist is not available or when the obstetrician is opposed to its use. It is not a suitable form of pain relief in the patient with cephalopelvic disproportion, when the fetal head is unengaged in the pelvis, in placenta praevia and in gross and uncontrolled nervousness. It should not be undertaken in the presence of local skin infection or of a coagulation abnormality due to disease or drugs. Gross hypovolaemia is another contraindication as severe hypotension may result from the block due to associated vasomotor paralysis.

Discussion has taken place about the suitability of extradural block in breech presentation or multiple pregnancy, though it is now generally accepted that there is no positive contraindication (Bowen-Simpkins and Fergusson, 1974) while abolition of inappropriate urges to push may avoid precipitate delivery of a small fetus through an incompletely dilated cervix. Where there has been a previous Caesarean section, some workers prefer to avoid a block in case a rupture of the scar might go unrecognised, though provided suitable precautions are taken there is no bar to extradural analgesia (Uppington, 1983). Another report (Kenney et al., 1978) points to the value of this type of analgesia in the presence of locked twins while it has been used also for Caesarean delivery of quadruplets (Datta et al, 1982).

Practical details of extradural block in labour

Block from the 10th thoracic to the 5th sacral segments is necessary for complete pain relief during labour. In practice the lower thoracic segments and perhaps the 1st lumbar are largely concerned with the appreciation of pain during the first stage of labour, and the 2nd sacral to the 4th sacral in the second stage. It would therefore be logical to use two catheters, one at the T.12/L.1 interspace and the other at L.4/5, or in the sacral extradural space. The two catheter technique (Potter and MacDonald, 1971) probably gives no better results, however, than a single catheter in either the L.1/2 or the

L.2/3 interspace, using gravity to aid the spread of the solution in the appropriate direction.

The analgesic drug most commonly employed in Britain for extradural injections in labour is bupivacaine. When injected through an indwelling catheter, volumes of the order of 5 to 8 ml suffice, and it has been shown that there is no advantage in the addition of adrenaline with these small doses (Reynolds and Taylor, 1970, 1971), but that systemic toxicity may arise if the total amount exceeds 320 mg (Reynolds et al., 1973). Strengths of 0.5 and 0.25 per cent solution have been most widely used, while good results have been claimed with 0.125 per cent in Belgium (Vanderick et al., 1974). Many workers now consider the optimal strength to be 0.375 per cent (Steel, 1968; Crawford, 1975b) as this provides the most efficient analgesia without motor block. The fact that etidocaine tends to cause motor paralysis in higher concentrations and poor or uncertain analgesia in more dilute solutions renders it less suitable than bupivacaine for extradural analgesia in obstetrics.

The choice of local analgesic agent for extradural analgesia in obstetrics is not difficult as bupivacaine is advantageous on a number of counts. Placental transfer is significantly less than in the case of lignocaine, prilocaine or mepivacaine, probably as a result of the greater protein binding of the first drug. Thus, although the maximal maternal blood levels are reached within 15 to 20 minutes of the extradural injection, the maximal levels in the umbilical vein are less than one-third of maternal blood levels in the case of bupivacaine (Thomas et al., 1969; Reynolds et al., 1973), but of the order of two-thirds when lignocaine is used (Thomas et al., 1968). Nor are the levels significantly different when adrenaline is added to the analgesic solution (Epstein and Coakley, 1967; Reynolds et al., 1973). Moreover the occurrence of tachyphylaxis with repeated injections of lignocaine may result in accumulation of the drug in maternal and fetal tissues (Moir and Willocks, 1966).

Prilocaine suffers the disadvantage that methaemoglobinaemia may occur in the mother and may cause diagnostic problems in the baby (Climie et al., 1967; Poppers and Mastin, 1970) due to cyanosis.

One disadvantage of bupivacaine as a local analgesic agent is the rather long period of latency as compared with lignocaine (Watt et al., 1968). In abdominal surgery, some workers (Howat, 1977) have sought to overcome this problem by the use of mixtures of bupivacaine and lignocaine, and it would seem to be logical that mixtures should be used in labour. Other workers have solved this problem of a rather prolonged latency by using 2-chloroprocaine which has a rapid time of onset, for the first injection (Villa and Marx, 1975). Moreover, since 2-chloroprocaine is rapidly metabolised it is not likely to cause problems as a result of placental transfer to the fetus. However, it is at present under review, following reports of prolonged sensory and motor deficits, following accidental intradural injection (Barsa et al, 1980; Covino et al, 1980; Ravindran et al, 1980; Reisner et al, 1980; Moore et al, 1982).

Extradural block may be used when surgical induction of labour is carried out (Caseby, 1974) or when the cervix is dilated to 5 or 6 cm in primigravidae or 3 to 4 cm in multiparae. The volume of solution required is between 5 and 8 ml in a single injection, and the effect may last for anything up to four hours, though a common finding is between two and three hours (Duthrie et al., 1968). The patient should be kept horizontal for relief of uterine pain, but when perineal analgesia is required the injection is better carried out with the patient sitting, and maintained in that position for five minutes, though the value of this has recently been disputed (Merry et al, 1983). Another approach is the continuous infusion of analgesic fluid via the catheter using a mechanical pump (Glover, 1977).

The technique of insertion of a catheter into the lumbar extradural space in labour is not very different from that used in other circumstances except that the pressure in the space may be positive during uterine contractions (Marx et al, 1962; Galbert and Marx, 1974; Messih, 1981). Is is therefore better to avoid methods of identification of the space which depend on the presence of a negative pressure. The loss of resistance technique using a syringe containing fluid or air is satisfactory.

Occasionally, difficulty is encountered when passing the tip of the catheter through the Tuohy needle even though it has slipped through quite easily during the preliminary preparation of equipment. It may be helpful to rotate the needle slightly, to use another catheter, or to ask the patient to extend the hips slowly (Crawford, 1978).

The catheter should not be advanced too far into the extradural space in case it takes a bizarre direction. Centimetre markings on both the needle and the catheter (Lee, 1962; Doughty, 1974) are useful here and a distance of 4 cm should be the limit of advance beyond the needle tip (Moir, 1976).

Full aseptic precautions are of course essential, and a bacterial filter should be used when injections are made. This has the added advantage that small particles of foreign matter such as glass, which can be a contaminant when the ampoule is opened, are barred from entry into the extradural space (Furgang, 1974; Crawford et al., 1975a). Aspiration of all solutions through an intradermal needle will also prevent injection of particulate material. In addition, the charged syringe may be enclosed within a sterile polypropylene bag (Cole, 1964).

In Britain, midwives are allowed to administer top-up injections provided that the first injection through the catheter has been given by a doctor. The midwife has of course to be properly trained in the technique. One of the reasons that the doctor is required to give the initial dose through the catheter is the fact that on rare occasions the tip of the catheter has punctured the dura (Moir and Hesson, 1965). Inadvertent intradural injection, with the possibility of a high or even a total spinal block might then cause a more profound and widespread zone of analgesia with accompanying hypotension requiring active resuscitative measures.

The patient must be observed carefully whenever the technique of extradural block is used. Blood-pressure measurements should be made at least every five minutes for the first 20 minutes following injection and at intervals between top-up doses. An intravenous infusion must be set up and care taken that the patient should avoid the supine position with the risk of caval compression by the gravid uterus. Lateral tilt of the bed or operating table or the use of a wedge under the right buttock minimises the risk when the patient must lie supine, when the lithotomy position is needed or during Caesarean section. If it is necessary for women to walk to the toilet following extradural block, they should be accompanied both because of possible hypotension and possible muscle weakness.

The nursing staff should be on their guard against retention of urine associated with the analgesia, and catheterisation should be performed if and when necessary. It may be wise to encourage patients to pass urine just before a top-up as sensation may then have returned.

Top-up doses of analgesic drug should be injected when the pains return, and when these are given by a midwife there must be a clearly understood policy. Written instructions by the doctor will include details of dose, the posture of the patient and the frequency of blood-pressure estimations. The midwife should check the dose and the drug with another person, and she must of course be properly trained in the technique. Ultimate responsibility for her actions is, however, always borne by the doctor concerned.

In labour and advanced pregnancy, smaller doses of analgesics than would be required in a normal woman must be used and, as a general rule, the systolic blood-pressure of the mother should be maintained above 90 mmHg. The incidence of post-lumbar puncture headache is fairly high in parturients, following either deliberate or accidental dural puncture, especially if a 16 or 18 gauge needle (e.g. a Tuohy needle) is employed.

Unfortunately pain relief during labour is not always complete and in all series of cases which have been published there has been described a small percentage of patients in whom the results have been unsatisfactory (Bromage, 1972; Crawford 1972b; Moore et al., 1974; Doughty, 1975). Unblocked segments have been described in up to 8 per cent of patients receiving a block (Moir and Willocks, 1967; Ducrow, 1971), the groin being the region where pain is sometimes experienced during an otherwise satisfactory block. This pain can often be relieved by the injection of a further 3 to 4 ml of analgesic solution with the patient lying on the side of the pain. Carbonated lignocaine may be used instead of the hydrochloride salt and this has been reported to be associated with a lower incidence of unblocked segments (Bromage, 1972), although this has been disputed (Moir et al., 1976).

Late complications

Spinal headache as a result of inadvertent dural puncture is even more distressing for the nursing mother than it is for the ordinary patient. Not only is it likely to interfere with her care of the baby if she has to receive analgesics or to remain in bed lying flat in the days following delivery, but it will detract from that feeling of contentment and well-being which normally follows parturition. Where the extradural catheter is in place it can be used for the single or repeated injection of Hartmann's solution to raise the extradural pressure and so reduce the leakage of cerebrospinal fluid. This is said to change the incidence from 73 to 21 per cent following dural puncture (Crawford, 1972d). The same solution can also be placed in the extradural space from the sacral canal by a single or by serial injection through a catheter. The use of an extradural blood patch is claimed to be even more effective (Ostheimer et al., 1974). Some doubts must, however, exist as the safety or the propriety of using this technique prophylactically whenever the dura is perforated, as a clot of the patient's own blood provides an excellent culture medium for bacteria gaining access through failure of aseptic technique or when blood-borne. Extradural infection has been described as having commenced 16 days after delivery, presumably as a result of bacteraemia secondary to high vaginal infection localising in an extradural haematoma (Crawford, 1975a). Bacteriological investigations of catheters placed in the extradural space show that they are not always as sterile as they are supposed to be (Hunt et al., 1977).

Neurological complications are discussed in Chapter 13. They can occur, independently of the analgesic technique, as a result of protrusion of an intervertebral disc (O'Connell, 1944), or of compression or traction on the lumbo-sacral plexus (Chalmers, 1949).

In recent years some doubt has been cast on the effects of maternal extradural block on the fetus. Some of the local analgesic drug is bound to pass into the fetal circulation (p. 264) and concern has been voiced about possible toxic effects. In a study of neurobehavioural responses of newborn infants, significantly lower scores were obtained when the mother had received extradural analgesia compared to a control group (Scanlon et al., 1964). It may be significant that the local analgesic drug used was either lignocaine or mepivacaine, both of which drugs pass more easily to the fetus than bupivacaine (p. 264). Other studies have shown that extradural analgesia is associated with less metabolic disturbance in the fetus than when pethidine is used for pain relief (Jouppila and Hollmen, 1976), while neurobehavioural responses of the newborn have not been affected when bupivacaine is used for maternal extradural block (Corke, 1977).

In two groups of comparable patients undergoing elective Caesarean section, one group was expertly managed under general anaesthesia, the other under extradural block. The subsequent well-being of both mothers and fetuses showed no marked difference (James et al., 1977).

Sacral block in labour

Continuous sacral analgesia (caudal analgesia), first introduced in the US in 1942 by Hingson and Edwards (Hingson and Edwards, 1942) has never been popular in obstetric practice in Britain, though it has its advocates. The sacral route has certain disadvantages. Considerably larger doses are necessary than when the lumbar approach is used and doses of up to 20 ml of 0.5 per cent bupivacaine may be required as an initial dose in the first stage of labour. Most anaesthetists would agree that correct placement of the needle is less certain in the case of the sacral canal than in the lumbar extradural space. Anatomical variations of the sacrum are common and it has been suggested that the sacral canal cannot be entered in up to 5 per cent of patients (Lindstrom and Moore, 1957; Carrie, 1972; Rubin, 1972).

A bizarre complication of sacral block is accidental injection into the presenting part of the fetus (Finster et al., 1965; Sinclair et al., 1965) and it has been recommended that sacral block should not be performed during the second stage of labour or when the fetal head is low in the pelvis (Moore, 1964; Bonica, 1970).

Accidental intrathecal injection is by no means impossible when the sacral approach is used. This is a possibility when a catheter is advanced to reach the upper sacral or lower lumbar region as the dural sac usually terminates at the level of the second piece of the sacrum. The presence of a wire stylet increases the possibility of this (Rubin, 1972). The authors have seen cerebrospinal fluid issue from a 40 mm needle inserted through the sacral hiatus. There is, therefore, no guarantee that accidental intradural injection will be avoided in sacral block.

There are, however, occasions when sacral block is indicated in obstetric practice. It may be appropriate when for some reason or other the lumbar extradural space cannot be found, or when a lumbar block has failed to include the sacral segments (Doughty, 1975). A single shot injection is also excellent for a low forceps extraction, when 20 to 30 ml of 1.5 per cent lignocaine forms a suitable solution.

Whenever sacral block is carried out the usual precautions must be taken against accidental intravascular or intradural injection, and when a catheter is used it must be firmly secured, and injection made through a bacterial filter.

Operative obstetrics

Extradural

Whether or not an extradural catheter is already in position when operative intervention becomes necessary, there are advantages in providing analgesia for the procedure by means of extradural block. For low forceps delivery it is necessary to block the sacral segments while for intrauterine manipulations, analgesia should extend as high as T.10. For Caesarean section, block up to T.6 or T.5 is recommended (Thorburn and Moir, 1980). The analgesic solution most commonly used in Britain is 0.5 per cent bupivacaine plain, but bupivacaine 0.75 per cent solution has its advocates on account of the more intense analgesia and motor block produced for operative surgery. The dose may be given in incremental amounts until the desired segmental level is reached. A supplementary dose of 1.5 ml of 0.5 per cent bupivacaine per segment between an existing level and T.6 has been suggested (Thorburn and Moir, 1980), while the use of incremental doses, in addition to preloading with intravenous fluids and avoidance of aorto-caval compression, is likely to lead to a reduction in the incidence of side-effects (Crawford, 1980). It is likely that a total dose of between 18 and 26 ml of 0.5 per cent bupivacaine will be required for Caesarean section (Thorburn and Moir, 1980). The authors have also obtained good results with a single shot of 20 to 24 ml of 1.5 per cent lignocaine with adrenaline 1:200 000. An intravenous line is essential, and preloading with up to 2000 ml of fluid is recommended. Hartmann's solution is often used (Lewis et al, 1983) but other workers employ polygelatin (Haemaccel) 500 ml with Hartmann's solution (Hallworth et al, 1982). Blood should be available if needed, and pressor drugs are occasionally required.

Intradural

Intradural spinal analgesia is an effective method for operative vaginal delivery and removal of retained placenta (Crawford, 1979) though in Caesarean section some fear the possibility of untoward cephalad spread with associated hypotension. Classically, hyperbaric solutions have been used to provide: (1) The so-called 'saddle block' (Adriani and Roma-Vega, 1946) which requires about 0.6 ml of solution with the patient sitting or in the lateral position with head-up tilt to provide sacral block for low forceps delivery. (2) Block up to T10 with 1.0 to 1.2 ml solution with the patient in the lateral position with slight head-down tilt suitable for intra-uterine manipulation or application of high forceps. (3) For Caesarean section block up to T5/6 is required; the volume should be increased to 1.6 ml, the patient being in the lateral position with some head-down tilt during injection though almost immediately afterwards placed on her back with a wedge.

Recently, there has been interest in the use of 0.5 per cent bupivacaine plain solution though it is clear that smaller doses are required in the pregnant patient at term than in the non-pregnant (Russell, 1983). Whereas a dose of 3 ml has been found unreliable in producing satisfactory conditions for lower abdominal surgery in the ordinary patient (Chambers et al, 1981), this dose has proved adequate for Caesarean section provided the patient is placed supine with a wedge soon after injection (Russell, 1983). It seems that as long as the patient at term is kept in the lateral position high levels of spread do not occur. This effect is different from that seen in non-pregnant patients when posture seems without much effect on the spread of plain solutions (see p. 191). It has been suggested that the slight hypobaricity of 0.5 per cent bupivacaine may encourage spread to the side uppermost during injection. Even spread may occur if the patient lies on her right side during injection and then is repositioned with a wedge under the right hip (Sprague, 1976).

As in the case of extradural block, pre-loading with intravenous fluids, the avoidance of aorto-caval compression and the administration of oxygen to the mother is likely to provide a smooth operative course. Blood for transfusion should always be available when Caesarean section is contemplated and the anaesthetist is entitled to skilled assistance whether regional or general techniques are employed.

The authors' experience of intradural block in obstetrics has been entirely favourable, though they are well aware that other workers are less enthusiastic. Certainly the technique can be accomplished more rapidly than when the extradural space has to be located; it is also advantageous when rapid onset of analgesia is required.

The selection of patients and the effect of pain relief, both general and regional on the mother and neonate, is discussed by Morgan (1983). All would agree that regional techniques should not be forced on patients who prefer general anaesthesia nor are regional methods suitable for hysterical patients or for those who are unable to make easy verbal contact with their attendants. Sympathetic management by both anaesthetist and surgeon is essential for the conscious patient. This, together with gentle technique, makes supplementary general anaesthesia unnecessary in the vast majority of anxious patients. Administration of oxygen to the mother throughout operation ensures oxygenation of both mother and fetus. Induction of general anaesthesia is not without risk, whether before or after delivery of the fetus, but in the opinion of the authors will very occasionally be necessary. Otherwise, agents such as diazepam 5 mg have been used after delivery (Crawford, 1980).

Extradural use of narcotic analgesic drugs in labour is discussed in Chapter 15.

REFERENCES

Aburel, E. B. (1930) Contributions à l'étude des voies nerveuses sensitives de l'uterus. *Comptes Rendus des Séances de la Société de Biologie* (Paris), **105**, 297–9.

Aburel, E. B. (1931) L'anesthésie locale continue (prolongée) en obstétrique. *Bulletin de la Société d'Obstétrique et Gynécologie* (Paris), **20**, 35–7.

Adams, R. C. Lundy, J. S. & Seldon, T. H. (1943) A technique for continuous caudal anesthesia: a preliminary report. *Proceedings of Staff Meetings of the Mayo Clinic*, **18**, 97.

Adamson, D. H. (1973) Continuous epidural anaesthesia in the community hospital. *Canadian Anaesthetists' Society Journal*, **20**, 687.

Adriani, J. & Roma-Vega, D. (1946) Saddle block anesthesia. *American Journal of Surgery*, **71**, 12–18.

Bailey, P. W. (1983) Epidural analgesia and forceps delivery: laying a bogey. *Anaesthesia*, **38**, 282.

Baptisti, A. (1939) Caudal anesthesia in obstetrics. *American Journal of Obstetrics and Gynecology*, **38**, 642.

Barsa, J. E., Batra, M., Fink, B.R. & Sumi, S. M. (1980) Correspondence. *Anesthesia and Analgesia*, **59**, 810.

Bonica, J. J. (1970 In Schnider, S. M. (ed.) *Obstetrical Anesthesia — Current Concepts and Practice*. Baltimore: Williams & Wilkins.

Bowen-Simpkins, P. & Fergusson, I. L. C. (1974) Lumbar epidural block and the breech presentation. *British Journal of Anaesthesia*, **46**, 420.

Brandstater, B. (1966) Epidural analgesia in obstetrics. *Acta Anaesthesiologica Scandinavica Suppl.*, **25**, 345.

Bromage, P. R. (1961) Continuous lumbar epidural analgesia for obstetrics. *Canadian Medical Association Journal*, **85**, 1136.

Bromage, P. R. (1972) Unblocked segments in epidural analgesia for relief of pain in labour. *British Journal of Anaesthesia*, **44**, 676.

Brown, S. E. & Vass, A. C. R. (1977) An extradural service in a district general hospital. *British Medical Journal*, **49**, 243.

Buley, R. J. R., Downing, J. W., Brock-Utne, J. G. & Cuerden, C. (1977) Right versus left lateral tilt for Caesarean section. *British Journal of Anaesthesia*, **49**, 1009.

Carrie, L. E. S. (1972) In Doughty, A. (ed.) *Proceedings of the Symposium on Epidural Analgesia in Obstetrics*, p. 99. London: Lewis.

Caseby, N. G. (1974) Epidural analgesia for the surgical induction of labour. *British Journal of Anaesthesia*, **46**, 747.

Chalmers, J. A. (1949) Traumatic neuritis in the puerperium. *Journal of Obstetrics and Gynaecology of the British Commonwealth*, **56**, 205.

Chambers, W. A., Edstrom, H. H. & Scott, B. D. (1981) Effect of baricity on spinal anaesthesia with bupivacaine. *British Journal of Anaesthesia*, **53**, 279.

Clark, R.B., Thompson, D. S. & Thompson, C. H. (1976) Prevention of spinal hypotension associated with Cesarean section. *Anesthesiology*, **45**, 670.

Cleland, J. G. P. (1933) Paravertebral anesthesia in obstetrics. *Surgery, Gynecology and Obstetrics*, **57**, 51.

Climie, C. R., McLean, S., Starmer, G. A. & Thomas, J. (1967) Methaemoglobinaemia in mother and foetus following continuous epidural analgesia with prilocaine. *British Journal of Anaesthesia*, **39**, 155.

Cole, P. V. (1964) Continuous epidural lignocaine — a safe method. *Anaesthesia*, **19**, 562.

Corke, B. C. (1977) Neurobehavioural responses of the newborn. The effect of different forms of maternal analgesia. *Anaesthesia*, **32**, 539.

Corke, B. C., Datta, S., Ostheimer, G. W., Weiss, J. B. & Alper, M. H. (1982) Spinal anaesthesia for Caesarean section. The influence of hypotension on neonatal outcome. *Anaesthesia*, **37**, 658.

Covino, B. G., Marx, G. F., Finster, M. & Zsigmond, E. K. (1980) Editorial. Prolonged sensory/motor deficits following inadvertent spinal anesthesia. *Anesthesia and Anesthesia and Analgesia*, **59**, 399.

Crawford, J. S. (1972a) Lumbar epidural block in labour — a clinical analysis. *British Journal of Anaesthesia*, **44**, 66.

Crawford, J. S. (1972b) The second thousand epidural blocks in an obstetric hospital practice. *British Journal of Anaesthesia*, **44**, 1277.

Crawford, J. S. (1978) *Principles and Practice of Obstetric Anaesthesia*, 4th edn. Oxford: Blackwell.

Crawford, J. S. (1972d) The prevention of headache consequent upon dural puncture. *British Journal of Anaesthesia*, **44**, 598.

Crawford, J. S. (1975a) Pathology in the extradural space. *British Journal of Anaesthesia*, **47**, 412.

Crawford, J. S. (1975b) Patient management during extradural anaesthesia for obstetrics. *British Journal of Anaesthesia*, **47**, 273.

Crawford, J. S. (1979) Experience with spinal analgesia in a British obstetric unit. *British Journal of Anaesthesia*, **51**, 531.

Crawford, J. S. (1980) Experiences with lumbar extradural analgesia for Caesarean section. *British Journal of Anaesthesia*, **52**, 821.

Crawford, J. S., Burton, M. & Davies, P. (1972) Time and lateral tilt at Caesarean section. *British Journal of Anaesthesia*, **44**, 477.

Crawford, J. S., Williams, M. E. & Veales, S. (1975) Correspondence. Particulate matter in the extradural space. *British Journal of Anaesthesia*, **47**, 807.

Curbelo, M.M. (1949) Continuous segmental peridural anesthesia by means of a ureteric catheter. *Anesthesia and Analgesia Current Researches*, **28**, 13.

Curelaru, I. & Sandu, L. (1982) Eugen Bogdan Aburel (1899-1975). *Anaesthesia*, **37**, 663-9.

Datta, S. & Brown, W. V. (1977) Acid-base states in diabetic mothers and their infants following general or spinal anesthesia for Cesarean section. *Anesthesiology*, **42**, 272.

Datta, S., Poreda, M., Naulty, J. S., Ostheimer, G. W., Greene, M. F. & Weiss, J. B. (1982) Epidural anesthesia for Cesarean delivery for quadruplets; acid-base and local anesthetic concentrations. *Regional Anesthesia*, **7**, 69.

Doughty, A. (1969) Selective epidural analgesia and the forceps rate. *British Journal of Anaesthesia*, **41**, 1058.

Doughty, A. (1974) A precise method of cannulating the lumbar epidural space. *Anaesthesia*, **29**, 63.

Doughty, A. (1975) Lumbar epidural analgesia — the pursuit of perfection. *Anaesthesia*, **30**, 741.

Downing, J. W., Coleman, A .J., Mahomedy, M. C., Jeal, D. E. & Mahomedy, Y. H. (1974) Lateral tilt table for Caesarean section. *Anaesthesia*, **29**, 696.

Drummond, G. B., Scott, S. E. M., Lees, M. M. & Scott, D. B. (1974) Effects of posture on limb blood-flow in late pregnancy. *British Medical Journal*, **4**, 587.

Ducrow, M. (1971) The occurrence of unblocked segments during continuous lumbar epidural analgesia for pain relief in labour. *British Journal of Anaesthesia*, **43**, 1172.

Duthrie, A. M., Wyman, J. B. & Lewis, G. A. (1968) Bupivacaine in labour. *Anaesthesia*, **23**, 20.

Ebner, H., Barcohana, J. & Brytoshun, A. K. (1960) Influence of postspinal hypotension on the fetal electrocardiogram. *American Journal of Obstetrics and Gynecology*, **80**, 569.

Eckstein, K. L. & Marx, G. F. (1974) Aorto-caval compression and uterine displacement. *Anesthesiology*, **40**, 92.

Edwards, W. B. & Hingson, R. A. (1942) Continuous caudal anesthesia in obstetrics. *American Journal of Surgery*, **57**, 459-64.

Epstein, B. S. & Coakley, C. S. (1967) Passage of lidocaine and prilocaine across the placenta. *Anesthesiology*, **28**, 246.

Finster, M. Poppers, P. J., Sinclair, J. C. Morishima, H. O. & Daniels, S. S. (1965) Accidental intoxication of the fetus with local anesthetic drug during caudal anesthesia. *American Journal of Obstetrics and Gynecology*, **92**, 922.

Flowers, C. E., Hellman, L. M. & Hingson, R. A. (1949) Continuous peridural anesthesia and analgesia for labour, delivery and Cesarean section. *Anesthesia and Analgesia* Current Researches, **28**, 181.

Furgang, F. A. (1974) Glass particles in ampoules. *Anesthesiology*, **41**, 525.

Galbert, M. W. & Marx, G. F. (1974) Extradural pressures in the parturient patient. *Anesthesiology*, **40**, 499.

Galley, A. H. (1949) Continuous caudal analgesia in obstetrics. *Anaesthesia*, **4**, 154.

Ghosh-Ray, G. C., Taylor, A. B. & Alberts, F. (1980) an integrated pain relief service for labour: cooperation between obstetricians, anaesthetists and midwives. *Anaesthesia*, **35**, 510.

Glover, D. J. (1977) Continuous epidural analgesia in the obstetric patient. A feasibility study using a mechanical infusion pump. *Anaesthesia*, **32**, 499.

Graffagnino, P. & Seyler, L. W. (1938) Epidural anesthesia in obstetrics. *American Journal of Obstetrics and Gynecology*, **35**, 587–602.

Gutsche, B. B., Cole, A. F. D., Hew, E. M., Pollard, A. & Virgant, S. (1982) Prophylactic intramuscular ephedrine before epidural anaesthesia for Caesarean Section. *Canadian Anaesthetists' Society Journal*, **29**, 148.

Hallworth, D., Jellicose, J. A. & Wilkes, R. G. (1982) Hypotension during epidural anaesthesia for Caesarean section: a comparison of intravenous loading with crystalloid and colloidal solutions. *Anaesthesia*, **37**, 53.

Hingson, R. A. & Edwards, W. B. (1942) Continuous caudal anesthesia during labor and delivery. *Anesthesia and Analgesia* Current Researches, **21**, 301.

Hingson, R. A. & Southworth, J. L. (1942) Continuous caudal anesthesia. *American Journal of Surgery*, **58**, 93.

Hoult, I. J. MacLennan, A. H. & Carrie, L. E. S. (1977) Lumbar epidural analgesia in labour — relation to fetal malposition and instrumental delivery. *British Medical Journal*, **1**, 14.

Howat, D. D. C. (1977) Anaesthesia for pancreatic and biliary surgery. *Proceedings of the Royal Society of Medicine*, **70**, 152.

Hunt, J. R., Rigor, B. M. & Collins, I. R. (1977) The potential for contamination of continuous epidural catheters. *Anesthesia and Analgesia*, **56**, 222.

James, F. M., Crawford, J. S., Hopkinson, R., Davies, P. & Naiem, H. (1977) *Anesthesia and Analgesia*, **56**, 228.

Jouppila, R. & Hollmen, A. (1976) The effect of segmental epidural analgesia on maternal and foetal acid-base balance, lactate, serum potassium and creatinine phosphokinase during labour. *Acta Anaesthesiologica Scandinavica*, **20**, 239.

Kenney, A., Koh, L. S. & Pole, Y. L. (1978) A case of locked twins managed under lumbar epidural analgesia. *Anaesthesia*, **33**, 32.

Kerr, M. G., Scott, D. B. & Samuel, E. (1964) Studies of the inferior vena cava in pregnancy. *British Medical Journal*, **1**, 532.

Kreis, A. (1900) Ueber Medullarnarkose bei Gebärenden. *Zentralblatt für Gynäkologie*, July, 747.

Laewen, A. (1910a) The utilisation of sacral anaesthesia in surgery. *Zentralblatt für Chirurgie*, **37**, 708.

Laewen, A. (1910b) Über die Verwendung des Novokains im Natriumbicarbonat Kochsalzlosungen zur lokales Anaesthesie. *Munchener Medizinische Wochenschrift*, **44**, 2044–6.

Lee, J. A. (1962) A new catheter for continuous extradural analgesia. *Anaesthesia*, **17**, 248.

Lees, M. M., Scott, D. B., Kerr, M. G. & Taylor, S. H. (1967a) The circulatory effects of recumbent postural change in late pregnancy. *Clinical Science*, **32**, 453.

Lees M. M., Scott D. B. and Kerr M. G. (1970). Haemodynamic changes associated with labour. *Journal of Obstetrics and Gynaecology of the British Commonwealth*, **77**, 29.

Lemmon, W. T. (1940) A method for continuous spinal anesthesia. *Annals of Surgery*, **3**, 141–4.

Lewis, M., Thomas, P. & Wilkes, R. G. (1983) Hypotension during spinal analgesia for Caesarean section. *Anaesthesia*, **38**, 250.

Lindström, C. & Moore, D. C. (1957) Trends in obstetrical anesthesia following the acceptance of a twenty-four hour physician anesthesia service. *Surgery, Gynecology and Obstetrics*, **65**, 63.

Lund, P. C. (1971) *Principles and Practice of Spinal Anesthesia*, p. 530. Springfield: Thomas.

Mair, J. C. (1939) The nature of the pain of labour. *Journal of Obstetrics and Gynaecology of the British Empire*, **46**, 409.

Marx, G. F., Cosmi, E. V. & Woolman, S. B. (1969) Biochemical status and clinical condition of mothers and infants at Cesarean section. *Anesthesia and Analgesia*, **49**, 986.

Marx, G. F., Uka, Y. & Orkin, L. R. (1962) Cerebrospinal fluid pressures during labor. *American Journal of Obstetrics and Gynecology*, **84**, 213.

Meeker, W. R. & Bonar, B. E. (1923) Regional anesthesia in gynecology and obstetrics. *Surgery, Gynecology and Obstetrics*, **37**, 816.

Merry, A. F., Cross, J. A., Mayadeo, S. V. & Wild, C. J. (1983) Posture and spread of extradural analgesia in labour. *British Journal of Anaesthesia*, **55**, 303.

Messih, M. N. A. (1981) Epidural space pressures during pregnancy. *Anaesthesia*, **36**, 775.

Moir, D. D. (1976) *Obstetric Anaesthesia and Analgesia*. London: Bailliére Tindall.

Moir, D. D. & Hesson, W. R. (1965) Dural puncture by epidural catheter. *Anaesthesia*, **20**, 373.

Moir, D. D. Willocks, J. (1966) Continuous epidural analgesia in incoordinate uterine action. *Acta Anaesthesiologica Scandinavica* Suppl., **23**, 144.

Moir, D. D. & Willocks, J. (1967) Management of incoordinate uterine action under continuous epidural analgesia. *British Medical Journal*, **3**, 396.

Moir, D. D., Slater, P. J., Thorburn, J., McLaren, R. & Moodie, J. (1976) Extradural analgesia in obstetrics — a controlled trial of carbonated lignocaine and bupivacaine hydrochloride, with and without adrenaline. *British Journal of Anaesthesia*, **48**, 129.

Moore, D. C. (1964) *Anesthetic Techniques for Obstetrical Anesthesia and Analgesia*. Springfield: Thomas.

Moore, D. C., Spierdyk, J., Van Cleef, J. D., Coleman, D. L. & Love, G. F. (1982) Four more cases of quite severe neurological sequelae after the use of 3 per cent chloroprocaine. *Anesthesia and Analgesia*, **61**, 155.

Moore, J., Murnaghan, G. A. & Lewis, M. A. (1974) A clinical evaluation of the material effects of lumbar extradural analgesia for labour. *Anaesthesia*, **29**, 537.

Morgan, H. (1983) Caesarean section under epidural analgesia. *British Journal of Hospital Medicine*, **30**, 179.

Noble, A. D. & de Vere, R. D. (1970) Epidural analgesia in labour. *British Medical Journal*, **2**, 296.

O'Connell, J. E. A. (1944) Maternal obstetrical paralysis. *Surgery, Gynecology and Obstetrics*, **79**, 374.

Ostheimer, G. N., Palahniuk, R. J. & Schnider, S. M. (1974) Correspondence. Epidural blood patch for the post-lumbar-puncture headache. *Anesthesiology*, **41**, 307.

Pitkin, G. P. (1927) Controllable spinal anesthesia. *Journal of the Medical Society of New Jersey*, **24**, 425.

Poppers, P. J. & Mastin, A. R. (1970) Maternal and foetal methaemoglobinaemia caused by prilocaine. *Acta Anaesthesiologica Scandinavica* Suppl., **37**, 258.

Posiero, J. J. (1967) Compression of the aorta or iliac arteries by the contracting human uterus during labour. In Caldeyro-Barcia, E. (ed.) *Effects of Labour on Fetus and Newborn*. New York: Pergamon.

Potter, N. & MacDonald, R. D. (1971) Obstetric consequences of epidural analgesia in multiparous patients. *Lancet*, **1**, 1031.

Ralston, D. H. & Schnider, S. M. (1978) The fetal and neonatal effects of regional anesthesia in obstetrics. *Anesthesiology*, **48**, 34.

Ralston, D. H., Schnider, S. M. & de Lorimer, A. A. (1974) Effect of equipotent ephedrine, metaraminol, mephentermine and methoxamine on uterine blood-flow in the pregnant ewe. *Anesthesiology*, **40**, 354.

Ravindran, R. S., Bond, V. K., Tasch, M. D., Gupta, C. D. & Luerssen, T. G. (1980) Prolonged neural blockade following regional analgesia with 2-chloroprocaine. *Anesthesia and Analgesia*, **59**, 447.

Reisner, L. S., Hocaman, B. N. & Plumer, M. H. (1980) Persistent neurologic deficit and adhesive arachnoiditis following intrathecal 2-chloroprocaine injection. *Anesthesia and Analgesia*, **59**, 452.

Reynolds, F. & Taylor, G. (1970) Maternal and neonatal blood concentrations of bupivacaine. *Anaesthesia*, **25**, 14.

Reynolds, F. & Taylor, G. (1971) Plasma concentrations of bupivacaine during continuous epidural analgesia in labour: the effect of adrenaline. *British Journal of Anaesthesia*, **43**, 436.

Reynolds, F., Hargrove, R. L. & Wyman, J. B. (1973) Maternal and foetal plasma concentrations of bupivacaine after epidural block. *British Journal of Anaesthesia*, **45**, 1049.

Robertson, D. N. S. (1963) The paraplegic patient in labour and pregnancy. *Proceedings of the Royal Society of Medicine*, **56**, 381.

Rolbin, S. H., Cole, A. F. D., Hew, E. M., Pollard, A. & Virgint, S. (1982) Prophylactic intramuscular ephedrine before epidural anaesthesia for Caesarean section: efficacy and actions on the foetus and newborn. *Canadian Anaesthetists' Society Journal*, **29**, 148.

Romine, J. C., Clark, R. B. & Brown, W. E. (1970) Lumbar epidural anaesthesia in labour and delivery: one year's experience. *Journal of Obstetrics and Gynaecology of the British Commonwealth*, **77**, 722.

Rubin, A. P. (1972) The choice between the lumbar and caudal route. In Doughty, A. (ed.) *Proceedings of the Symposium on Epidural Analgesia in Obstetrics*, p. 91. London: Lewis.

Rucker, M. P. (1930) Epidural anesthesia in obstetrics. *Anesthesia and Analgesia, Current Researches*, **9**, 67.

Russell, I. F. (1983) Spinal anaesthesia for Caesarean section: the use of 0.5 per cent bupivacaine. *Anaesthesia*, **37**, 346

Scanlon, J. W., Brown, W. U., Weiss, J. B. & Alper, M. H. (1974). Neurobehavioral responses of newborn infants after maternal epidural anesthesia. *Anesthesiology*, **40**, 121.

Schlimpert, H. (1911) Über lokal extradural Anaesthesie. *Deutsche Medizinische Wochenschrift*, **37**, 719.

Schlimpert, H. & Schneider, K. (1910) Sacral anaesthesia in gynaecology and obstetrics. *Münchener Medizinische Wochenschrift*, **57**, 2561–5.

Schnider, S. M., de Lorimer, A. A., Asling, J. H. & Morishima, H. O. (1968) Vasopressors in obstetrics. I. Correction of fetal acidosis with ephedrine during spinal hypotension. *American Journal of Obstetrics and Gynecology*, **102**, 911.

Scott, D. B. (1968) Inferior vena caval occlusion in late pregnancy and its importance in anaesthesia. *British Journal of Anaesthesia*, **40**, 120.

Sinclair, J. C., Fox, H. A., Lentz, J. F. Fued, C. L. & Murphy, J. (1965) Intoxication of the fetus by a local anaesthetic. *New England Journal of Medicine*, **273**, 1173.

Sprague, D. H. (1976) Effects of position and uterine displacement on spinal anesthesia for Cesarean section. *Anesthesiology*, **44**, 164.

Steel, G. C. (1968) Bupivacaine: a comparison with lignocaine in epidural block. *Proceedings of the Royal Society of Medicine*, **61**, 1157.

Stoekel, W. (1909) Concerning sacral anaesthesia. *Zentralblatt für Gynäkologie*, **33**, 1.

Taylor, A. B. W., Abukhalil, S. H., El-Guindi, M. M., Tharian, B. & Watkins, J. A. (1977) Lumbar epidural analgesia in labour: a 24-hour service provided by obstetricians. *British Medical Journal*, **2**, 370.

Thomas, R. C. (1944) Caesarean section under spinal anaesthesia. *Journal of Obstetrics and Gynaecology of the British Empire*, **51**, 324.

Thomas, J., Climie, C. R. & Mather, L. E. (1968) Placental transfer of lignocaine following lumbar epidural administration. *British Journal of Anaesthesia*, **40**, 965.

Thomas, J., Climie, C. R. & Mather, L. E. (1969) Maternal plasma levels and placental transfer of bupivacaine following epidural analgesia. *British Journal of Anaesthesia*, **41**, 1035.

Thorburn, J. & Moir, D. D. (1980) Epidural analgesia for elective Caesarean section. Technique and its assessment. *Anaesthesia*, **35**, 3.

Tuohy, E. B. (1945) Continuous spinal anesthesia: a new method utilising a ureteric catheter. *Surgical Clinics of North America*, **25**, 834.

Uppington, J. (1983) Epidural analgesia and previous Caesarean section. *Anaesthesia*, **38**, 336.

Vanderick, C., Geerinckx, K., van Steenberge, A. L. & de Muylder, E. (1974) Bupivacaine 0.125 per cent in epidural block analgesia during childbirth. Clinical evaluation. *British Journal of Anaesthesia*, **46**, 838.

Vasicka, A. & Hutchison, H. T. (1963) Fetal response to induction, augmentation and correction of labour by oxytocin. *American Journal of Obstetrics and Gynecology*, **85**, 8.

Villa, E. A. & Marx, G. F. (1975) Chloroprocaine — bupivacaine. Sequence for obstetrical extradural analgesia. *Canadian Anaesthetists' Society Journal*, **22**, 76.

Watt, M. J., Ross, D. M. & Atkinson, R. S. (1968) A double-blind trial of bupivacaine and lignocaine. (Latency and duration in extradural blockade.) *Anaesthesia*, **23**, 331.

Wollmann, S. B. & Marx, G. F. (1968) Acute hydration for prevention of hypotension of spinal anaesthesia in obstetrics. *Anesthesiology*, **29**, 374.

13

Complications and sequelae

The most common complications during an operation conducted under central neural blockade are hypotension with cardiovascular depression, respiratory depression, sometimes going on to respiratory arrest, and, in the case of extradural block, total spinal due to accidental dural puncture. Convulsions may be seen occasionally following the intravascular injection of local analgesic solution. Headache may complicate dural puncture, either deliberate in intradural block, or accidentally during a proposed injection into the extradural space.

Headache

The typical headache which may follow lumbar puncture or spinal analgesia is diffuse, sometimes throbbing, and may be accompanied by stiffness of the neck. Its onset is likely to be 12 to 24 hours after the lumbar puncture and it may last up to a week. Occasionally it may go on for several weeks. It is not directly related to cerebrospinal fluid pressure or the volume of fluid lost or withdrawn (Handler et al, 1982).

Estimates of the incidence of headache after spinal analgesia range between 3 and 30 per cent (Tourtellotte, 1964; Crawford, 1979), with an average of 13 per cent according to other observers (Abouleish, et al, 1975b), while the condition is by no means unknown following simple lumbar puncture. Its occurrence is influenced by age, sex, type of operation performed, technique of spinal analgesia employed, and the measures taken for its prevention (Moore, 1955). This complication cannot be completely avoided however skilled and experienced the anaesthetist may be. Headache is, and always has been, a sequel frequent and disabling enough to intrude itself into any general picture of spinal analgesia. Indeed, prominent reference is made to this unpleasant complication in the first two records of operations carried out under spinal analgesia by

Bier (Bier, 1899) and Tuffier (Tuffier, 1899), and it cannot be affirmed that the prediction of the latter 'the explanation of it will come later' has been completely fulfilled even now after 85 years. But there is almost universal agreement that the frequency and severity of any headache depends principally on the size of the lumbar puncture needle used (Frumin, 1969; Tourtellotte and Henderson, 1972; Gerner, 1980; Ekstein et al, 1982). Headache after inadvertent dural puncture with a Tuohy needle while trying to place a catheter in the extradural space has been estimated to be 70 to 75 per cent (Crawford, 1972b; Craft et al, 1973). Other workers report a slightly lower incidence of headache with the Tuohy needle (Crawford, 1972a).

Observations during operations on the brain under local analgesia, (Symonds, 1946) show that the brain itself is insensitive but that pain is caused by traction on structures which support and anchor it, particularly the dura mater round the base of the brain, and the tentorium. Pulling on the blood vessels is also painful. This resembles the state of affairs within the abdominal cavity where, although the main structures are insensitive, pain may be elicited by traction on the anchoring mesentery and blood vessels. Other experiments show that headache can be caused by anything which increases the amplitude of arterial pulsations within the cranium, e.g. inflammation or febrile conditions, and is due to abnormal stretching of the arterial wall (Symonds, 1946). Whatever the primary cause may be, it is probable that the headache which follows a spinal analgesic is mediated through one or other of these two mechanisms, but the factors responsible for putting them into action are different in the two cases.

There are three quite distinct causes of headaches after spinal analgesia. The first is the continued escape of cerebrospinal fluid through the hole in the dura into the extradural space. This accounts for the great majority of these headaches; and the complication here has nothing to do with the spinal analgesia *per se*, since it is just as likely to follow a simple lumbar puncture. The second cause is the development of an aseptic inflammatory meningeal reaction to the injected solution, possibly to the introduction of a minute amount of antiseptic from the skin, a few skin cells, contamination of the lumbar puncture needle or local analgesic solution with starch powder from the anaesthetist's gloves (Dunkley and Lewis, 1977), or to a drop or two of blood: and occasionally this reaction is severe enough for the stretched walls of the engorged vessels to cause pain. The third cause, inflammatory reaction to the introduction of organisms, is the rarest, yet the only serious one. Some rise in cerebrospinal fluid pressure coexists with the last two causes of headache. It is misleading, however, in these cases to refer to 'high pressure' headache, since, as will be seen later, the cerebrospinal fluid pressure can be raised greatly without causing symptoms.

The indictment of the continued escape of cerebrospinal fluid as *the* cause of headache after lumbar puncture is convincing. That there must be some loss is self-evident. The pressure within the dural sac is of the order of say 150 mm water, the pressure in the lumbar extradural space is sub-atmospheric (Macintosh and Mushin, 1947); some escape of fluid, therefore, inevitably occurs after lumbar puncture, and this will continue until the hole becomes occluded. By an ingenious experiment Franksson and Gordh (Franksson and Gordh, 1946), have demonstrated that in an average case the escape is about 10 ml an hour. There is plenty of evidence that the hole in the dura takes some time to heal and a period of three weeks has been proved by radio-isotope myelography (Liebermann et al, 1971). It is not uncommon to find, at autopsy, that the hole resulting from lumbar puncture many days previously has not healed, but in these cases the reparative processes may have been deficient. Leakage of CSF on to the skin surface, following unsuccessful attempts to enter the extradural space, has been reported (Jawalekar and Marks, 1981). During operation for a prolapsed intervertebral disc one of us has seen fluid escape through a lumbar puncture hole in the dura made 36 hours previously. If the outward leak is severe enough the volume of fluid in the cisterns around the base of the brain becomes depleted: when the patient sits up the brain is no longer adequately cushioned and the drag on the pain-sensitive structures — the tentorium and large vessels — results in headache. The characteristic feature of this type of headache is that it bears a constant relation to posture; it is alleviated by lying down, aggravated by sitting up. Drainage of 20 ml of cerebrospinal fluid from a volunteer standing upright causes immediate headache (Kunkle et al, 1943).

Correlation between the size of the needle and the incidence of headache is convincing (Ekstein et al, 1982; Moore, 1982; Charlton, 1983). In one series of cases (Phillips et al, 1969) when a needle gauge 20 was used, the incidence of headache was 14 per cent, in another (Sears, 1959), needle gauge 25, the incidence was 3.5 while in a third in which an extremely fine 32 gauge needle was used, the percentage of headache was reduced to 1.4 per cent (Frumin, 1969). A post-lumbar puncture headache rate of less than 1 per cent has been claimed by Gerner (Gerner, 1980) using a 25 gauge needle and mobilisation of the patient within half an hour. Such narrow needles are of course most easily inserted if they are passed through a 19 gauge needle or introducer (Slattery et al, 1980; Casey, 1983).

But the belief that escape of fluid is responsible for headache is not based on the effect of posture only. The headache can be relieved immediately, though temporarily, by the intrathecal injection of saline. The pressure of cerebrospinal fluid in the dural sac in these cases is indeed low — almost invariably below 50 mm water, sometimes unrecordable. Nevertheless, it is meaningless to refer to a 'low pressure' headache since the condition is greatly aggravated if the intracranial pressure is increased by straining, or by gentle compression of the jugular veins. This no doubt causes the anchoring structures of the brain to be put still further on the stretch. In contrast to dural punctures elsewhere, cisternal puncture is rarely followed by headache. In the sitting patient the intradural hydrostatic pressure at this level is negligible, and the pressure in the extradural space is not negative as in the thoracic and lumbar regions; there is no reason, therefore, why there should be a continued escape of fluid through the puncture hole. Post-lumbar puncture headache is more frequent at high altitudes than at sea level (Safar and Tenicela, 1964; Vacanti, 1972).

Conditions causing loss of body fluids, such as diarrhoea, vomiting, haemorrhage, sweating and lactation, tend to make the condition worse so that it is relatively frequent in obstetric patients especially in those delivered spontaneously. Indeed there is a good case for applying forceps to prevent straining during labour pains in those patients who have been unfortunate enough to have their dura punctured by a 16 to 18 gauge needle in an attempt to produce extradural block (Garrett and Bolsin, 1982). Other workers, however, disagree with this (Brownridge, 1983).

Very rarely, post-lumbar puncture headache may be due to a cerebral tumour (Alfery et al, 1979), while a fatality occurring 15 days after a lumbar puncture using a 25 gauge needle has been reported, due to herniation of the uncus against the tentorium cerebelli (Eerola et al, 1981). Severe and prolonged headache should always be treated seriously.

Prevention

The aim both of the technique of lumbar puncture and of the subsequent care of the patient should be to encourage the early closure of the defect in the dura. The main contribution the anaesthetist can make towards this is the prophylactic use of the smallest possible needle (Tourtellotte and Henderson, 1972). Not only is the rate of fluid loss through a small hole very much less than through a large one, but the smaller hole heals very much more quickly. The needle should be introduced so that the bevel is parallel to the longitudinal fibres of the dura which are thus separated and not sectioned. Multiple punctures of the dura should be avoided, but if the point of the needle becomes blocked these can be made unwittingly since successful puncture is not proclaimed by issue of fluid. Anything which raises the cerebrospinal fluid pressure at the site of puncture will encourage loss and reduce the opportunity of healing. Coughing and straining are to be avoided. It was for a long time the custom to encourage the patient to remain recumbent for 12 to 24 hours after intradural analgesia, but recent work suggests that the results of posture are equivocal (Smith et al, 1980; Handler et al, 1982) or useless (Jones, 1974; Carbaat and Van Crevel, 1981). Another practice, the adoption of the prone position for several hours each day to reduce leakage of CSF (Brocker, 1958) has also been shown to be of doubtful benefit (Smith et al, 1980; Handler et al, 1982). The use of a fine needle, e.g. 25 gauge, together with scrupulous cleanliness are the only certain ways of minimising these headaches. (The whole problem is well discussed by Handler et al (1982).)

Diagnosis

This presents no difficulty. The pain is most severe in the occipital region and in the back of the neck. It may spread to the shoulders in the distribution of the cervical nerves. The patient finds sitting up intolerable and soon discovers that he is reasonably comfortable only when lying down; often the horizontal position relieves the pain altogether. External stimuli in the form of strong light or loud noise prove disturbing and add an element of irritability to the reigning depression. The patient dislikes movement, and is completely incapable of sustained effort involving muscular power. Thus reading is out of the question, and a man may have to interrupt shaving three or four times to lie flat for a few minutes.

Treatment

Once headache is established the results of active treatment are disappointing: but fortunately the slothfulness which accompanies the disability speeds recovery. The accepted pain-relieving drugs are strikingly ineffective. The intrathecal injection of saline affords passing relief but, as a therapeutic measure, the procedure is not to be recommended since it leaves an additional hole in the dura through which leakage can take place. The suggestion of Dr Robert Hingson is a more rational one (Rice and Dabbs, 1950). A catheter is introduced into and left in the extradural space from either the lumbar or sacral region (Crawford, 1972b). Saline is injected as required to give 'a head of pressure' around the dura, 30 to 60 ml being an average dose, given through a catheter and repeated as required. Several injections may be necessary (Smith, 1979). The intrathecal pressure is thus raised and the symptom relieved until the hole in the dura heals. Care must be taken, however, not to injure the dura with the large needle through which the catheter is introduced! The patient should be encouraged to drink freely since this increases formation of cerebrospinal fluid. Alternatively, it has been suggested that 15 ml/kg/hour of bland fluid should be given intravenously to stimulate the choroid plexuses to secrete an excess of cerebrospinal fluid (Birkahahn and Heifetz, 1969). The regime described above, under the heading of prevention, should be followed to promote early healing of the dura: for once this is accomplished any deficiency in the volume of cerebrospinal fluid is soon made good, and recovery is complete. The application of a tight abdominal binder has its advocates (Mosavy and Shafei, 1975).

Many drugs have been recommended at one time or another for the relief of this disability, a fact tending to confirm that the problem is far from solved. Simple analgesics should be given liberally, such as soluble aspirin or paracetamol, but in some patients their effects are disappointing. The use of antidiuretic drugs to promote fluid retention provides a large circulating volume for the choroid plexuses to work on and so, by increasing cerebrospinal fluid formation, influences headache. This method has its advocates (Asbell, 1949; Pfeiffer, 1953; Aziz et al, 1968; Wolfson and Siker, 1970). Synthetic argenine vasopressin or DDAVP (Desmopressin) has 10 times the antidiuretic effect of vasopressin in its natural form and is free from pressor side-effects (Widerlov and Lindström, 1979; Cowan et al, 1980; Handler et al, 1982). Results, however, are not encouraging (Durward and Harrington, 1976; Hansen and Hansen, 1980).

A method of treatment which is said to be effective (Philbin et al, 1970; Sikh and Agawal, 1974) and is certainly harmless is the inhalation of 5 to 6 per cent CO_2 in oxygen from the Magill circuit

(Mapleson A.) of an anaesthetic machine for periods of 10 minutes, repeated daily if necessary. There is of course evidence that a rise in $PaCO_2$ causes an increase in cerebral blood flow (Rich et al, 1953) and it may be supposed that this results in a rise in cerebrospinal fluid pressure.

An aseptic meningeal reaction severe enough to cause headache, although formerly common, is now rare. When it does occur the condition clears up within a day or two without treatment, but in the meantime the patient may have to put up with a fairly severe headache which is unaffected by posture. Some degree of head retraction and malaise may arouse fears of septic meningitis: and if lumbar puncture is done to exclude this, it will be found that the fluid is under slight pressure and that the cell count is raised. It is wrong to refer to this condition as a high pressure headache. The discomfort is not influenced by posture nor relieved by withdrawal of fluid. It is extremely doubtful whether mere rise in pressure of cerebrospinal fluid does cause headache. Symonds (Symonds, 1946) reports a case in which saline was injected intrathecally and the patient's normal pressure of 170 mm water raised to, and maintained at, 550 mm water for some minutes without causing symptoms: and there are pathological states which result in similar high pressures yet do not cause headache.

A more recent suggestion is the extradural blood patch which results when a small volume of the patient's own blood is injected under careful sterile conditions, into the extradural space close to the level of the dural puncture. This was originally described by Gormley in 1960, who used 2 to 3 ml of blood (Gormley, 1960). His imitators have often used larger volumes of blood, ranging up to 10 ml (Di Giovanni and Dunbar, 1970; Ostheimer et al, 1974; Walpole, 1975; Doctor et al, 1976) and even 20 ml (Crawford, 1980). Rarely, two injections of blood are required. While the success rate claimed is high (Abouleish et al, 1975a) so that four out of five patients complaining of headache are cured (Abouleish, 1978), it is not without its own complications which include fever, back pain, ataxia, root pains (Cornwall and Dolan, 1975) and even facial palsy (Abouleish et al, 1975a). The results in the hands of other investigators have not been as satisfactory (Palahniuk and Cumming, 1979) while blood patch given prophylactically, before the onset of headache, has proved disappointing (Palahniuk and Cumming, 1979). This may be due to the leakage of blood into the intradural space although in dogs, deliberate injection of blood into the theca causes no neurological deficits (Ravindran et al, 1981). If the patient complains of pain during the injection it is probably wise to pause (Crawford, 1980). A previous blood patch does not appear to make subsequent lumbar puncture or location of the extradural space more difficult (Abouleish et al 1975b) although it has been suggested that fibrous adhesions between the wall of the vertebral canal and the dura may limit upward extension of a subsequent block (Rainbird and Pfitzner, 1983). The controlled blood patch is a very different entity from the extradural haematoma due to the trauma of repeated lumbar punctures or to blood dyscrasia, which may cause dangerous compression of the cord. However, injection of autologous blood into the extradural space may be followed by transient neck and backache, tinnitus, temporary radiculitis, abdominal cramps and temporary pyrexia (Rainbird and Pfitner, 1983).

Although a good deal is known about post-lumbar puncture headache, the whole picture is not yet clearly defined and there is no remedy which can be guaranteed to be effective in every case. Why, when apparently identical techniques are followed, is one patient stricken while another remains immune? There is a general impression that headache develops more readily in neurotics, and in patients subject to migraine, and it may be that in these a small stimulus provokes an excessive response. It would appear, too, that the symptom follows minor rather than severe operations: what is more certain is that patients in the first group tend to be ambulatory, while those who have had extensive operations have something more compelling than headache on which to focus their attention. The whole problem of post-lumbar puncture headache is fully and excellently dealt with by Brownridge (1983), who favours blood patch in intractable cases.

Severe post-lumbar puncture pain in the back, associated with flaccid paralysis and sensory loss, possibly due to such a haematoma, demands myelography and, if necessary, laminectomy without delay.

Dry puncture

Here, resistances similar to those offered by the ligamentum flavum and dura may be felt, but cerebrospinal fluid does not flow. Despite this, the anaesthetist may assert that he is satisfied the point of the needle lies within the dura. In these and similar trying situations in anaesthesia generally there is a temptation and a tendency to blame the unfortunate patient for some abnormality which exonerates the anaesthetist from any blame for failure. It has been suggested that the needle penetrates the dura only to enter an area devoid of cerebrospinal fluid. It is reassuring that these anomalous cases are encountered with greater frequency during one's noviciate, and that care and experience decrease their number. There is, however, one well recognised exception. If a second lumbar puncture is carried out to investigate the cause of a post-lumbar puncture headache, a very low pressure of cerebrospinal fluid, or even true dry tap is sometimes recorded.

Poor flow of CSF

Occasionally puncture of the dura is disappointingly rewarded by a few hesitant drops of cerebrospinal fluid. This may be due to a component of the cauda equina lying against the bevel of the needle, blocking it. If the needle is rotated, or pushed a little further in, or slightly withdrawn, the flow may be improved. Nevertheless, sometimes these obvious manoeuvres do not improve matters. Fluid (e.g. a local analgesic solution) can be injected freely, but attempts at aspiration are unsuccessful. Various unconvincing explanations are given for this state of affairs, but the fact remains that if a spinal analgesic solution is now injected in the usual way, there is a high probability that the extent of the resultant analgesia will be disappointing. *If fluid does not drip freely, or is not easily aspirated, the anaesthetist is strongly advised to withdraw the needle and try another space.* This decision is hard to make when difficulty has been encountered in making a dural puncture at all. An unsuccessful attempt may already have been made and the anaesthetist is sorely tempted to rest on his laurels when a few drops of cerebrospinal fluid issuing from the needle acclaim that the fault is no longer his.

Abnormalities in the form of a firm attachment of the arachnoid to the conus medullaris and/or nerve roots of the cauda equina are not uncommon. It is possible that the very slow but nevertheless sure dripping of fluid is due to the needle, after it passes through the dura, entering a loculus which communicates through a very small opening with the general subarachnoid cavity. This would account, too, for the ineffectiveness of aspiration. If for one reason or another the anaesthetist decides to make the best of things as they are, he should inject a considerably larger dose of local analgesic solution than he otherwise would. In this way, despite the mechanical obstruction and rapid absorption into local venous plexuses, enough may find its way to the appropriate nerve roots to provide a satisfactory field of operation.

After injection the plunger should be kept depressed for some time with the needle *in situ* to prevent reflux of fluid, locally under considerable pressure, through the hole in the dura into the extradural space.

Patchy analgesia; unblocked segments (see Ch. 9)

The spinal that does not 'take'

All experienced workers have encountered this occasionally even though accepted procedure has apparently been followed. Reflection, however, usually discloses some flaw in technique. In 1907 Alfred E. Barker wrote that for successful spinal analgesia it is necessary 'to enter the lumbar dural sac effectually with the point of the needle, and to discharge through this, all the contemplated dose of the drug, directly and freely into the cerebrospinal fluid, below the termination of the cord' (Barker, 1907). Failure to follow the details of this advice is the commonest cause of a poor result.

Other causes of failure are faults in the tilt of the vertebral canal, inadequate dosage, contamination of the local analgesic solution with alkali, high alkalinity of the cerebrospinal fluid causing inactivation and precipitation of the local analgesic agent (Cohen and Knight, 1947), and impatience to commence the operation. An attempt to compensate for deficient analgesia by giving an intravenous barbiturate may result in an uncontrollable patient; it is generally wiser to admit failure and administer full general anaesthesia.

The broken needle

If the needle should break during attempted lumbar puncture, the proximal part should, if possible, be left in place to serve as a guide to the distal end. If this cannot be done, a second needle should be inserted along the track of the broken one to serve as a guide to its location. Removal under X-ray control should be attempted right away (Lahey, 1929; Maxson, 1938; Eng and Zorotovitch, 1977). As all needles, if they fracture, usually do so near the hub, they should never be inserted to their maximal depth.

Surgical emphysema

Subcutaneous surgical emphysema in the supra-clavicular region has been reported (Laman and McLeskey, 1978) and was presumably due to the injection of too much air when eliciting the 'loss of resistance' test. It should not be necessary to inject more than 3 ml· of air using this test. Venous air embolism has also been reported (Naulty et al, 1982).

Retching and vomiting

These distressing reflexes are most commonly due to visceral afferent stimuli. They are certainly encountered less frequently by surgeons who, once the abdomen is open, infiltrate freely with local analgesics the cardiac end of the stomach to block afferent fibres in the vagus. We have known the situation respond dramatically to the intravenous injection of atropine 0.25 to 0.5 mg and /or the inhalation of oxygen. Anti-emetic agents have been recommended both in the premedication, where chlorpromazine has been used (Ratra et al., 1972) and during the operation. But if the condition does not yield to these simple treatments then the patient must be anaesthetised. A small dose of intravenous thiopentone relieves the condition at once and the peaceful state can be maintained by quite light general anaesthesia. Scrupulous care must be taken to prevent the aspiration of gastric contents.

Hiccups

Hiccups can mar an otherwise excellent spinal block just as it can spoil operating conditions during otherwise satisfactory general anaesthesia. The cause is unknown, though it is frequently associated with traction on the mesentery or handling the stomach, so that the condition is rarely seen if the vagi have been infiltrated, as above. Its effects during abdominal surgery can be embarrassingly inconvenient. So many 'cures' have been reported that none are to be relied on. The use of curare-like drugs except in paralysing doses is ineffective. Deepening the level of general anaesthesia with a volatile agent affords the best chance of restoring peace and quiet to the heaving abdomen.

Circulatory collapse

A sudden fall in blood-pressure, with or without hypoventilation or apnoea, requires prompt management. This situation can generally be prevented by an alert anaesthetist since the common cause is extensive vasomotor paralysis together with hypoxia of the vital centres. Any pillow must be removed. The rate of infusion should be increased and the legs raised. Oxygen must be brought to the alveoli, while pressor drugs should not be totally forgotten.

Bronchospasm

This has been reported in a patient with chronic asthma in whom the block, to enable a termination of pregnancy to be performed, ascended too high (T.5). The bronchospasm was relieved by aminophylline and hydrocortisone (Mallamparti, 1981).

Backache

After operation the patient may complain of a pain in the region of the lumbar puncture just as he may complain of similar pain after general anaesthesia. The lithotomy position may itself be the cause due to the stretching of the ligaments of the pelvic girdle and vertebral column. Our experience leads us to believe that backache is transient and not a serious sequel. It would probably be advantageous if all patients undergoing surgery had the small of the back supported by a suitable firm pillow.

Cardiac complications

Because the central nervous system is the primary target for local analgesic toxicity (Liu et al, 1983), the convulsive dose is many times lower than the dose required to seriously embarrass the heart. This applies to the less lipid soluble, less protein bound agents as well as to the more lipid soluble and protein bound drugs. Sudden cardiac arrest has occurred during central neural blockade with etidocaine (Prentiss, 1979; Albright, 1979) and with other drugs. Prinzmetal's variant angina has also been seen and is due to spasm of the coronary arteries and not to hypotension; the treatment should therefore be nitroglycerine (Krantz et al, 1980). Mild acute chest discomfort during a block may be of oesophageal origin (Moon, 1980).

Convulsions associated with extradural block (see Ch. 9.)

Respiratory arrest

Hypoventilation, sometimes progressing to apnoea (Scott, 1981), has been reported many times after extradural blockade (see Ch. 4). The cause is not always obvious although the accidental injection of a large amount of local analgesic solution into the intradural space undoubtedly accounts for some cases. Apnoea certainly occurs, not infrequently, after true extradural block and its onset may be delayed for 20 to 30 minutes after the extradural injection (Holmboe and Kongsrud, 1982). The anaesthetist must be on the look-out for this potentially disastrous complication which, if it is recognised in time, can be so satisfactorily treated by positive pressure respiration. Under no condition is the old adage 'the price of safety is eternal vigilance' more true. Pulmonary embolism during intradural block has been reported (Berry, 1982) and a fatal case occurred in the practice of one of the authors following the application of an Esmarch bandage to an injured lower limb.

Paralysis of the 6th cranial nerve

This is a rare sequel and leads to double vision from inactivation of the external rectus muscle of the eyeball. The disability usually makes its appearance between the third and twelfth day after operation (or after simple lumbar puncture), though onset may be delayed for anything up to three weeks. Paresis is never complete, and it is neurologically distinct from the total paralysis which may be seen after trauma, as in fracture of the skull. The prognosis is good, 50 per cent of cases recovering spontaneously within a month. It has been reported where a considerable loss of cerebrospinal fluid is known to have occurred (Bryce-Smith and Macintosh, 1951) and if this plays a major part in its aetiology it is not surprising that paresis is almost invariably preceded by disabling headache. If the cause is mechanical it seems reasonable to suppose that vigorous hydration of the patient suffering from headache may prevent the onset of paresis. Bilateral nerve involvement has been reported (Bryce-Smith and Macintosh, 1951). Paralysis of every cranial nerve except the 1st and 10th has been attributed to spinal analgesia, while transient tinnitus and deafness may occur. Diplopia has been seen after general anaesthesia and after the use of muscle relaxants (Kennedy and Lockhart, 1952; Norman, 1955). Paralysis of the 6th nerve together with headache treated by blood patch may result in relief of the headache without immediate improvement of the diplopia (Heyman et al, 1982). Spinal analgesia has also been followed by paralysis of the trigeminal nerve (Lee and Roberts, 1978).

Retention of urine

This occurs somewhat more frequently after spinal than after general anaesthesia. If the injection has been made in the lumbar region the concentration of local analgesic drug is necessarily high in the sacral area, and the small size of the parasympathetic fibres which control micturition make them particularly vulnerable to local analgesics. Given a little time the condition usually yields to the familiar and time-honoured remedies so well known to the nursing profession.

Meningitis

Formerly this was commonly assumed to be due to faulty asepsis (Garrod, 1946; Kennedy et al, 1950), but meningitis has been reported following techniques which could not easily be criticised in this respect (Neumark et al, 1980). A case of a severe meningeal reaction was thought to be due to contamination of the equipment by detergent (Seigne, 1970). Chalk from the anaesthetist's gloves may also act as an irritant (Dunkley and Lewis, 1977). Contamination with antiseptics (Cope, 1954) and the pH of the injected solution have also been blamed. The whole armamentarium of spinal analgesia should be autoclaved or sterilised by gamma radiation.

Horner's syndrome

This has been reported to occur following both extradural lumbar and sacral analgesia, many of the patients being in advanced pregnancy (Mohan et al, 1973; Collier, 1975; Evans et al, 1975; Mohan and Potter, 1975a; Mohan and Potter, 1975b; Carrie and Mohan, 1976; Skaredoff and Datta, 1981; Clayton, 1983). Its onset may be delayed (Hertz et al, 1980) while it may be unilateral.

Neurological sequelae of intradural and extradural block

Intradural and extradural analgesia are not employed in pain relief so frequently today as they might be because of the fear of causing neurological sequelae, and the additional fear of the medico-legal consequences of such sequelae. There is no doubt that transient and relatively unimportant post-spinal disabilities occur (Vandam and Dripps, 1954, 1956a; Phillips et al, 1969), but also on record are a distressing number of more serious lesions. These include spinal cord and nerve root damage, transverse myelitis (Birkahahn and Rosenberg, 1977), adhesive arachnoiditis, bulbar involvement, cauda equina lesions and paraplegia (Kennedy et al, 1950). There are those who hold that such problems arise more frequently after intradural than after extradural block (Foldes et al, 1956; Lund, 1966) but we do not share this opinion as quite a large number of workers have reported neurological problems after extradural block (Braham and Saia, 1958; Davies et al, 1958; Urquhart-Hay, 1969; Harrison, 1975; Desnoyers et al, 1976).

Lesions may involve the whole cord causing permanent motor loss and sensory analgesia below the site of the lesion. In other rare cases, those parts of the cord supplied by the anterior spinal artery are infarcted, so that the patient so afflicted has motor loss and analgesia below the site of the lesion although the sensations of touch, vibration and position are largely spared (*Lancet*, Annotation, 1958; Wells, 1966; Silver and Buxton, 1974). In patients with less serious complaints there may be small areas of skin where sensation is abnormal or lost, and minor motor disturbances confined to the legs and perineum, with sometimes loss of sphincter control and impotence. There may be sensory and motor abnormalities confined to the distribution of one or more spinal nerves or the cauda equina may bear the brunt of the damage. Electromyographic studies may enable lesions of the lower motor neuron type, suspected as having been caused by the method of analgesia, to be differentiated from myopathic or neurological abnormalities present before the operation (Marinacci and Courville, 1958; Goodgold and Eberstein, 1972).

Aseptic meningitis has followed spinal analgesia (Seigne, 1970) and so has chemical damage to the cord from the injection of solutions contaminated with antiseptics (Cope, 1954) or detergent (Winkleman, 1952). Haematoma formation in the extradural space has caused signs and symptoms due to compression of the cord or its nerve roots (Seglov, 1967; Gingrich, 1968; Butler and Green, 1970; Halpern and Cohen, 1971; Pavlin et al, 1979; Ballin, 1981; Brem et al, 1981; Edelman and Wingard, 1980; Garrett and Bolsin, 1982; Newrick and Read, 1982; Scott, 1982), and blood clot under tension may arise from numerous attempts at lumbar puncture (Lerner, et al, 1973). Subarachnoid haematoma can also cause problems (Brem et al, 1981; Mayumi and Dohi, 1983). Spinal puncture is probably unwise in those patients with defective blood clotting whether due to a coagulopathy or to the administration of low dose heparin in an attempt to prevent postoperative thrombophlebitis (Rao and El-Etr,

1982; Odoom et al, 1983). Severe pain in the back with paraplegia, immediately following the operation, suggests the formation of such a haematoma so that the advice of a neurosurgeon and a radiologist should be urgently sought so that myelography and possible decompression can be carried out without delay. It does not take very long for the damage caused by compression to become permanent. Very rarely, an extradural abscess has come to light (Loarie and Fairley, 1978) and such lesions may be due to infection elsewhere in the body (Crawford, 1975).

It has been suggested that the lesions suffered by the cord or its nerve roots are more likely to be due to the ill-effects of ischaemia associated with hypotension in diseased or even in normal arteries, rather than to the injection of local analgesic solution (Bromage, 1976). We are still uncertain as to the role of the vasoconstrictor often added to the solutions injected into the intradural or extradural space in the genesis of lesions of the cord, but we ourselves have employed adrenaline in a strength of 1:200 000 or 1:250 000 in many hundreds of extradural blocks, without incident, and are happy to continue doing so. Any position of the patient on the operating table which stretches the cord, such as the lateral with lateral flexion of the spine, may contribute to ischaemic damage.

Intracranial complications very rarely occur and may include subdural haematoma (Edelman and Wingard, 1980; Jonsson et al, 1983), cerebral uncus herniation (Eerola et al, 1981) and intracranial haemorrhage (Mantia, 1981). It is possible that the intracranial pressure changes thought to be responsible for the post-spinal headache may be the cause of the subdural haematoma (Jonsson et al, 1983). If diffuse neurological signs or symptoms follow dural puncture and are resistant to treatment, careful neurological examination should not be delayed; surgical evacuation of a haematoma can lead to complete recovery (Jonsson et al, 1983).

Unfortunately the cause of post-spinal neurological sequelae is often unknown so that in the absence of a precise aetiology preventive steps cannot be taken. Even when experienced and careful workers have followed an apparently impeccable technique, disaster has sometimes resulted. Phantom limb pain during intradural block has been reported, requiring general anaesthesia for its relief (Mackenzie, 1983).

Neurological complications after operation, totally unrelated to spinal injection, are well documented in patients given general anaesthesia or no anaesthetic at all (Horsley, 1909; Elkington, 1936; *Anesthesiology*, Current comment, 1948; Ciliberti, 1948; Thomas and

Dwyer, 1950; Sinclair, 1954; Leatherdale, 1959; Teague and Urquhart-Hay, 1974; Crawford, 1975; Newbery, 1977; Economacos, 1978; Schreiner et al, 1983), and in obstetric patients such sequelae, post-partum, unrelated to anaesthesia are seen from time to time (O'Connell, 1944; Chalmers, 1949; Neumark et al, 1980). Multiple sclerosis has followed spinal analgesia (Fleiss, 1949), while spinal stroke (*Lancet*, Editorial, 1974; Silver and Buxton, 1974), haematoma and extradural abscess can all occur spontaneously, bearing no relation to any technique of regional analgesia (Crawford, 1975). Rare complications associated with but not due to central neural blockade include temporary neurological deficit associated with a large intracranial arterio-venous malformation (Wark, 1977) and neurological complications erroneously attributed to spinal analgesia have been documented by Nicholson and Eversole (1946), Wilson et al (1949), Vandam and Dripps (1956b) and Sadove et al (1961). Intraspinal epidermoid tumour has been reported from a core of skin carried in by a lumbar puncture needle with an ill-fitting stylet (Batnitzky et al, 1977; *Lancet*, Annotation, 1977). The employment of an introducer or a disposable needle might prevent similar occurrences in the future.

Extradural spinal cord tumour with associated paraplegia is another such complication (Hirlekar, 1980) and the tumour may be metastatic (Hillman, 1965; Schreiner et al, 1983). Transverse myelitis following block has been reported (Birkahahn and Rosenberg, 1977). A patient maintained in the lithotomy position with the legs widely abducted may suffer from femoral neuropathy (Schreiner et al, 1983; Tondare et al, 1983). In this position, abduction must not be extreme.

We must frankly acknowledge that we do not know the cause of many of these tragedies and too often we theorise as to their exact nature (Kane, 1981). For example, unexplained hemiplegia with retrobulbar neuritis in a fit young patient undergoing operation for the cure of his hydrocoele under intradural block has been reported (Ghate et al, 1981); the signs came on soon after the operation. Cutaneous cerebrospinal fluid leakage after dural puncture must be a rare occurrence; such a case lasting 48 hours has been reported (Jawalekar and Marks, 1981).

Chloroprocaine has its advocates in the US but reports of harm to the cord have been reported following its intradural injection (Ravindran et al, 1980; Reisner et al, 1980; Moore et al, 1982b). Prolonged block has followed the extradural injection of 1 per cent solution of etidocaine (Ramanathan et al, 1978).

Patients with lumbar spinal stenosis, narrowing of intervertebral foramina or nerve tunnels are especially at risk (Chaudhari et al, 1978; Critchley, 1982) so that preoperative questioning and neurological examination of the patient are most important. Ultrasound measurement of the spinal canal may not always be able to exclude this abnormality (Davis, 1982). A narrow canal makes extradural bleeding potentially more dangerous (Ballin, 1981).

The present authors who have a fairly lengthy experience of the techniques are of the opinion that either intradural or extradural analgesia, wisely chosen and skilfully administered, are reasonably safe and satisfactory procedures when indicated and bear comparison with any other method of pain relief.

REFERENCES

Abouleish, E. (1978) Epidural blood patch for the treatment of chronic post-lumbar puncture cephalalgia. *Anesthesiology*, **49**, 291.

Abouleish, E., de la Vega, S., Blendinger, J. & Tio, Y. (1975a) Long-term follow up of epidural blood patch. *Anesthesia and Analgesia*, **54**, 459.

Abouleish, E., Wadhwa, R. K., de la Vega, S., Tan, R. H. & Lim, Y.N.T. (1975b) Regional analgesia following epidural blood patch. *Anesthesia and Analgesia*, **54**, 634.

Albright, G. A. (1979) Cardiac arrest following regional anesthesia with bupivacaine and etidocaine. *Anesthesiology*, **51**, 285.

Alfery, D. D., Marsh, M. L. & Shapiro, H. M. (1979) Postspinal headache or intracranial tumour after obstetric anesthesia. *Anesthesiology*, **51**, 92.

Anesthesiology (1948) Current comment: paraplegia following inhalation anesthesia. *Anesthesiology*, **9**, 439.

Asbell, N. (1949) Postspinal headache: treatment with desoxycorticosterone acetate. *Journal of the Medical Society of New Jersey*, **46**, 433.

Aziz, H., Pearce, J. & Miller, E. (1968) Vasopressin in the prevention of lumbar puncture headaches. *British Medical Journal*, **4**, 677.

Ballin, N. C. (1981) Paraplegia following epidural analgesia. *Anaesthesia*, **36**, 952.

Barker, A. E. (1907) Clinical experiences with spinal analgesia in 100 cases. *British Medical Journal*, **1**, 665.

Batnitzky, S., Keucher, T. R., Mealey, J. & Campbell, R. L. (1977) Epidermoid tumour following lumbar puncture. *Journal of the American Medical Association*, **237**, 148. Annotation (1977) Lumbar puncture and epidermoid tumours. *Lancet*, **1**, 635.

Berry, A. J. (1982) Acute pulmonary embolism during spinal anesthesia. *Anesthesiology*, **57**, 57.

Bier, A. (1899) Versuche über Cocainiserung des Ruckenmarkes. *Deutsche Zeitschrift für Chirurgie*, **51**, 361.

Birkahahn, H. J. & Heifetz, M. (1969) Letter. *British Medical Journal*, **1**, 782.

Birkahahn, H. J. & Rosenberg, B. (1977) Transient iatrogenic transverse myelitis. *Anaesthesia*, **32**, 680.

Braham, M. C. & Saia, S. (1958) Neurological complications of epidural anaesthesia. *British Medical Journal*, **2**, 657.

Brem, S. S., Hafler, D. A., Van Uitert, R.L., Ruff, R. L. & Reichert, W. H. (1981) Spinal subarachnoid hematoma: a hazard of lumbar puncture resulting in reversible paraplegia. *New England Journal of Medicine*, **303**, 1020.

Brocker, R. J. (1958) Technic to avoid spinal tap headache. *Journal of the American Medical Association*, **168**, 261.
Bromage, P. R. (1976) Correspondence. *Anaesthesia*, **31**, 947.
Brownridge, P. (1983) The management of headache following accidental dural puncture in obstetric patients. *Anaesthesia and Intensive Care*, **11**, 4.
Bryce-Smith, R. & Macintosh, R. R. (1951) Sixth nerve palsy after lumbar puncture and spinal analgesia. *British Medical Journal*, **1**, 275.
Butler, A. B. & Green, D. C. (1970) Haematoma following epidural anaesthesia. *Canadian Anaesthetists' Society Journal*, **17**, 635.
Carbaat, P. A. T. & Van Crevel, H. (1981) Lumbar puncture headache: controlled study on the preventive effects of 24 hour bed rest. *Lancet*, **2**, 433.
Carrie, L. E. S. & Mohan, J. (1976) Horner's syndrome following obstetric extradural block. *British Journal of Anaesthesia*, **48**, 611.
Casey, W. F. (1983) Correspondence. *British Medical Journal*, **286**, 144.
Chalmers, J. A. (1949) Traumatic neuritis of the puerperium. *Journal of Obstetrics and Gynaecology of the British Commonwealth*, **56**, 205.
Charlton, J. E. (1983) Correspondence: hazards of lumbar puncture. *British Medical Journal*, **286**, 392.
Chaudhari, L. S., Kop, B. R. & Dhruva, A. J. (1978) Paraplegia after epidural analgesia. *Anaesthesia*, **33**, 722.
Ciliberti, B. J. (1948) Paraplegia following inhalation anesthesia for subtotal gastrectomy: a case report. *Anesthesiology*, **9**, 439.
Clayton, K. C. (1983) The incidence of Horner's syndrome during lumbar extradural for elective Caesarean section and provision of analgesia during labour. *Anaesthesia*, **38**, 583.
Cohen, E. N. & Knight, R. T. (1947) Hydrogen ion concentration of the cerebrospinal fluid and its relationship to anesthetic failure. *Anesthesiology*, **8**, 594.
Collier, C. B. (1975) Horner's syndrome following obstetrical extradural block analgesia. *British Journal of Anaesthesia*, **47**, 1342.
Cope, R. W. (1954) The Woolley and Roe case: Woolley and Roe v. the Ministry of Health and others. *Anaesthesia*, **9**, 249.
Cornwall, R. D. & Dolan, W. M. (1975) Radicular back pain following lumbar epidural patch. *Anesthesiology*, **42**, 692.
Cowan, J. M. A., Durward, W. F., Harrington, H. et al (1980) D.D.A.V.P. in prevention of headache after lumbar puncture. *British Medical Journal*, **1**, 244.
Craft, J. B., Epstein, B. S. & Coakley, C. S. (1973) Prophylaxis of dural puncture headaches with epidural saline. *Anesthesia and Analgesia*, **52**, 228.
Crawford, J. S. (1972a) Observations on 1000 epidurals given in labour. In Doughty, A. (ed.) *Proceedings of the Symposium on Epidural Analgesia in Obstetrics*, p. 83. London: Lewis.
Crawford, J. S. (1972b) Prevention of headache consequent on dural puncture. *British Journal of Anaesthesia*, **44**, 598.
Crawford, J. S. (1975) Pathology in the extradural space. *British Journal of Anaesthesia*, **47**, 417.
Crawford, J. S. (1979) Experiences with spinal analgesia in a British obstetrical unit. *British Journal of Anaesthesia*, **51**, 531.
Crawford, J. S. (1980) Experiences with an epidural blood patch. *Anaesthesia*, **35**, 513.
Critchley, E. M. R. (1982) Annotation. *British Medical Journal*, **284**, 1588.
Davies, A., Soloman, B. & Levene, A. (1958) Paraplegia following epidural anaesthesia. *British Medical Journal*, **2**, 654.
Davis, P. (1982) Lumbar spinal stenosis. *British Medical Journal*, **285**, 893.
Desnoyers, Y., Bisson, L. & Sindon, A. (1976) Paraplegia following transurethral surgery. *Canadian Anaesthetists' Society Journal*, **23**, 440.
Di Giovanni, A. J. & Dunbar, B. S. (1970) Epidural injection of autologous blood for post lumbar puncture headache. *Anaesthesia and Analgesia*, **49**, 268.

Doctor, N., De Zoysa, S., Shah, R., Modi, K. & Hussain, S. Z. (1976) The use of the blood patch for post spinal headache. *Anaesthesia*, **31**, 794.
Dunkley, B. & Lewis, T. T. (1977) Meningeal reaction to starch powder in cerebrospinal fluid. *British Medical Journal*, **2**, 1391.
Durward, W. F. & Harrington, H. (1976) Headache after lumbar puncture. *Lancet*, **2**, 1403.
Economacos, G. (1978) Neurological complications after spinal analgesia. *Anaesthesia*, **33**, 374.
Edelman, J. D. & Wingard, D. W. (1980) Subdural hematoma after lumbar dural puncture. *Anesthesiology*, **52**, 166.
Eerola, M., Kaukinen, L. & Kaukinen, S. (1981) Fatal brain lesion following spinal anaesthesia. *Acta Anaesthesiologica Scandinavica*, **25**, 115.
Ekstein, K., Rogacev, Z. et al (1982) Prospectiv vergleichende Studie Koofsschmerzen bei jungen Patientien. *Der Anaesthesist*, **31**, 57.
Elkington, J. C. (1936) Meningitis serosa circumscripta spinalis — spinal arachnoiditis. *Brain*, **59**, 181.
Eng, M. & Zorotovitch, R. A. (1977) Broken needle complication with a disposable spinal introducer. *Anesthesiology*, **46**, 147.
Evans, J. M., Ganci, C. A. & Watkins, G. (1975) Horner's syndrome as a complication of epidural block. *Anaesthesia*, **30**, 774.
Fleiss, A. M. (1949) Multiple sclerosis appearing after spinal anesthesia. *New York State Journal of Medicine*, **49**, 1076.
Foldes, F. F., Colovinzenzo, J. W. & Birch, J. H. (1956) Epidural anesthesia: a reappraisal. *Anesthesia and Analgesia*, **35**, 33; and **35**, 89.
Franksson, C. & Gordh, T. (1946) Headache after spinal anaesthesia and a technique for lessening its frequency. *Acta Chirurgica Scandinavica*, **94**, 443.
Frumin, M. J. (1969) Spinal anesthesia using a 32 gauge needle. *Anesthesiology*, **30**, 599.
Garrett, C. P. O. & Bolsin, S. N. (1982) Subdural haematoma complicating spinal anaesthetic. *British Medical Journal*, **285**, 1047.
Garrod, L. P. (1946) The nature of meningitis following spinal anaesthesia and its prevention. *British Medical Bulletin*, **4**, 106.
Gerner, R. H. (1980) Posture and headache after lumbar puncture. *Lancet*, **2**, 33.
Ghate, S. V., Kulkarni, S. G. & Sarate, G. S. (1981) Hemiplegia and retrobulbar neuritis after subarachnoid block. *Canadian Anaesthetists' Society Journal*, **28**, 283.
Gingrich, T. F. (1968) Spinal epidural hematoma following continuous epidural anesthesia. *Anesthesiology*, **29**, 162.
Goodgold, J. & Eberstein, A. (1972) *Electrodiagnosis and Neuromuscular Diseases*. Baltimore: Williams & Wilkins.
Gormley, J. B. (1960) Treatment of postspinal headache. *Anesthesiology*, **21**, 565.
Halpern, S. W. & Cohen, D. D. (1971) Hematoma following epidural anesthesia. *Anesthesiology*, **35**, 641.
Handler, C. E., Perkin, G. D., Smith, F. R. & Rose, F. C. (1982) Posture and lumbar puncture headache: a controlled trial in 50 patients. *Journal of the Royal Society of Medicine*, **75**, 404.
Hansen, P. V. & Hansen, J. H. (1980) Desmopressin (D.D.A.V.P.) in lumbar puncture. *British Medical Journal*, **1**, 1146.
Harrison, P. (1975) Paraplegia following epidural anaesthesia. *Anaesthesia*, **30**, 778.
Hertz, R., Chiovari, C. A. & Marx, G. (1980) Delayed Horner's syndrome following obstetrical extradural block. *Anesthesia and Analgesia*, **59**, 299.
Heyman, H. J., Salem, M. R. & Klimov, I. (1982) Persistent 6th cranial nerve paresis following blood patch for post-dural puncture headache. *Anesthesia and Analgesia*, **61**, 948.
Hillman, K. (1965) Epidural anaesthesia in obstetrics: a second look at 26 127 cases. *Canadian Anaesthetists' Society Journal*, **12**, 4.
Hirlekar, G. (1980) Paraplegia after epidural analgesia associated with an extradural spinal tumour. *Anaesthesia*, **35**, 363.

Holmboe, J. & Kongsrud, F. (1982) Delayed respiratory arrest after bupivacaine. *Anaesthesia*, **37**, 60.

Horsley, V. (1909) Chronic spinal meningitis: its differential diagnosis and surgical treatment. *British Medical Journal*, **1**, 513.

Jawalekar, I. & Marks, G. F. (1981) Cutaneous cerebrospinal fluid leakage following attempted extradural block. *Anesthesiology*, **54**, 348.

Jones, R. J. (1974) The role of recumbency in the prevention and treatment of post-spinal headache. *Anesthesia and Analgesia*, **53**, 788.

Jonsson, L. O., Einarsson, P. & Olsson, G. L. (1983) Subdural haematoma and spinal anaesthesia. *Anaesthesia*, **38**, 144.

Kane, R. E. (1981) Neurological deficits following epidural and spinal anesthesia. *Anesthesia and Analgesia*, **60**, 150.

Kennedy, F., Effron, A. S. & Perry, G. (1950) The gross spinal cord paralysis caused by spinal anesthesia. *Surgery, Gynecology and Obstetrics*, **91**, 385.

Kennedy, R. J. & Lockhart, G. (1952) Paresis of the abducens nerve following spinal anesthesia. *Anesthesiology*, **13**, 189.

Krantz, E. M., Viljoen, J. F. & Gilbert, M. S. (1980) Prinzmetal's variant angina during extradural anaesthesia. *British Journal of Anaesthesia*, **52**, 945.

Kunkle, E. C., Ray, B. S. & Wolff, H. G. (1943) Experimental studies on headache. *Archives of Neurology and Psychiatry*, **49**, 323.

Lahey, F. H. (1929) The removal of broken spinal needles. *Journal of the American Medical Association*, **93**, 518.

Laman, E. N. & McLeskey, C. H. (1978) Supraclavicular subcutaneous emphysema following lumbar epidural anesthesia. *Anesthesiology*, **48**, 219.

Lancet (1958) Annotation. **2**, 515; and (1967) **2**, 143.

Lancet (1974) Editorial. Spinal stroke. **2**, 1299.

Lancet (1977) Annotation. Lumbar puncture and epidermoid tumours. **1**, 635.

Leatherdale, R. A. L. (1959) Spinal analgesia and unrelated paraplegia. *Anaesthesia*, **14**, 274.

Lee, J. J. & Roberts, R. B. (1978) Paralysis of the fifth cranial nerve following spinal anesthesia. *Anesthesiology*, **48**, 210.

Lerner, S. M., Guttermann, P. & Jenkins, F. (1973) Epidural hematoma and paraplegia after numerous lumbar punctures. *Anesthesiology*, **39**, 550.

Liebermann, L. R., Tourtellotte, W. W. & Newkirk, J. A. (1971) Prolonged post lumbar puncture cerebrospinal fluid leakage from the subarachnoid space demonstrated by radio-isotope myelography. *Neurology*, **21**, 925.

Liu, P. L., Feldman, H. S., Giasi, R. et al (1983) Comparative central nervous system toxicity of lidocaine, etidocaine, bupivacaine and tetracaine in awake dogs following rapid intravenous administration. *Anesthesia and Analgesia*, **62**, 375.

Loarie, D. J. & Fairley, H. B. (1978) Epidural abscess following spinal anesthesia. *Anesthesia and Analgesia*, **57**, 351.

Lund, P. L. (1966) *Peridural Analgesia and Anaesthesia*, Springfield: Thomas.

Macintosh, R. R. & Mushin, W. W. (1947) Observations on the epidural space. *Anaesthesia*, **2**, 100.

Mackenzie, N. (1983) Phantom limb pain during spinal anaesthesia. *Anaesthesia*, **38**, 886.

Mallamparti, S. R. (1981) Bronchospasm during spinal anesthesia. *Anesthesia and Analgesia*, **60**, 839.

Mantia, A. M. (1981) Clinical report of the occurrence of an intracranial hemorrhage following post-lumbar puncture headache. *Anesthesiology*, **55**, 684.

Marinacci, A. A. & Courville, C. C. (1958) Electromyogram in evaluation of neurological complications in spinal anesthesia. *Journal of the American Medical Association*, **168**, 1337.

Maxson, L. H. (1938) *Spinal Anesthesia*, p. 172. Philadelphia: Lippincott.

Mayumi, T. & Dohi, S. (1983) Spinal subarachnoid hematoma after lumbar puncture in a patient receiving antiplatelet therapy. *Anesthesia and Analgesia*, **62**, 777.

Mohan, J. & Potter, J. M. (1975a) Horner's syndrome complicating lumbar and sacral extradural block. *Anaesthesia*, **30**, 769.

Mohan, J. & Potter, J. M. (1975b) Pupillary constriction and ptosis following caudal epidural analgesia. *Anaesthesia*, **30**, 769.

Mohan, J., Lloyd, J. W. & Potter, J. M. (1973) Pupillary constriction following extradural analgesia. *Injury*, **5**, 151.

Moon, G. J. (1980) Chest pain of esophageal origin during spinal anesthesia. *Anesthesiology*, **53**, 510.

Moore, D. C. (1955) *Complications of Regional Anesthesia*, ch. 20. Springfield: Thomas.

Moore, D. C. (1982) Factors influencing spinal anesthesia. *Regional Anesthesia*, **7**, 20.

Moore, D. C., Thompson, G. E. & Crawford, R. D. (1982a) Long-acting local anesthetic drugs and convulsions with hypoxic acidosis. *Anesthesiology*, **56**, 230.

Moore, D. C., Spierdijk, J., van Kleef, J. D. et al (1982b) Four more cases of quite severe neurological sequelae after the use of 3 per cent chloroprocaine. *Anesthesia and Analgesia*, **61**, 155.

Mosavy, S. H. & Shafei, M. (1975) Prevention of headache consequent on dural puncture in obstetric patients. *Anaesthesia*, **30**, 807.

Naulty, J. S., Ostheimer, G. W., Datta, S., Knapp, R. & Weiss, J. B. (1982) Incidence of venous air embolism during epidural catheter insertion. *Anesthesiology*, **57**, 410.

Neumark, J., Feichtinger, W. & Gassner, A. (1980) Epidural block in obstetrics followed by meningoencephalitis. *Anesthesiology*, **52**, 518.

Newbery, J. M. (1977) Paraplegia following general anaesthesia. *Anaesthesia*, **32**, 78.

Newrick, P. & Read, D. (1982) Subdural haematoma as a complication of spinal anaesthesia. *British Medical Journal*, **285**, 341.

Nicholson, M. J. & Eversole, U. H. (1946) Neurologic complications of spinal anesthesia. *Journal of the American Medical Association*, **132**, 679.

Norman, J. E. (1955) Correspondence on nerve palsy following general anaesthesia. *Anaesthesia*, **10**, 87.

O'Connell, J. E. A. (1944) Maternal obstetrical paralysis. *Surgery, Gynecology and Obstetrics*, **79**, 374.

Odoom, J. A. & Sih, I. L. (1983) Epidural analgesia and anti-coagulant therapy. *Anaesthesia*, **38**, 254.

Ostheimer, G. W., Palahniuk, R. J. & Schnider, S. M. (1974) The epidural blood patch. *Anesthesiology*, **41**, 307.

Palahniuk, R. J. & Cumming, M. (1979) Prophylactic blood patch does not prevent post lumbar puncture headache. *Canadian Anaesthetists' Society Journal*, **26**, 132.

Pavlin, A. J., McDonald, J. S., Child, B. & Rusch, V. (1979) Acute subdural hematoma: an unusual sequel to lumbar puncture. *Anesthesiology*, **51**, 338.

Pfeiffer, R. I. (1953) Treatment of postspinal headache. *American Journal of Obstetrics and Gynecology*, **65**, 21.

Philbin, D. M., Baratz, R. A. & Patterson, R. W. (1970) The effect of carbon dioxide on plasma antidiuretic hormone levels during intermittent positive pressure breathing. *Anesthesiology*, **33**, 345.

Phillips, O. C., Ebner, H., Nelson, A. T. & Black, M. H. (1969) Neurological complications following spinal anesthesia with lidocaine. A prospective view of 10 440 cases. *Anesthesiology*, **30**, 284.

Prentiss, J. E. (1979) Cardiac arrest following caudal anesthesia. *Anesthesiology*, **50**, 51.

Rainbird, A. & Pfitzner, J. (1983) Restricted spread of analgesia following epidural blood-patch. *Anaesthesia*, **38**, 481.

Ramanathan, S. Chalon, J., Richards, M. et al (1978) Prolonged spinal nerve involvement after epidural anesthesia with etidocaine. *Anesthesia and Analgesia,* 57, 361.

Rao, T. L. K. & El-Etr, A. A. (1982) Anticoagulation following placement of epidural catheter. An evaluation of neurological sequelae. *Anesthesiology,* 55, 618.

Ratra, C. K., Badola, R. P. & Bhargava, B. (1972) A study of factors concerned in emesis during spinal anaesthesia. *British Journal of Anaesthesia,* 44, 1208.

Ravindran, R. S., Tasch, M. D., Baldwin, D. J. & Hendrie, M. (1981) Subarachnoid injection of autologous blood in dogs unassociated with neurological deficits. *Anesthesia and Analgesia,* 60, 603.

Ravindran, R. S., Bond, J. K., Tasch, M. D. et al (1980) Persistent neurological deficit and adhesive arachnoiditis following intrathecal 2-chloroprocaine *Anesthesia and Analgesia,* 59, 447.

Reisner, L. S., Hochman, R. N. & Plumer, M. H. (1980) Neurological deficits following epidural or spinal anesthesia. *Anesthesia and Analgesia,* 59, 452.

Rice, G. G. & Dabbs, C. H. (1950) The use of peridural and subarachnoid injections of saline solution in the treatment of severe postspinal headache. *Anesthesiology,* 11, 17.

Rich, M., Scheinberg, P. & Belle, M. S. (1953) Relationship between cerebrospinal fluid pressure changes and cerebral blood flow. *Circulation,* 1, 389.

Sadove, M. S., Levin, M. J. & Rant-Sejdinaj, I. (1961) Neurological complications of spinal anaesthesia. *Canadian Anaesthetists' Society Journal,* 8, 405.

Safar, D. & Tenicela, R (1964) High altitude physiology in relation to anesthesia and inhalation therapy. *Anesthesiology* 25, 515.

Schreiner, E., Lipson, S. F., Bromage, P. R. & Camporesi, E. M. (1983) Neurological complications following general anaesthesia. *Anaesthesia,* 38, 226.

Scott, D. B. (1981) Toxicity caused by local anaesthetic drugs. *British Journal of Anaesthesia,* 53, 553.

Scott, D. B. (1982) Subdural haematoma complicating spinal anaesthetic. *British Medical Journal,* 285, 1048.

Sears, R. T. (1959) Spinal analgesia using a 32 gauge needle. *British Medical Journal,* 1, 755.

Seglov, J. M. (1967) Spinal epidural hematoma: a report of two cases. *Pacific Medicine and Surgery,* 75, 169.

Seigne, T. D. (1970) Aseptic meningitis following spinal analgesia. *Anaesthesia,* 25, 402.

Sikh, S. S. & Agawal, G. (1974) Post-spinal headache. *Anaesthesia,* 29, 297.

Silver, J. R. & Buxton, T. H. (1974) Spinal stroke. *Brain,* 97, 539.

Sinclair, R. N. (1954) Ascending spinal paralysis following hysterectomy under general anaesthesia. *Anaesthesia,* 9, 286.

Skaredoff, M. N. & Datta, S. (1981) Horner's syndrome during epidural anaesthesia for elective Caesarean section. *Canadian Anaesthetists' Society Journal,* 28, 82.

Slattery, P. J., Rosen, M. & Rees, G. A. D. (1980) An aid to identification of the subarachnoid space with a 25 g needle. *Anaesthesia,* 35, 391.

Smith, B. E. (1979) Prophylaxis of epidural 'wet-tap' headache. *Anesthesiology,* Suppl., 51, 304.

Smith, F. R., Perkin, G. D. & Rose, F. C. (1980) Posture and headache after lumbar puncture. *Lancet,* 1, 1245.

Symonds, C. (1946) Headache. *Guy's Hospital Gazette,* 60, 202.

Teague, C. A. & Urquhart-Hay, D. (1974) Spinal thrombophlebitis after prostatectomy with hypotensive anaesthesia: a case report. *New Zealand Medical Journal,* 80, 654.

Thomas, P. & Dwyer, C. S. (1950) Postoperative flaccid paralysis: a case report. *Anesthesiology,* 11, 635.

Tondare, A. S., Nadkarmi, A. V., Sathe, C. H. & Dave, J. V. (1983) Femoral neuropathy: a complication of the lithotomy position under spinal anaesthesia. *Canadian Anaesthetists' Society Journal*, **30**, 84.

Tourtellotte, W. W. (1964) *Post-lumbar Puncture Headaches*, Springfield: Thomas.

Tourtellotte, W. W. & Henderson, W. G. (1972) Evidence for efficiency of a small needle. *Headache*, **12**, 75.

Tuffier, T. (1899) Analgésie chirurgicale par l'injection sous-arachnoidienne lombaire de cocain. *Comptes Rendus des Séances de la Société de Biologie*, **51**, 882.

Urquhart-Hay, D. (1969) Paraplegia following epidural analgesia. *Anaesthesia*, **24**, 461.

Vacanti, J. J. (1972) Postspinal headache and air travel. *Anesthesiology*, **37**, 358.

Vandam, L. D. & Dripps, R. D. (1954) Long term follow-up of 10 089 patients who received spinal anesthetics. *Journal of the American Medical Association*, **161**, 586.

Vandam, L. D. & Dripps, R. D. (1956a) Long term follow-up of 10 098 spinal anesthetics. *Surgery* (St Louis), **38**, 463.

Vandam, L. D. & Dripps, R. D. (1956b) Exacerbation of pre-existing neurological disease after spinal anesthesia. *New England Medical Journal*, **255**, 843.

Walpole, J. B. (1975) Blood patch for spinal headache. *Anaesthesia*, **30**, 783.

Wark, H. J. (1977) An unusual complication of an inadvertent dural tap. *Anaesthesia*, **32**, 336.

Wells, C. E. C. (1966) Clinical aspects of spinovascular disease. *Proceedings of the Royal Society of Medicine* **59**, 790; and *Lancet*, annotations, (1958) **2**, 515; and (1967) **2**, 143.

Widerlov, E. & Lindström, L. (1979) D.D.A.V.P. and headache after lumbar puncture. *Lancet*, **1**, 548.

Wilson, G., Rupp, C. & Wilson, W. W. (1949) The dangers of intrathecal medication. *New York Medical Journal*, **140**, 1076.

Winkleman, N. W. (1952) Neurological symptoms following accidental intraspinal detergent infection. *Neurology*, **2**, 284.

Wolfson, B. & Siker, E. S. (1970) Postpneumoencephalography headache. *Anaesthesia*, **25**, 328.

14

Spinal analgesia and intractable pain

When intractable pain from malignant disease becomes intolerable, one must consider the possible beneficial results from an injection of a neurolytic drug to block pain impulses from the affected area. At the same time it is undesirable to block nerve fibres other than sensory, and indeed not to cause a sensory loss over an area wider than necessary. Because the spread of a solution injected intradurally is more controllable than when it is injected extradurally, the major interest has been in intradural injection, when neurolytic agents are employed.

Phenol, 5 per cent in glycerine and 7.5 per cent in iophendylate (Myodil) have been recommended (Maher, 1955; Nathan and Scott, 1958), as have ammonium sulphate in 6 per cent solution (Hand, 1944) and chlorocresol (Maher, 1963). These are all hyperbaric solutions. Absolute alcohol, a hypobaric injection, has been used since 1931 (Dogliotti, 1931). Because pain impulses reach the spinal cord via the posterior roots, the aim is to use gravity so that the neurolytic agent reaches the posterior roots but avoids the anterior roots with the motor fibres. When hyperbaric solutions are used, the patient is placed in a semi-supine position for the intradural injection. He is rotated into the semi-prone position prior to alcohol injection.

Following a detailed history and examination of the patient the segments to be blocked are identified. It is usual to attempt block on one side only in any one session. Lumbar puncture is performed at the appropriate level, the patient carefully positioned, and the injection made. The volume of the injected solution must be the minimum to obtain the desired result. Thus 5 to 7 per cent phenol in glycerine may be given as an initial injection of 0.2 ml with further increments of 0.1 ml as judged by the patient's response, to a maximum of 1 ml. (Swerdlow, 1978). Larger doses may be dangerous; 3 ml 6 per cent phenol in glycerine injected in the cervical region has been followed by respiratory arrest (Holland and

Youssef, 1979). Phenol in iophendylate and chlorocresol can be used in a similar manner. Absolute alcohol may be injected in increments of 0.5 ml up to a maximum of 5 ml (Swerdlow, 1978).

These injections are most satisfactory when given in the lumbar region. At levels above T.6, there is a risk of paralysis of nerves to the arm, or of cranial nerves, and the extradural route may be considered, as may injection into the extracranial subdural space (Mehta and Maher, 1977).

Pain in the perineum or rectum is difficult to treat because of the risk to the bowel and bladder function when neurolytic agents are used. After lumbar puncture in the sitting position, the patient is tilted backwards to make an angle between 15 and 20 degrees with the table, and 5 per cent phenol in glycerine injected, taking at least one minute for the injection; the position is maintained for at least half an hour. The neurolytic solution tends to move slowly along the posterior aspect of the subarachnoid space, avoiding the 2nd, 3rd and 4th sacral nerves which innervate the bladder and which lie in the anterior part of the compartment (Mehta, 1973).

Before attempting any of these injections the operator must be convinced that the likely benefit to the patient outweighs the disadvantages. Risk of untoward paralysis can never be excluded.

Because of the dangers of neurolytic drugs, other workers have investigated the use of mechanical methods. Some of these afford a measure of pain relief without the patient being subjected to the risk of nerve paralysis.

Ice-cold saline was described by Hitchcock (1967). Eighty to 90 ml of cerebrospinal fluid is withdrawn and replaced by the saline which has been for some time in a refrigerator. The supernatant fluid is hypertonic but is painful on injection so that general anaesthesia is necessary. A solution of 12 per cent saline at normal temperature is probably just as effective (Lloyd, 1976).

The technique of barbotage has been recommended (Lloyd et al., 1972; Lloyd, 1973). Twenty ml of cerebrospinal fluid is alternately withdrawn and injected. This simple technique is painless and of value in the amelioration of pelvic and lower limb pain. It can be combined with cooling of the cerebrospinal fluid before replacement.

The injection of steroids into the extradural space has been reported to relieve dorsal root pains such as pain after herpes zoster and pain following trauma (Forrest, 1978; Perkins and Hanlon, 1978). Lasting and profound analgesia has followed the intradural injection of 3 mg of synthetic beta-endorphin with 15 per cent glucose in 3 ml of solution (Shimoji et al, 1977; Illis and Sedgwick, 1978; Oyama et al, 1981; Oyama, 1983).

The extradural injection of narcotic analgesic drugs has the advantage of a long duration of action from a single dose, with the possibility of continuous analgesia when a catheter is used (see Ch. 9).

Stimulation techniques also have a place. Transcutaneous stimulation can be applied, or electrodes can be implanted over the dorsal columns of the cord and activated by the use of a radio frequency (Shealy et al., 1972). Electrodes can also be passed into the extradural space via a Tuohy needle. Stimulation techniques have the advantage that they cause no permanent damage to nerve structures, although they are only effective for a limited period of time in a percentage of patients.

The treatment of intractable pain is a complex subject, and spinal techniques are only one method available. Results are often temporary and disappointing, although excellent pain relief is afforded in a number of patients. The reader is referred to the many comprehensive reviews on the subject (Lloyd, 1976; Swerdlow et al, 1978; Lloyd, 1980; Swerdlow, 1981; Mehta, 1982).

REFERENCES

Dogliotti, A. M. (1931) Traitement des syndromes douloureux de la péripherie par l'alcolisation des racines posterieures. *Presse Médicale*, 39, 1249.
Forrest, J. B (1978) Management of dorsal root pain with epidural steroids. *Canadian Anaesthetists' Society Journal*, 25, 218.
Hand, L. V. (1944) Subarachnoid ammonium sulphate therapy for intractable pain. *Anesthesiology*, 5, 354.
Hitchcook, E. R. (1967) Hypothermic irrigation for intractable pain. *Lancet*, 1, 1133.
Holland, A. J. C. & Youssef, M. (1979) A complication of subarachnoid phenol blockade. *Anaesthesia*, 34, 260.
Illis, L. S. & Sedgwick, E. M. (1978) Spinal cord stimulation. *British Journal of Hospital Medicine*, 20, 682.
Lloyd, J. W. (1973) Barbotage of the cerebrospinal fluid for the relief of intractable pain. *Proceedings of the Royal Society of Medicine*, 66, 543.
Lloyd, J. W. (1976) The management of intractable pain. In Lee, J. A. & Bryce-Smith, R. (eds) *Practical Regional Analgesia*, Amsterdam: Excerpta Medica.
Lloyd, J. W. (1980) Intractable pain conditions which require treatment. *British Medical Journal*, 2, 432.
Lloyd, J. W., Hughes, J. T. & Davies-Jones, G. A. B. (1972) The relief of severe intractable pain by barbotage of the cerebrospinal fluid. *Lancet*, 1, 354.
Maher, R. M. (1955) Relief of pain in incurable cancer. *Lancet*, 1, 18.
Maher, R. M. (1963) Intrathecal chlorocresol in the treatment of pain in cancer. *Lancet*, 1, 965.
Mehta, M. (1973) *Intractable Pain*. London: Saunders.

Mehta, M. (1982) Chronic pain. In Atkinson, R. S. & Hewer, C. L. (eds) *Recent Advances in Anaesthesia and Analgesia*, 14, Edinburgh: Churchill Livingstone.

Mehta, M & Maher, R. M. (1977) Injection into the extra-arachnoid subdural space. *Anaesthesia*, 32, 760.

Nathan, P. W & Scott, T. G. (1958) Intrathecal phenol for intractable pain. *Lancet*, 1, 895.

Oyama, T. (1983) Beta-endorphin for the treatment of pain. (Abstracts) *Third Asean Congress of Anesthesiologists* (Bangkok), p. 51.

Oyama, T., Toshiro, J., Yamaya, R., Ling, N. & Guillemin, R. (1981) Profound analgesia with beta endorphins in man. *Lancet*, 1, 122.

Perkins, H. M. & Hanlon, P. R. (1978) Epidural injections of local anesthetics and steroids for relief of pain secondary to herpes zoster. *Archives of Surgery*, 113, 253.

Shealy, C. N., Mortimer, J. T. & Hagfors, N. R. (1972) Dorsal column electroanalgesia. *Journal of Neurosurgery*, 32, 560.

Shimoji, K., Matsuki, M., Shimizu, H., Iwane, T., Takahashi, R., Maruyama, M. & Masuko, K. (1977) Low-frequency, weak extradural stimulation in the management of intractable pain. *British Journal of Anaesthesia*, 49, 1081.

Swerdlow, M. (1978) Intrathecal neurolysis. *Anaesthesia*, 33, 733.

Swerdlow, M. (1981) *The Therapy of Pain*. Lancaster: MTP Press.

Swerdlow, M., Mehta, M. & Lipton, S. (1978) The role of the anaesthetist in chronic pain management. *Anaesthesia*, 33, 250.

15

Narcotic analgesic drugs in the extradural and intradural space

The discovery of opiate receptors in the central nervous system (Pert and Snyder, 1973; Pert et al, 1976) was soon followed by experimental work in animals (Yaksh and Rudy, 1976) which showed that morphine injected intrathecally did produce analgesia by a local effect. This action is predominantly on pre- and post-synaptic membranes of laminae 2 and 5 of the spinal cord horn as proposed by Rexed (Rexed, 1952; Rexed, 1954). Lamina 2 corresponds to the substantia gelatinosa (Ralston, 1981). Pain is inhibited and there may be some interference with hot and cold sensation and also with bladder function (Bromage et al, 1982). Clinical applications in man showed that small doses of intradural morphine produce effective and prolonged analgesia, whether injected intradurally (Wang et al, 1979) or extradurally (Behar et al, 1979).

Publication of this work stimulated interest so that many clinicians claimed successful use of spinal opioids in their practice. The rapid development from basic scientific experiment to widespread clinical use without controlled trials, knowledge of the best drug, best volume and the factors which determine the incidence of side-effects, has been commented upon by thoughtful writers (Winnie, 1980; Morgan, 1982), while the present state of knowledge of dose-response has been summarised by Bullingham et al (1982).

Opioids have been injected extradurally more commonly than intradurally, but consideration of the latter route is fundamental since molecules of the drug must cross from the extradural to the intradural space to produce their effect on receptors in the spinal cord. Opioid injected into the intradural space is immediately diluted by cerebrospinal fluid and must ascend to spinal cord level since it will not be effective locally when injected in the lumbar region among the nerves of the cauda equina. It has been calculated (Bullingham et al, 1982) that the resultant cord concentrations of the narcotic analgesic drug will be many times that seen after normal parenteral use, even bearing in mind the small dose injected.

Of the narcotic analgesic drugs in common clinical use, all are lipophilic except morphine. This has important implications in terms of brain/plasma or neural substance/cerebrospinal fluid distribution coefficients. Morphine is the narcotic analgesic which has been most commonly employed by anaesthetists for extradural or intradural injection, but because of its low lipophilicity its distribution differs from that of other drugs. The concentration in the neural substance will be less than that in the cerebrospinal fluid with the consequence of slow drug removal and the possibility of continued rostral spread. Other narcotic analgesics which are more lipid soluble pass into the lipids of the cord more readily and so are less likely to travel rostrally in the cerebrospinal fluid with the danger of respiratory depression. The intrathecal opioid is removed by diffusion into the cord substance and absorption into blood flowing through the cord; transference across the thick dense membrane of the dura mater is negligible by comparison. However, the more lipophilic agents have a slower rate of dissociation from the receptor than morphine, a major factor in determination of the duration of analgesia (Bullingham, 1981).

Narcotic analgesic drugs injected into the extradural space must first pass to the intradural space before reaching the spinal cord. There is no proven action in the extradural space itself. The dura mater, an inert, relatively thick barrier compared to lipid membranes, maintains a concentration gradient of at least a hundredfold (Cousins et al, 1979). Systemic absorption also begins at once with a plasma profile similar to that which follows intramuscular injection (Weddel and Ritter, 1981). It should be remembered also that there is no barrier to drainage to the cerebral veins at the base of the brain with the possibility of consequential respiratory depression. Systemic absorption may itself make a contribution to systemic analgesia, but it also lowers the concentration gradient across the dura mater so that less drug reaches the neuraxis. The more lipophilic drugs will be absorbed faster but will also undergo quicker dural transfer. It is interesting to note that the dose of extradurally administered narcotic analgesic has tended to increase with operator experience (Chambers et al, 1981) while some authors have gone so far as to suggest that the extradural dose of morphine required to produce effective analgesia is close to that required by intravenous medication (Bromage et al, 1980).

Selection of the intrathecal route requires injection of a dose which is large relative to that needed in the cord since there is a desirability to create a reservoir. Selection of the extradural space requires creation of a much larger depot outside the dura mater, but cerebrospinal fluid concentrations are relatively low, whereas the significant levels obtained in the systemic circulation prevent cord levels from declining rapidly while at the same time possibly activating supraspinal mechanisms which have a synergistic action with the local effect. Bullingham et al (1982) indeed go so far as to suggest that good results might be achieved if injection of a very small dose (e.g. pethidine 1 mg) was made intradurally with a larger dose (e.g. pethidine 75 mg) intramuscularly.

Whatever drug and dose is chosen it should be appreciated that higher dosage produces greater intensity of both analgesia and side-effects, while severe chest and upper abdominal pain require larger doses than lower abdominal pain when the drug is injected in the lumbar region. The intensity of both analgesia and side-effects is enhanced by the addition of adrenaline, 1:200 000 to the solution (Bromage et al, 1983).

A number of narcotic analgesic drugs have been employed to provide extradural analgesia. Morphine (Graham et al, 1980; Johnston and McCaughey, 1980; Magora et al, 1980; Reiz and Westberg, 1980) has the longest effect but is most likely to give rise to respiratory depression. It has been used in doses of 2 to 4 mg in a volume of 10 ml dextrose or saline to treat various types of both acute and chronic pain. Diamorphine has been used extradurally in a dose of 0.1 mg/kg in 10 ml (Jacobson et al, 1983). Methadone (Welch and Hrynaszkiewicz, 1981) has been used in a dose of 5 to 6 mg with top-up doses of 4 mg in volumes up to 20 ml of saline for postoperative pain relief. Various workers have employed pethidine (Perris, 1980). Fentanyl (Wolfe and Nicholas, 1979; Wolfe and Davies, 1980) has the shortest duration of action of those narcotic analgesics which have been studied. Because of this short action it has been used in a continuous infusion (Bailey and Smith, 1980). Pain from upper abdominal or thoracic surgery was more adequately controlled than with intramuscular papaveretum in a recent study (Welchew and Thornton, 1982) in which a loading dose of 200 μg in 12 ml saline given via a lumbar extradural catheter was followed by an infusion of 60 μg/h.

Narcotic analgesic drugs injected intradurally or extradurally have the advantage that neither motor nor autonomic nerves are affected. Motor function is preserved so that patients retain active use of their limbs, while the cardiovascular stability which occurs is advantageous. The analgesic effect, while not so complete as that following injection of local analgesic drugs, is prolonged in its duration, an advantage in the management of postoperative and chronic pain. Extradural fentanyl has been used for minor surgery with success (Herrera–Hoyos, 1983) though it was combined with an intravenous infusion of etomidate for sedation.

Side-effects

The most serious complication which may develop is severe respiratory depression, which may not be manifest for several hours (Glynn et al, 1979; Davies et al, 1980). Naloxone will reverse this depression (Jones and Jones, 1980), but clearly this can only be given in time if the patient is monitored continuously. Naloxone does not reverse the analgesia.

Other side-effects which have been reported including itching, which may especially occur in the distribution of the trigeminal nerve, nausea and dizziness, urinary retention (Petersen et al, 1982) and temporary inability to ejaculate in males (Torda et al, 1980). There is evidence that phenoxybenzamine in four divided doses of 10 mg before and after operation may reduce the incidence of postoperative urinary retention (Evron et al, 1983).

Pain relief in obstetrics

The fact that spinal narcotic analgesics produce analgesia without concomitant sympathetic and motor block, and without central depression, makes their use particularly attractive in obstetric practice. Unfortunately, clinical results have been disappointing. Extradural morphine in a dose of 2 mg has been unsatisfactory (Husemeyer et al, 1980; Crawford, 1981), perhaps because of rapid removal due to increased vascularity of the space in pregnancy, though some workers have obtained better results (Booker et al, 1980).

Pethidine (Perriss, 1979; Perriss, 1980; Perriss and Malins, 1981) and fentanyl (Carrie et al, 1981) have been more satisfactory, though often with doses large enough for systemic absorption to occur to levels which might be expected following intramuscular injection. Possible respiratory depression of the newborn has also to be considered (Carrie et al, 1981).

At the present time it does not seem likely that spinal narcotic analgesics will replace the well-tried and successful use of local analgesic drugs for extradural block in obstetrics.

Postoperative pain relief

For a number of reasons, the conventional method of providing postoperative analgesia by use of intramuscular opioids is far from satisfactory (*British Medical Journal*, Editorial, 1978). Extradural or intradural narcotic analgesia, administered while the patient is in the operating suite, may hopefully provide a prolonged period of pain relief without the need for frequent supplementary injections. Success has been reported by a number of authors (Bailey and Smith, 1980; Bromage et al, 1980; Graham et al, 1980; Mathews and Abrams, 1980; Chambers et al, 1981; Gjessing and Tomlin, 1981; Weddel and Ritter, 1981; Kaufman, 1983). It is clear, however, that patients managed in this way require good postoperative observation in case respiratory depression should occur even several hours after administration of the analgesic.

Acute trauma

Morphine has been successfully used when injected extradurally for relief of pain associated with acute trauma to the thorax (Johnston and McCaughey, 1980). Analgesia produced in this way, combined with other appropriate measures for the treatment of chest injuries, may obviate the need for mechanical ventilation of the lungs in these patients.

Chronic pain

Patients with chronic pain are sometimes managed by the use of serial injections of a narcotic analgesic drug via an indwelling extradural catheter (Howard et al, 1981). Such a technique is effective for the dull, constant ache of cancer, but the risk of side-effects must be balanced against the benefit obtained. The risks of infection (Wenningsted-Torgard et al, 1982) may be worth taking in a patient who has a terminal illness, while subcutaneous tunnelling to an exit 8 cm from the mid-line reduces the risk and aids stability of the catheter (Howard et al, 1981). With suitable precautions some patients can be managed at home. Another interesting development is the use of a subcutaneous reservoir system connected to an extradural catheter (Coombs et al, 1982). Although open operation is necessary for its insertion, once in place, top-up increments are no harder to give than a subcutaneous injection. Nevertheless, the dangers of respiratory depression should be considered whenever extradural narcotic analgesic drugs are employed (Mehta, 1982).

REFERENCES

Bailey, P. W. & Smith, B. E. (1980) Continuous epidural infusion of fentanyl for postoperative analgesia. *Anaesthesia*, 35, 1002.
Behar, M., Magora, F., Elshwang, D. & Davidson, J. T. (1979) Epidural morphine in treatment of pain. *Lancet*, 1, 527.
Booker, P. D., Wilkes, R. G., Bryson, T. H. L. & Beddard, J. (1980) Obstetric pain relief using epidural morphine. *Anaesthesia*, 35, 377.
British Medical Journal (1978) Editorial. Postoperative pain. *British Medical Journal*, 2, 517.
Bromage, P. R., Camporesi, E. M. & Chestnut, D. (1980) Epidural narcotics for postoperative analgesia. *Anesthesia and Analgesia*, 59, 473.
Bromage, P. R., Camporesi, E. M., Durant, A. C. & Nielson, C. H. (1982) Non-respiratory side effects of epidural morphine. *Anesthesia and Analgesia*, 59, 61, 473, 490.
Bromage, P. R., Camporesi, E. M., Durant, P. A. & Nielsen, C. H. (1983) Influence of epinephrine as an adjuvant to epidural morphine. *Anesthesiology*, 58, 257.
Bullingham, R. E. S. (1981) Synthetic opiate analgesics. *British Journal of Hospital Medicine*, 25, 59.
Bullingham, R. E. S., McQuay, H. J. & Moore, R. A. (1982) Extradural and intrathecal narcotics. In Atkinson, R. S. & Hewer, C. L. (eds) *Recent Advances in Anaesthesia and Analgesia*, 14; ch. 10. Edinburgh: Churchill Livingstone.
Carrie, L. E. S., O'Sullivan, G. M. & Seegobin, R. (1981) Epidural fentanyl in labour. *Anaesthesia*, 36, 965.
Chambers, W. A., Sinclair, C. J. & Scott, D. B. (1981) Extradural morphine for pain after surgery. *British Journal of Anaesthesia*, 53, 921.
Coombs, D. W., Saunders, R. L., Gaylor, M. & Pareau, M. G. (1982) Epidural narcotic infusion reservoir: implantation techniques and efficacy. *Anesthesiology*, 56, 469.
Cousins, M. J., Mather, L. E., Glynn, C. J., Wilson, P. R. & Graham, J. R. (1979) Selective spinal analgesia. *Lancet*, 1, 1141.
Crawford, J. S. (1981) Experiences with epidural morphine in obstetrics. *Anaesthesia*, 36, 207.
Davies, G. K., Tolhurst-Cleaver, C. L. & James, T. L. (1980) Respiratory depression after intrathecal opiates. *Anaesthesia*, 35, 1080.
Evron, S., Sadovsky, E. & Magora, F. (1983) The effect of phenoxybenzamine on the postoperative urinary retention after epidural morphine analgesia. (Abstracts) *Scientific Meeting of the European Academy of Anaesthesiology* (Stockholm).
Gjessing, J. & Tomlin, P. J. (1981) Postoperative pain control with intrathecal morphine. *Anaesthesia*, 36, 268.
Glynn, C. J., Mather, L. E., Cousins, M. J., Wilson, P. R. & Graham, J. R. (1979) Spinal narcotics and respiratory depression. *Lancet*, 2, 356.
Graham, J. L., King, R. & McCaughey, W. (1980) Postoperative pain relief using epidural morphine. *Anaesthesia*, 35, 158.
Herrera-Hoyos, J. O. (1983) Correspondence. *Anaesthesia*, 38, 509.
Howard, R. P., Milne, L. A. & Williams, N. E. (1981) Epidural morphine in terminal cancer. *Anaesthesia*, 36, 51.
Husemeyer, R. P., O'Connor, M. C. & Davenport, H. T. (1980) Failure of epidural morphine to relieve pain in labour. *Anaesthesia*, 35, 161.
Jacobson, L., Phillips, P. D., Hull, C. J. & Conacher, I. D. (1983) Extradural versus intramuscular diamorphine. *Anaesthesia*, 38, 10.
Johnston, J. R. & McCaughey, W. (1980) Epidural morphine: a method of management of multiple fractured ribs. *Anaesthesia*, 35, 155.
Jones, R. D. M. & Jones, G. B. (1980) Intrathecal morphine — naloxone reverses respiratory depression but not analgesia. *British Medical Journal*, 281, 645.

Kaufman, L. (1983) Reflections on spinal analgesia. II. Pain relief. *British Journal of Parenteral Therapy*, **4**, 14.

Magora, F., Olshwang, D., Eimerl, D., Shorr, J., Katzenelm, R., Coter, S. & Davidson, J. T. (1980) Observations on extradural morphine analgesia in various pain conditions. *British Journal of Anaesthesia*, **52**, 247.

Mathews, E. T. & Abrams, L. D.(1980) Intrathecal morphine in open heart surgery. *Lancet*, **2**, 543.

Mehta, M. (1982) Chronic pain. In Atkinson, R. S. & Hewer, C. L. (eds) *Recent Advances in Anaesthesia and Analgesia*, 14; ch. 11. Edinburgh: Churchill Livingstone.

Morgan, M. (1982) Editorial. *Anaesthesia*, **37**, 527.

Perriss, B. W. (1979) Epidural opiates in labour. *Lancet*, **2**, 422.

Perriss, B. W. (1980) Epidural pethidine in labour. A study of dose requirements. *Anaesthesia*, **35**, 380.

Perriss, B. W. & Malins, A. F. (1981) Pain relief in labour using epidural pethidine with adrenaline. *Anaesthesia*, **36**, 631.

Pert, C. B. & Snyder, S. H. (1973) Opiate receptors: demonstration in nervous tissue. *Science*, **179**, 1011.

Pert, C. B., Kuhar, M. J. & Snyder, S. H. (1976) Opiate receptors: autoradiographic localization in rat brain. *Proceedings of the National Academy of Science* (USA), **73**, 3729.

Petersen, T. K., Husted, S. E., Rybro, L., Shurizek, B. A. & Wernberg, M. (1982) Urinary retention during i.m. and extradural morphine analgesia. *British Journal of Anaesthesia*, **54**, 1175.

Ralston, H. J. (1981) The synaptic organisation of the Macaque dorsal horn. In Brown, A. G. & Rethelyi, M. (eds) *Spinal Cord Sensation*. Edinburgh: Scottish Academic Press.

Reiz, S. & Westberg, M. (1980) Side effects of epidural morphine. *Lancet*, **2**, 203.

Rexed, B. (1952) The cytoarchitectonic organization of the spinal cord in the cat. *Journal of Comparative Neurology*, **96**, 415.

Rexed, B. (1954) A cytoarchitectonic atlas of the spinal cord in the cat. *Journal of Comparative Neurology*, **100**, 297.

Torda, T. A., Pybus, D. A., Liberman, H., Clark, M. & Crawford, M. (1980) Experimental comparison of extradural and i.m. morphine. *British Journal of Anaesthesia*, **52**, 939.

Wang, J. K., Nauss, L. A. & Thomas, J. E. (1979) Pain relief by intrathecally applied morphine in man. *Anesthesiology*, **50**, 149.

Weddel, S. J. & Ritter, R. R. (1981) Serum levels following epidural administration of morphine and correlation with relief of postsurgical pain. *Anesthesiology*, **54**, 210.

Welch, D. B. & Hrynaszkiewicz, A. (1981) Postoperative analgesia using epidural methadone. Administration by the lumbar route for thoracic pain relief. *Anaesthesia*, **36**, 1051.

Welchew, E. A. & Thornton, J. A. (1982) Continuous thoracic epidural fentanyl. *Anaesthesia*, **37**, 309.

Wenningsted-Torgard, K., Heyn, J. & Willunsen, L. (1982) Spondylitis following epidural morphine. *Acta Anaesthesiologica Scandinavica*, **26**, 649.

Winnie, A. P. (1980) Epidural and intrathecal opiates. New uses for old drugs. *Anesthesiology*, **7**, 8.

Wolfe, M. J. & Davies, G. K. (1980) Analgesic action of epidural fentanyl. *British Journal of Anaesthesia*, **52**, 357.

Wolfe, M. J. & Nicholas, A. D. G. (1979) Selective epidural analgesia. *Lancet*, **2**, 150.

Yaksh, T. L. & Rudy, T. A. (1976) Analgesia mediated by a direct spinal action of narcotics. *Science*, **192**, 1357.

16

Do's, don'ts and doubtfuls

Do's

If the spinal block is high — or in any emergency — remove head pillows, raise the legs, infuse fluid intravenously and give oxygen. These measures are the best treatment for collapse, and the ones most calculated to prevent its onset. The main threat of high block comes from suboxygenation: this results from a combination of the almost inevitable fall in blood-pressure and diminished respiratory exchange, and itself leads to a greater fall in blood-pressure and to a further decrease in respiratory efficiency — a vicious circle which, if not interrupted, can end fatally.

A block is sometimes desirable because a comparatively bloodless field is likely to result, while on other occasions the technique should be avoided so that any oozing will be evident at the time. After spinal analgesia, intradural or extradural, the surgeon should make sure that any potential bleeding points are ligated: otherwise reactionary haemorrhage can occur.

Always allow plenty of time if you propose to give an extradural block. A sense of hurry and the meticulousness necessary for this technical procedure do not go well together. A surgeon who is frequently kept waiting for his patient while the anaesthetist is giving such a block may, quite naturally, develop a dislike for this form of pain relief.

When engaged in the delicate task of locating the extradural space, give your maximal attention to the task in hand, otherwise the 'end-point' may be missed, resulting possibly in dural puncture.

Always take great care with extradural injection after inadvertent dural puncture as very high block may result.

If you are unsure of the exact location of the tip of your needle or catheter, do give a 'test dose', e.g. 2 ml of 0.5 per cent of bupivacaine with adrenaline. Injected into the theca, this will cause relaxation of anal tone and tingling or paresis of the feet; injected into a vessel, tachycardia will result from the adrenaline (Peters, 1983).

Do consider the treatment of intractable headache after dural puncture, especially in obstetric patients, by extradural blood patch (Brownridge, 1983).

Don'ts

Do not inflict unnecessary discomfort on your patient. If a difficult lumbar puncture is expected, or if the patient is specially nervous or anxious, do not hesitate to give an intravenous analgesic, e.g. diamorphine 2 to 5 mg or a benzodiazepine, e.g. midazolam 2.5 to 10 mg before using the needle. If the block is considered to be necessary, it may be desirable to precede it by full general anaesthesia.

Never procure a central neural blockade unless you have an intravenous infusion running freely, or a cannula in place to which such an infusion can be instantly connected.

In assessing the level of the block do not say to the patient 'tell me if you feel any pain'. A look at the patient's face will give all the information you need. An ether-soaked swab or an ethyl chloride spray is often better for this purpose than a needle point.

Do not use a 25 or similar gauge needle for eliciting the 'loss of resistance' test before extradural injection. A 20 to 16 gauge needle is more efficient for this purpose.

Do not allow tactless chatter if your patient is conscious. Anaesthetic or surgical 'shop-talk', not intended for the ears of the patient, may be remembered.

Do not try to 'cover' an inadequate block by repeated injections of a barbiturate alone. Admit to yourself that the block is unsatisfactory and proceed to give a suitable general anaesthetic.

Do not allow glove powder to contaminate the inside of the syringe or it may stick and complicate the location of the extradural space, thus increasing the risk of dural puncture.

Do not employ central neural blockade for patients who are opposed to it or for operations performed by surgeons who are prejudiced against it, unless you consider it to be the safest method of pain relief: the results will seldom be completely satisfactory. There are some patients who are quite unsuitable for any technique of regional analgesia just as there are some surgeons for whose operations it is almost always likely to be considered less than perfect.

In an emergency do not have faith in drugs. Rely on removing the head pillow and raising the legs, and administering oxygen — if necessary by artificial ventilation.

Never place ampoules in alcohol, spirit or antiseptics of any sort. This dangerous practice has been dealt with extensively in a previous edition of this book (Macintosh, 1957). If ampoules and apparatus cannot be sterilised by gamma radiation, they should be autoclaved.

Do not give a high block to patients suspected of having certain vascular diseases, particularly cerebral arteriosclerosis or coronary ischaemia. Efficient circulation through the vessels in question is dependent on a good *vis a tergo*, or, in other words, on the maintenance of a good head of pressure. With high segmental analgesia some fall in blood-pressure must be counted on: if this is severe enough to cause marked slowing of the rate of flow through the vessels, already narrowed and possibly irregular, thrombosis may result.

Be healthily suspicious of any container of 'sterile' water to be used in spinal analgesia, and distrust completely a container which has already been opened.

Do not use 'sterile' local analgesic solution from a stock bottle to make a skin weal through which the spinal needle is to be passed. Open and use another ampoule of analgesic solution for the purpose. The anaesthetist should be as careful before administering a spinal block as the orthopaedic surgeon is before opening the knee-joint, as regards his aseptic technique.

Doubtfuls

It is commonly stated that a spinal analgesic should not be given to patients suffering from diseases of the central nervous sytem. It may be politic to accept this view, since any exacerbation may be blamed not on the natural course of the disease, but on the administration. Nevertheless, we find it difficult to believe that spinal analgesia will cause any more harm than the lumbar puncture which is made as a routine in the investigation of these diseases. We know of occasions when a spinal analgesic has been given to a patient suffering from tabes and to another suffering from syringomyelia, and there has been no suggestion that either was any the worse for the experience. We have knowledge of large numbers of extradural blocks given for laminectomy in surgery of the intervertebral disc and have not seen harm resulting from this method of pain relief.

We do not know anything to suggest that a lesion of the central nervous system is likely to respond more unfavourably to a spinal than to a general anaesthetic. Nevertheless, in the event of a flare-up the anaesthetist who has chosen spinal analgesia would probably find himself more exposed to litigation. In these circumstances, we feel it prudent to confine the administration to anaesthetists of experience who are convinced of the benefits of the method to the patient and who are prepared to explain their reasoning to the patient or his friends. In the absence of these two factors we consider it wise to sidestep central neural analgesia if there are no pressing contraindications to other forms of pain relief (Crawford et al, 1981).

We have no personal knowledge of the effect of spinal analgesia in shock, but we are under the impression that it is a blunderbuss method, incapable of refinement. A professional anaesthetist confronted with a shocked patient would choose a general anaesthetic: for the depth of this can be controlled and varied to suit the changing condition of the patient and the surgeon's requirements. There can be no doubt that if the patient is fit enough to stand spinal analgesia, he is fit enough for a general anaesthetic properly administered. On the other hand, an ill patient can easily die if the general anaesthetic is not given skilfully. In an emergency, therefore, where an experienced anaesthetist is not available, it may be justifiable to give a spinal analgesic provided hypovolaemia has been reversed, and particular attention paid to keeping the legs raised, to giving oxygen throughout and to the avoidance of so-called stimulating medicaments.

Whether vasopressor drugs have any merit in spinal analgesia is an old controversy. Some anaesthetists use them as a routine, others avoid them and yet achieve satisfactory results. We include ourselves in the latter group: but in making this statement we think it right to stress that if respiratory function becomes in any way depressed oxygen should be given by either spontaneous or artificial ventilation. The procedures should be limited to reasonably fit subjects, and avoided studiously in patients suffering from recent acute coronary disease or cerebrovascular accident. There is no reason why a 'low' block, i.e. one confined to the cauda equina for an operation on the legs or perineum, should not be given to an ill patient. An example of a very unfit patient who may be more safely dealt with by intradural block, especially if unilateral, than by general anaesthesia, is the old and decrepit and possibly diabetic patient with arteriosclerosis who has to have a leg amputated. We would subscribe to the view that block confined to the sacral and lumbar roots subjects the patient to minimal physiological insults, respiratory, haemodynamic or metabolic (Davis and Lawrenson 1981; Nightingale and Marstrand, 1981; Stefansson et al, 1982).

REFERENCES

Brownridge, P. (1983) The management of headache following accidental dural puncture in obstetric patients. *Anaesthesia and Intensive Care*, **11**, 4.

Crawford, J. S. et al (1981) Correspondence. *Anaesthesia*, **36**, 821.

Davis, F. M. & Lawrenson, V. G. (1981) Spinal anaesthesia or general anaesthesia for emergency hip surgery. *Anaesthesia and Intensive Care*, **9**, 352.

Macintosh, R. R. (1957) *Lumbar Puncture and Spinal Analgesia*, p. 133, 2nd edn. Edinburgh: Livingstone.

Nightingale, P. J. & Marstrand, T. (1981) Subarachnoid anaesthesia with bupivacaine for orthopaedic procedures in the elderly. *British Journal of Anaesthesia*, **53**, 369.

Peters, C. G. (1983) Correspondence. *Anaesthesia*, **38**, 72.

Stefansson, T., Wickstrom, I. & Haljamie, H. (1982) Effects of neurolept and epidural analgesia on cardiovascular function and tissue metabolism. *Acta Anaesthesiologica Scandinavica*, **26**, 386.

Index

'A' fibres
  afferents, 99
  alpha fibres, 100
  delta fibres, 99
  efferents, 99
  gamma fibres, 99
Abdominal operations, 247
  caudal analgesia, infants/children and, 232
  gynaecological, 247
  intradural analgesia, 191–193, 200–201
    motor nerves to abdominal wall and, 192
    splanchnic nerves and, 192
  lower abdomen *see* Lower abdominal operations
  upper abdomen *see* Upper abdominal operations
Abdominal tumour, 225
Acetazolamide, CSF formation and, 89
Acid-base status, 122
Aconite, 6
Action potential, 99
Adhesive arachnoiditis, 292
Adrenal glands, 111
  cortex, 111–112
  medulla, 112
  suppression of cortical function by sedatives, 145
Adrenaline BP, 11, **136**, 293
  with amethocaine hydrochloride, 125
  with bupivacaine, 131, 136, 264, 313
  cardiovascular system and, 106
  with etidocaine, 134
  historical aspects, 15, 28
  intradural analgesia and, 202
  with lignocaine, 127
  with narcotic analgesics, 308
  placental transfer and, 264
  with prilocaine, 129
Afferent fibres, spinal ganglion, 52

Age, spinal analgesia and, 106
  spread of solutions and, 225
Alcohol
  absolute, 302
  withdrawal symptoms, 144
Allergic reactions, 119
Allocaine, 124
Alpha adrenergic drugs, 108, 262
Alpha adrenergic receptors, phenylephrine hydrochloride and, 139
Alphadolone acetate, 145
Alphaxalone, 145
Althesin, **145**, 245
Alveolar dead-space, 103
Ambu rescuscitator, 243
American Society of Regional Anesthesia, 32
Amethocain hydrochloride BP, 101, 118, **125–126**, 154
  addition of vasoconstrictor agents, 136, 202
  historical aspects, 15
  hyperbaric, 125, 136, 202
  intradural analgesia, 125, 191, 199, 202
  isobaric solution, 125
Amidases, hepatic, 119
Amide-linked local analgesic agents, **126–135**
Aminophylline, 289
Ammonium sulphate, 302
Amnesia, use of sedatives and, 142, 143, 144
Amputation, leg, 249, 316
Amylocaine, 118
Anaemia, 253
Anaesthetic face mask, 243
Anal operations, 248
Anal sphincter muscle tone, 209
Anaphylactoid reactions, 142
Anastomotic breakdown, 111, 249

319

320 INDEX

Anatomy, **38–85**
Anethaine, 125
Angioneurotic oedema, 24
Ankle jerk reflexes, 209
Ankylosing spondylitis, 252
Anterior abdominal wall
  motor innervation, intradural analgesia and, 192
  muscle tone, 209
Anterior columns of cord, 52
Anterior median fissure, 51
Anterior primary division, spinal nerve, 51
Anterior root, spinal nerve, 52
Anterior spinal artery, 53, 292
  thrombosis, 53
Anticoagulants, 253
Anti-emetic agents, 288
Anti-hypertensive agents, 139
Antioxidant, 130
Antiseptic contamination, meningitis and, 291
Aorto-caval compression, 219, 261–62
Apnoea, 104, 288, 290
  lignocaine toxicity and, 244
  total spinal and, 244
Aqueduct of midbrain, 76
Aqueduct of Sylvius, 89–90
Arachnoid granulations, CSF circulation and, 91
Arachnoid mater, **55**
Arachnoid villi, CSF circulation and, 91
Aramine, **138–139**
Argenine vasopressin (DDAVP), 283
Arm operations, 210
1-Arterenol, **140**
Arteries of Adamkiewicz, 53
Arteriosclerosis, 225
Aseptic meningitis, 292
  chemical, CSF pressure and, 96
Aspirin, 283
Atherosclerotic patients, leg amputation in, 249
Ativan, 143
Atropine, 108, 111, 140, 243, 246, 288
Autologous blood injection, 285
Autonomic blockade, 98
Autonomic fibres, spinal nerves, 51
Autonomic nervous system, 98
'Auto-observation' of intradural analgesia, 16–17
Azygos system, 54

'B' fibres, 99
Back deformity, 253
Back pain, severe, 293

Backache
  chronic, 253
  lithotomy position and, 289
Bacterial filter, 154, 222, 265, 269
Barbotage
  historical aspects, 12
  intractable pain relief and, 303
  intradural analgesia and, 12, 195–198, 200
  sitting position and, 198
Benzodiazepines, **142–143**
Beta blockade, 106
Beta eucaine, 28
Beta stimulation, adrenaline absorption and, 106
Bladder
  function, narcotic analgesics and, 306
  prolonged dilatation, 251
  wall, 110
Bleeding time, dextran and, 142
Blood clotting, defective, 252, 292
  obstetric analgesia and, 263
Blood pressure
  monitoring, 244
  sudden fall, 288
  see also Hypotension
Blood supply, spinal cord, 53–54
Blood transfusion, 27, 248
Bloodless field, 247, 313
Bone surgery, 132
Bowel anastomosis, 111
Bowel sounds, 111
Bradycardia, 243
Breast operations, 210
Broken needle, 287
Bronchospasm, 250
Bucking, local infiltration at cardia and, 198–199
Bulbar involvement, 292
Bupivacaine hydrochloride BP, 100, 119, **130–134**, 264
  addition of vasoconstrictor agents, 131, 136, 202, 264
  allergic reaction, 119
  barbotage and, 200
  bone surgery and, 132
  carbonated form, 132
  cardiac arrest and, 132
  cardiovascular toxicity, 135
  convulsions and, 132
  endoscopic prostatic resection and, 133
  extradural analgesia
    historical aspects, 17
    labour pain, 131, 134, 135

general surgery, 134
gynaecological operations, 134, 201
hip surgery, 133
hyperbaric solution, 125, 133, 136, 199, 202
hypobaric solution, unilateral block and, 200
intradural analgesia, 133, 188, 191, 199–200, 201, 202
  historical aspects, 17
  latency, 200, 264
  lower limb surgery, 133–201
  mixed with lignocaine, 264
  neurobehavioural responses of newborn and, 268
  neurological sequelae, 133
  obstetric analgesia, 270–71
  0.5 per cent solution, 199, 200, 270
  0.75 per cent solution, 270
  perineal operations, 133
  postoperative analgesia, 134
  sodium metabisulphite addition, 132
  systemic toxicity, 131
  test dose, 313
Butethanol, 125
'Butterfly' needle, 156, 182, 243

'C' fibres, 99
Caesarean section, 247, 249
  extradural block, 266, 268, 269
  historical aspects, 256–257
  intradural block, 270, 271
  previous section, rupture of scar and, 263
Caisson disease, 6
Cap, prevention of sepsis and, 52
Caramelisation, autoclaving and, 154
Carbocaine, 130
Carbonated salts, 128
  bupivacaine, 132
  lignocaine, 128, 220, 267
  prilocaine, 220
Cardiac
  arrest, 106, 233
    bupivacaine and, 132
  complications, 105–8, 219, 289
  compression, 219
  contractility, dopamine and, 140
  end of stomach, infiltration with local analgesic, 288
  output, contraindications and, 253
  preload, contraindications and, 252, 253
Cardiovascular
  collapse, **219**
  disease, dosage and, 226
  system, **105–109**
    obstetric patients, 261–263
    preload, 105
    venous return, 261–263
  toxicity, 135
Catecholamines, circulating, 112
Catheters, extradural analgesia and, 154, **220–223**
  accidental dural puncture, 221
  accidental intravascular cannulation, 215, 223, 231
  advantages, 222
  bacterial filter, 222
  dead space in hub of needle and, 221
  fixation, 222
  Huber point and, 220, 221
  knotted catheter, 223
  obstetrics, 222, 265
  postoperative analgesia and, 222
  respiration and, 104
  slicing off tip of catheter, 222
  technical difficulties, 221
  'tenting' of dura and, 221
  testing position in extradural space, 223
Cauda equina, **64–66**
  intradural analgesia and, 189
  lesions, 292
Caudal analgesia, 59, 68, 69, 224
  continuous, 18, 19
  infants/children, 19, 232–233
  obstetrics, 268
Central nervous system disorder, 253, 315–316
Central neural blockade, physiology, **98–112**
  autonomic blockade and, 98
Cerebellomedullary cistern, CSF circulation, 90, 91
Cerebellum, 76
Cerebral complications, 248
Cerebral tumour, post-lumbar puncture headache and, 281
Cerebral uncus herniation, 281, 293
Cerebrospinal fluid, **88–97**
  bloodstained, **183**
  circulation, **89–92**
  composition, **92–93**
  formation, 89
  function, 93
  poor flow of, 286–287
  pressure, 95–97
    factors influencing, 96–97

Cerebrospinal fluid (cont.)
  hydrostatic pressure and, 95
  leakage and, 96
  Queckenstedt's test and, 96
 source, 88
 volume, 94
Cerebrospinal fluid leakage
  CSF pressure and, 96
  cutaneous, 294
Cerebrovascular insufficiency, 253
Chalk from gloves, meningitis and, 291
Chemical damage to cord, 292
Chest
  injury, mechanical ventilation and, 310
  pain, 308
Chlorhexidine, 152
Chlormethiazole, **144–145**, 243
  anticonvulsant action, 144
Chlorocresol, 302
Chloroprocaine hydrochloride, **124–125**, 224, 227, 265, 294
  accidental intradural injection, 265
  mixtures with long-acting agent, 227
Chlorpromazine, 288
Choroid plexus, 88
Chronic asthma, 289
Chronic lung disease, 250
Chronic obstructive airways disease, 103
Chronic respiratory disease, 103, 250, 289
Cinchocaine hydrochloride BP, 118, **126–127**, 258
  historical aspects, 13
  intradural analgesia, 188, 191, 199, 200, 201
  hyperbaric, 126, 191, 199, 200
  1:1500 solution, 199
Circumcision, 249
  children, 252
  postoperative pain, 232, 252
Cisterna magna, 62
Cisterna pontis, 62
Cisternal puncture, 281
Cisterns at base of brain, 62
Citanest, 128
Classification of nerve fibres, 98–99
Coca, 21
Cocaine hydrochloride BP, 118, **123**, 245
  historical aspects, 6, 21–23, 29
  substitution of by other drugs, 9
Coeliac plexus, 52, 78, 79, 98
Colon
  breakdown of anastomosis, 249
  operations, 242, 249

Colpoperineorrhaphy, 251
Colporrhaphy, posterior, sacral block and, 231
Complications, **278–295**
  backache, 289
  broken needle, 287
  bronchospasm, 289
  cardiac, 248, **289**
  cerebral, 248
  circulatory collapse, 288–289
  convulsions see Convulsions
  dry puncture, 285–286
  failure, 287
  headache see Headache
  hiccups, 288
  Horner's syndrome, 291
  meningitis see Meningitis
  paralysis of 6th cranial nerve, 290
  paralysis of trigeminal nerve, 290
  poor flow of CSF, 286–287
  respiratory arrest, **289–290**
  retching, 288
  retention of urine, 291
  surgical emphysema, 287–288
  venous air embolism, 288
  vomiting, 288
Compound sodium lactate solution see Hartmann's solution
Consciousness, 77
Continuous caudal analgesia, 18, 19
  obstetrics, 258
Continuous extradural block, 250–252
  functional residual capacity and, 251
  physiotherapy and, 251
  postoperative atelectasis and, 250
  plus 'one-shot' intradural block, 216
Continuous spinal analgesia, 13, 18, 145
Contraindications, 183–184, **252–253**
Conus medullaris, 69
Convulsions, 218–219, 278
  bupivacaine and, 132
  metabolic acidosis and, 218
Coronary disease, 139, 140
  acute, recent, 316
Cough reflexes, active, 250
Cranial sensory nerves, 77
Cranial subarachnoid space, 76
Cremophor EL, 145
Cross-matching, 142
Crura of diaphragm, 78
Curare, 15
Cutaneous cerebrospinal fluid leakage, 294
Cutaneous sensibility, 84
Cystectomy, total, 249
Cystoscopy, sacral block and, 231

Deafness, 290
Decicain, 125
Deep vein thrombosis, 248
Dehydration, 252
Delirium tremens, 144
Denticulate ligaments, 63, 64, 69
　spread of local analgesic solution and, 192
Detergent contamination, meningitis and, 291
Dextran, 108, 141–142
Dextrose
　5 percent, 141
　with saline, 141
Diabetic patients
　amputation of leg, 249
　hypoglycaemia, 112
Diamorphine, 145, 204, 243, 308
Diazemuls, 143, 245
　cost, 143
Diazepam, **143**, 243
　after delivery, 271
　rectal, 143
Dibucaine, 13, 118, 126
Differential sympathetic block, 106
Di-isopropylphenol, **145**
　continuous infusion, 145
Dikain, 125
Diprivan, **145**
Direct vein anaesthesia, 25
Disoprofol, **145**
Disposable sets for sterile pack, 155
Distanest, 128
Dixon's law, 13
Dopamine, 109, **140**
Dorsal root pains, 303
Dosage
　for extradural injection, 225, **226–227**
　for intradural analgesia, 200–201
Dose response curves, 226
Double vision, 290
Drip indicator, 214
Drugs, **153–155**
Dry puncture, **285–286**
Duncaine, 127
Dura mater, **54–55**
　damage, median approach and, 164
　inadvertent puncture, 68, **216–217**, 233, 267
　　by extradural catheter, 220–223, 266
　　mid-thoracic region, 210
　　median dorsal fold, 212
Dural sac, 66
　young children, 232
Duranest, 134

Efferent fibre, spinal nerves, 52
Efferent sympathetic nerves, 52
Elderly patients, 249
　amputation of leg, 249
Endocrine system, **111–112**
Endoscopic prostatic resection, 133
Endotracheal insufflation anaesthesia, 26
Enflurane, 242
Ependyma, 88
Ephedrine BP, 108, **138**, 204
　historical aspects, 15
　hypotension and, 15, 138
　obstetrics, 138, 262
　tachyphylaxis, 138
Epidural space *see* Extradural space
Epinephrine, **136**
Epistaxis, 245
Equipment, 151–158
Ergotamine tartrate, 141
Esmarch bandage, 290
Ester-linked local analgesic agents, **123–126**
Ether and air, 242
Ethocaine, 124
Etidocaine hydrochloride **BP**, 100, 119, **134–135**, 264, 289, 294
　cardiovascular toxicity, 132, 135
　dosage, 227
　lipid solubility, 134
　obstetric analgesia, 134, 135
　prolonged spinal nerve involvement, 219
　protein binding, 134
Etomidate, **145**, 243, 309
　suppression of adrenocortical function, 145
Extradural abscess, 293, 294
Extradural analgesia, **17–19, 208–236**
　abdominal tumour, spread (of solution) and, 225
　accidental dural puncture, 68, **216–217**, 233
　　by extradural catheter, 220–223
　age, spread of solution and, 225
　anal sphincter relaxation and, 234
　approach to extradural space, 210–211
　arteriosclerosis and, 225
　cardiovascular collapse and, **219**
　catheters *see* Catheters, extradural analgesia and
　caudal, 18–19, 224
　choice between intra and extradural block, 234–236

complications, 216–217
continuous caudal analgesia, 18, 231
continuous plus 'one-shot' intradural block, 216
convulsions and, **218**
degenerative vascular disease, spread of solution and, 225
direction of needle bevel, 216, 224
dosage, 225, **226–227**
dose response curves, 226
drip indicator, 214
drug toxicity, 216
extradural space identification *see* Extradural space, identification of
facial pallor and, 233
glass syringe with ceramic/metal piston, 214
gravity, spread of solutions and, 224
height of patient, spread of solution and, 225
hypotension and *see* Hypotension
Iklé syringe, 212
indications, 208
laminectomy following, 219
legs, warm to palpation, 234
level of sensory block, application of bursts of electric current and, 234
Macintosh spring-loaded needle, 212
marked needle, 215
massive spread, 217–219
neurological complications, 236
numb legs and, 233
obstetrics, 135, 224–225, 236, **256–271**
Odom's indicator, 213
opiate receptors in spinal cord and, 19
Oxford balloon, 213
Oxford Epidural Space Detector, 214
para-oesophageal infiltration of local analgesic, 226
patchy analgesia, **215, 220**
phrenic nerve roots and, 210
pinprick sensitivity, 234
'pins and needles' in legs and, 233
plastic disposable syringes, 214
postoperative analgesia, 236
radioisotope tracers, spread (of solutions) and, 224
radio-opaque solutions, spread of solutions and, 224
rate of injection, 215, 216
respiratory depression, 216
sacral injection, 18, 19, **227–232** *see also* Sacral block
sacrococcygeal membrane, injection through, 211
signs of successful lumbar block, **233–234**
silicone oil, syringe lubrication and, 215
site of injection, spread of solutions and, 224
speed of injection, spread of solutions and, 224
spina bifida occulta and, 219
spread of solutions in extradural space, 101, **224–226**
spread up subdural space, 225
subdural extra-arachnoid injection, 218
surgical emphysema and, 215
syringes, recommended, 214
tendon reflexes and, 233
test dose *see* Test dose
total central neural blockade, 217
total spinal block, 215, 217
toxic effects, 218
Tuohy needle and, 212
uncooperative patient, 208
venous air embolism and, 215
volume injected, spread of solutions and, 224
Extradural blood patch, 267, 284–285, 313
pain during injection, 285
Extradural space, 57–60, 68, 69
identification of, **211–216**
dimpling of dura, 212
hanging drop method, 212, 251
median dorsal fold and, 212
Oxford Extradural Space Detector, 214
indicator, 154
posterior boundaries, 71
Extradural spinal cord tumour, 294
Extradural veins, 53–54

Falx cerebri, 54
Felypressin, 136
Femoral aortography, 249
Femoral neuropathy, 294
Fentanyl, 308, 309
continuous infusion, 308
extradural, 309
Fibrinolytic effects, 109, 248
Filum terminale, 51, 54, 66
Foramen magnum, 54, 59, 77, 91
Foramina of Luschka, 76, 92
CSF circulation, 90
Foramen of Magendie, 76, 92
CSF circulation, 90
Foramina of Monro, 89

INDEX

Fourth ventricle, 76
  CSF circulation, 90
Fourth World Congress, 259
Fracture of the skull, 290
Free airway, 245
Frusemide, CSF formation and, 89
Functional residual capacity (FRC), 104, 251

Gamma radiation, 155
Gastric emptying time, 111
Gastrointestinal tract, **110–111**
Gelatins, **142**
Gelofusin, 142
General anaesthesia, 243
Genitourinary system, **109–110**
Glass fragments, sepsis prevention and, 153
Glass spine, 10, 192
Glass syringe with ceramic/metal piston, 214
Gloves, prevention of sepsis and, 152
Glucose
  hyperbaric solutions and, 199
  5 per cent, 244
Gown, sterile, 152
Gravocaine, 13
Grey rami communicantes, 52, 98
Groin operations, 189, 200
Guedel pharyngeal airway, 245
Gynaecological operations
  abdominal, 247
  bupivacaine and, 134
  perineal, 247

Haemaccel, 142
Haematoma
  extradural, 285, 294
  formation, compression of cord and, 292–293
    decompression, 293
    myelography, 293
    severe back pain and, 293
  subarachnoid, 292
  subdural, surgical evacuation, 293
Haemorrhage
  homeostatic response, 244
  reactionary, 313
Haemorrhoidectomy
  intradural analgesia, 191
  maintenance of sphincter tone, 231
  postoperative pain relief, 251
Halothane, 242
Hand operations, 210
Hartmann's solution, 108, 141, 244, 262, 267, 270

Headache, 236, **278–285**
  antidiuretic drugs and, 283
  aseptic inflammatory meningeal reaction and, 279, 284
  back of neck, 282
  cerebral tumour and, 281
  cisternal puncture and, 281
  CO_2 in oxygen inhalation from Magill circuit and, 283
  coughing and, 282
  CSF cell count, 284
  diagnosis, **282**
  diarrhoea and, 281
  extradural blood patch treatment, 284–285, 314
    pain during injection, 285
  following intradural analgesia, 10
  haemorrhage and, 281
  head retraction, 284
  high altitude and, 281
  'high pressure', 280, 284
  incidence, 278
  inflammatory reaction to introduction of organisms, 279–280
  lactation and, 281
  'low pressure', 281
  migraine and, 285
  multiple punctures of dura and, 282
  in neurotics, 285
  obstetric patients, 267, 281
  occipital region, 282
  posture and, 280, 282
  prevention, **281–282**
  rise in $PaCO_2$, treatment and, 284
  septic meningitis, 284
  severe/prolonged, 281
  simple analgesics, 283
  size of lumbar puncture needle and, 279
  with stiffness of neck, 278
  straining and, 282
  sweating and, 281
  synthetic argenine vasopressin (DDAVP) and, 283
  tentorium and, 280
  treatment, **282, 285**
    choroid plexus stimulation, 283
    drugs, 283
    head of pressure around dura, 283
    intrathecal injection of saline, 283
  vomiting and, 281
Hemiplegia, unexplained, 294
Hemineurin, **144**
Heminevrin, **144**
Hepatitis B antigen, sterilisation and, 155

Hernia repair, 247, 249
Heroin, 243
Herpes zoster, 303
Hiccups, 288
High spinal block, 77, 106
  apnoea following, 104
  intradural, 189
Hip surgery, 243, 248
  bupivacaine and, 133
  fixation of fracture, 248
  intradural analgesia and, 189, 200
  postoperative pain relief, 251
  total replacement, 248
Historical aspects, **4–32**
  biographies, 19–32
Horner's syndrome, 291
Huber pointed needle, 259
  introduction of catheter and, 220, 221
Human serum albumin, IV infusion, 142
Hydrocoele, 249
Hydrocortisone, 289
Hydroxyethyl starch, 142
Hyoscine, 145, 246
Hyperbaric medicine, 20
Hyperbaric solutions, 101, **198–199**
  addition of glucose, 199
  intradural analgesia, **198–199**
Hyperglycaemic response of surgical stress, 112
Hypertensive heart disease, 140
Hyperthyroidism, 112, 137, 140
Hypnomidate, **145**
Hypnovel, **143–144**
Hypobaric solutions, 199
Hypogastric nerves, 110
Hypoglycaemia, 112
Hypotension, 106–107, 108, 243, 278
  ephedrine and, 138
  extradural analgesia and, 216, 233
  ischaemia with neurological sequelae and, 293
  total spinal analgesia and, 15
Hypothermia, CSF formation and, 89
Hypoventilation, 288
Hypovolaemia, 252, 316
  dosage and, 226

Iklé syringe, 212
Immunosuppression, 112
Impotence, post-spinal, 292
Inclination of vertebral column, 195
Indications, 247–250
  in robust young adults, 247
  single-handed doctors, 249
Indwelling needle, 243

Inferior articular processes, 74
Inferior splanchnic nerves, 111
Inotropin, **140**
Insulin
  response to, 112
  syringe, 154
Interanalgesic interval, 123
  analgesic potency and, 123
Intercostal
  nerves, 84
  paralysis, 80, 103
  spaces, 59
Interlaminar foramen, 45, 71, 72
Interlaminar space, 71
  lumbar puncture technique and, 161
Intermediate duration of action, agents of, 121
Intermedio-lateral horn, 52
Intermittent positive pressure ventilation, 243
Interspinous ligament, **73**
  anatomy, 46, **49**
  cystic degeneration, false positive sign and, 49, 164
Interstitial fluid of brain, 93
Interventricular foramina (of Monro), CSF circulation and, 89
Intervertebral disc, **49–51**, 73
  prolapsed, 50, 51, 280
  neurological complications and, 268
Intervertebral foramen, 73, 74, 76
  narrowing of, 295
Intestinal tone, 111
Intra-abdominal perforation, 111
Intracranial arterio-venous malformation, 294
Intracranial haemorrhage, 293
Intracranial sinuses, 53
Intractable pain, 302–304
  barbotage and, 303
  cooling of CSF and, 303
  dangers of neurolytic drugs, 303
  electrodes in extradural space, 304
  extradural analgesia, 210
  ice cold saline, 303
  injection into extracranial subdural space, 303
  malignant disease and, 302
  narcotic analgesic drugs and, 309, 310
  in perineum, 303
  in rectum, 303
  steroid injection, 303
  transcutaneous stimulation, 304
  untoward paralysis and, 303
Intradural analgesia, **188–204**
  barbotage, 195–198, 200

Intradural analgesia (*cont.*)
    sitting position and, 191, 198–200
  baricity, posture and, 189–195
  in children, 11–12
  choice of analgesic drug, **200–201**
  choice between intra- and extradural block, 234–236
  concentration of analgesic drug, 200–201
  dose of analgesic drug, **200–201**
  early use in Britain, 10
  establishment in UK, 27
  first use of, 8–9
  historical aspects, 4–17
  hyperbaric solutions, **198–199**
  Jonnesco's technique, 17
  Labat's technique, 12
  level of sensory blockade, application of bursts of electric current and, 234
  obstetrics, 121, **256–271**
  opiate receptors, spinal cord and, 19
  plain solutions, 191, **199–200**
  postoperative sequelae, 17, 278–295
  sacral nerves and, 191
  spread of local analgesic solution, 101, 189
    inclination of vertebral column and, 195
    turbulent currents and, 196–198
  for surgeon, 204
  unilateral block, 200, 316
  in U.S., 12
  vasoconstrictor agents, **202**
  volume, degree of spread and, **198**
Intradural space, 60–62
Intraspinal epidermoid tumour, 294
Intravenous fluids, **141**
  brandy, 11
  historical aspects, 11, 15
Intravenous sedative, 143
Introducer, 294
Irritable bronchial tree, 250
Isotonic saline, 141, 244

Jonnesco's technique, 17, 30
  postoperative sequelae, 17

Keller's operation, sacral block and, 231
Kerocain, 124
Ketamine, 232, 243
Kidney operations, 242
Knee jerk reflex, 209

Laminectomy, 219, 248, 285
  extradural analgesia, 208
  in surgery of intervertebral disc, 315

Laryngospasm, 250
Lateral columns of cord, 52
Lateral approach *see* Paramedian approach
Lateral position, 242
Lateral ventricles, CSF circulation, 89
Leg operations *see* Lower limb surgery
Levophed, **140**
Lidocaine USP, 127
Ligamenta denticulata, 62–64, 69
Ligamentum flavum, **46–48**, 71, 73, 74, 75, 76
  extradural analgesia and, 210
  lumbar puncture technique and, 160
Lignocaine hydrochloride BP, 119, **127–128**
  addition of vasoconstrictor agents, 202
  carbonated salts, 128, 220
    obstetric analgesia and, 127, 267
  caudal analgesia in infants/children, 232
  extradural analgesia, 17, 135
  hyperbaric, 128, 202
  intradural analgesia, 199, 202
  mixed with bupivacaine, 264
  obstetrics, 127, 135, 267
  patchy analgesia and, 220
  5 per cent in glucose, 199
  placental transfer, 264, 268
  postoperative analgesia, 127
  tachyphylaxis, 127, 264
  toxic effect, 244
Lipid solubility, 102
  etidocaine, 134
Lipiodol, 29
Litigation, 316
Lithotomy position, 289
Liver, **109**
Local infiltration analgesia, 28
Local analgesic agents, **118–123**
  actions on nerve fibres, 98–102
  action potential and, 99
  carbonated salts, 128
  duration of action, 121
  'interanalgesic interval', 123
  nodes of Ranvier and, 99
  Swedish, 119
  tachyphylaxis, 122, 123
  toxic effects, 121–122
    acid-base status and, 122
Long duration of action, agents of, 121
Lorazepam, **143**
Lower abdominal pain, 308
Lower abdominal operations, 247
  extradural analgesia, 208
  intradural analgesia, 200

Lower abdominal operations (cont.)
  postoperative pain relief, 251
Lower limb surgery, 189, 191, 200, 247, 316
  bupivacaine, 133
  elderly patients, 249
  intradural analgesia, 133
  orthopaedic, 252
  postoperative pain relief, 251, 252
  sacral block and, 231
Lumbago, extradural sacral cocaine injection, 29
Lumbar convexity, 192
Lumbar intervertebral joints, 45
Lumbar enlargement, blood supply, 53
Lumbar puncture, 159
  contraindications, 183–184
  needles, 28, 156
  technique *see* Lumbar puncture technique
Lumbar puncture technique, **159–185**
  in bed, 162
  lateral route *see* Paramedian approach
  lumbo-sacral approach, 178–179
  median approach, 163–164
  paramedian approach, 163, 164–177
  position of patient, 159–162
    sitting up, 160
  site of puncture, 162–163
    Tuffier's line and, 162
    vertebra prominens and, 163
  spinal needle director, 179–183
Lumbar spinal stenosis, 295
Lumbar vertebra, **39–45**
Lumbo-sacral angle, sacral injection and, 231
Lumbo-sacral approach, 178–179
Lumbo-sacral joint, 66
Lumbo-sacral plexus, traction neurological complications and, 268

Ma huang, 15
Macintosh balloon, 154
Macintosh spinal needle, 214
Macintosh spring-loaded needle, 212
Magnesium sulphate, 16
Malignant hyperpyrexia, 124, 126
Management during operation *see* Patient management
Marcain, 130
Marcaine, 130
Marked needle, 215
Mask, prevention of sepsis and, 152
Meaverin, 130
Median aperture *see* Foramen of Magendie

Median approach, 163–164
  hanging drop test, 163
  loss of resistance test, 163
Meningeal infection, 151
  CSF pressure and, 96
Meninges, **54–57**
  nerve supply, 57
Meningitis, **291**
  aseptic, 96, 292
  chalk from gloves and, 291
  detergent contamination and, 291
Mephentermine sulphate BP, 108, **139**
Mephine, **139**
Mepivacaine hydrochloride, 119, **130**
  antioxidant, 130
  hyperbaric, 125
  intradural analgesia, 188, 199, 200
  obstetrics, 130
  placental transfer, 264, 268
Mesentery traction, hiccups and, 288
Metabolic acidosis
  CSF formation and, 89
  convulsions and, 218
'Metameric anaesthesia', 30
Metaraminol bitartrate, **138–139**
Metastatic extradural spinal cord tumour, 294
Methadone, 308
Methaemoglobin
  lignocaine and, 127
  o-toluidine and, 129
  prilocaine and, 129
Methedrine, **138**
Methoxamine hydrochloride BPC, 108, **139–140**
  obstetrics, 140
Methyl-amphetamine, **138**
Methyl guanine, 15
Methyl paraben, 121
Metycain, 18
Midazolam, **143–144**
  amnesia and, 144
  anticonvulsant activity, 143
  anxiolytic activity, 143
  induction time, 144
  thrombophlebitis and, 144
Mid-thoracic region, extradural analgesia, 210
Migraine, 285
Mission hospitals, 249
Mixed spinal nerves, 52
Monoamine oxidase inhibitors, 136, 138, 139
Morphine, 111, 145, 244, 306, 308
Motor fibres, spinal nerve, 51
Motor loss, permanent, 292

Multiple sclerosis, 294
Muscle tone, 100
Myelogram, **184–185,** 285, 293
Myocardial disease, 139
Myocardial infarction, 253
Myocardium, effects of spinal block, 105
Myotomes, 84
Naloxone, 309
Narcotic analgesics, **145, 306–310**
  acute trauma, 310
  brain/plasma distribution coefficient, 307
  chest pain, 308
  chronic pain, 310
  continuous infusion, 308
  infection risk, injection via indwelling catheter and, 310
  lipophilicity, 307
  lower abdominal pain, 308
  neural substance/CSF distribution coefficient, 307
  obstetric pain relief, 309
  postoperative observation, respiratory depression and, 310
  postoperative pain relief, 310
  respiratory depression and, 307, 309, 310 of newborn, 309
  side effects, 308, 309, 310
  subcutaneous reservoir system, 310
  systemic absorption, 307
  upper abdominal pain, 308
Nasal catheter, 243
Nasopharyngeal airway, 245
Neck stiffness, 278
Needle director, 6, 164, 179–183
Needles, 153–155, **156–158**
Neocaine, 12, 124
Neophryn, **136–137**
Neosynephrine, **136–137**
Nerve fibres, classification, 98–99
Nerve roots, 51–52
  damage, 292
Nerve tunnels, narrowing of, 295
Nervi erigentes, 110
Nesacaine, **124–125**
Neuroglia, 51
Neurological sequelae, **291–295**
  anterior spinal artery and, 292
  electromyographic studies, 292
  haematoma formation, compression of cord and, 292–293
  intracranial complications, 293
  ischaemia associated with hypotension and, 293
  medico-legal consequences, 291

  transient post-spinal disabilities, 291
  ultrasound measurement of spinal canal and, 295
  unrelated to spinal injection, 293–294
Neurolytic solutions, 57
Newborn, respiratory depression, 309
Nitroglycerine, 289
'No touch' technique, 153
Nodes of Ranvier, 99
Noradrenaline acid tartrate BP, **140**
Norepinephrine, **140**
Novocaine, 118, 124
Nucleus pulposus, 73
  protrusion in disc prolapse, 50
Nupercaine, 13, 118, 126

Obesity, 210, 250
  difficulties of lumbar puncture and, 82–83
  respiration and, 103
'Objective observation', intradural analgesia, 17
Obstetric analgesia, 124, 125, 142, 224–225, 236, 247, **256–271**
  accidental dural puncture, 267, 269
    by catheter tip, 266
  afferent nerve pathways of labour pains and, 258
  antacids and, 260
  aorti-caval compression, avoidance of, 270, 271
  bacterial filter, 265, 269
  bilateral paravertebral block, 258
  blood pressure measurement, 266
  breech presentation, 263
  bupivacaine, 131, 134, 135
  Caesarean section, 12, 247, 249, 266, 268, 269
    intradural, 270, 271
    previous section, rupture of scar and, 263
    single shot, 270
  cardiac distress, 263
  cardiovascular system in obstetric patients and, 261–263
  catheters, extradural analgesia and, 222
  caudal analgesia, 130, 268
    continuous, 258
  centimetre markings on needle and catheter, 265
  cephalopelvic disproportion, 263
  coagulation abnormality, 263
  compression of inferior vena cava, 261, 262

Obstetric analgesia (cont.)
  latent, 261
  overt, 261
  spread of analgesia and, 225
  supine position and, 266
 'controllable spinal anaesthesia', 257
 diastolic pressure and, 261
 ephedrine as vasopressor, 138, 262
 etidocaine, 134, 135
 extradural block, 208, 224–225, 259–261
   lumbar, 258–259
   operative procedures, 260, 269–270
   practical details, 263–267
   practised by obstetricians, 260
   sacral (caudal) block, 257–258
 extradural haematoma, bacteraemia and, 268
 extradural infection, 267–268
 fall in arterial pressure, spinal block and, 262
 fetal effects, 268
   acidosis, 261, 262
   arterial oxygen tension, 261
   trauma to head and, 256
 forceps extraction, 247, 269, 270
 H2 antagonists, 260
 heart rate and, 261
 high forceps, 270
 historical aspects, **256–257**
 hypotension, 262
   Apgar scores and, 262
 hypovolaemia, 262, 263
 hysterical patients, 271
 inadvertent intradural injection, 266
 incremental doses, 270
 inhalation of vomitus, mortality/morbidity and, 256
 insertion of catheter into extradural space, 220, 265
   loss of resistance, technique and, 265
 intradural analgesia, 12, **256–271**
   operative delivery, 270
 intrauterine manipulations, 269, 270
 intravenous infusion, 266, 271
 late complications, 267–268
 lateral position, 262
 lateral tilt of bed/operating table, 266
 leakage of CSF following, 267
 lignocaine, 127, 267
 lithotomy position, 266
 locked twins, 263
 low forceps delivery, 269, 270
 mechanical pump, continuous infusion catheter and, 265

 mepivacaine, 130
 methoxamine and, 140
 midwives, extra-dural block and, 266
   supervision, 260
 Minnitt's nitrous oxide and air, 256
 multiple pregnancy, 263
 narcotic analgesics and, 271, 309
 nerve supply of uterus and, **259**
 neurobehavioural responses of newborn infants and, 268
 neurological sequelae, 260, 268, 294
 open drop chloroform, 256
 operative obstetrics, 269–271
 oxygen administration, 271
 pain relief service by obstetricians, 260
 perineal analgesia, 265
 peripheral resistance, 261
 phenylephrine hydrochloride and, 139
 placenta praevia and, 263
 placental blood flow and, 261
 Posiero effect, 262
 post-lumbar puncture headache and, 267, 281
 pre-eclampsia and, 263
 quadruplets, 263
 relaxation of pelvic floor, 256
 removal of retained placenta, 270
 respiratory distress, 263
 retention of urine, catheterisation and, 266
 sacral block, 258, **268–269**
 saddle-block, 257, 270
 shortage of anaesthetists and, 260
 slow painful labour, 263
 stroke volume and, 261
 supine hypotensive syndrome of pregnancy and, **261**
 supine position, 266
 supplementary general anaesthesia, 271
 surgical induction of labour, 265
 systolic pressure and, 261
 techniques of regional block, historical aspects, 256–257
 tilting patient to one side, 262
 tone of uterine muscle and, 256
 top-up doses of analgesic drug, 266
 total spinal block, 266
 trial of labour, 263
 Tuohy needle and, 265
 two catheter technique, 263
 unblocked segments, 267
 uncontrolled nervousness, 263
 volume of solution, 265
 wedge under buttock, 262, 266

INDEX 331

Odom's indicator, 213
Operator preparation, 152-153
Opiate receptors, CNS, 19, 306
Opioids, 306
Orthopaedic operations, 134
O-toluidine, 129
Ouabain, CSF formation and, 89
Oxford balloon, 213
Oxford Epidural Space Detector, 214
Oxygen dissociation curve, 129
Oxygen inhalation, retching/vomiting and, 288
Oxygen administration, 243

Pacchionian bodies, CSF circulation and, 91
Pain
  chest, 308
  dorsal root, 303
  intractable *see* Intractable pain
  postoperative *see* Postoperative pain
  down thigh, 71
  following trauma, 303
  upper abdominal, 308
Pantocaine, 125
Pantokain, 125
Papaveretum, 145, 244, 308
Para-aminobenzoic acid, 119
  allergic reaction, 119
Paracetamol, 283
Paralytic ileus, 111
Paramedian approach, 49, 163, 164-177
  thoracic region, 164
Para-oesophageal infiltration of local analgesic, 226
Paraplegia, 292
  severe back pain and, 293
  spontaneous vaginal delivery and, 259
Paravertebral ganglia, 52
Paravertebral spaces, 59
Passive hyperaemia, 25
Patchy block, 215, 220
  obstetrics, 267
Patient management, **242-246**
  anaesthetic face mask, 243
  apnoea, total spinal and, 244
  assisted or controlled respiration, 243
  blood pressure, 244
  bradycardia with hypotension, 243
  free airway, 245
  general anaesthesia, 243
  Guedel pharyngeal airway, 245
  homeostatic response to haemorrhage and, 244
  indwelling needle/'butterfly', 243
  intermittent positive pressure ventilation, 243
  nasopharyngeal airway, 245
  respiration, 243
  spraying of naris with 4 percent cocaine, 245
  tracheal intubation, 242, 245
  transtracheal analgesia, 246
Pelvic floor repair, sacral block and, 231
Pelvic operations, 208
Penis engorgement, 110
Pentobarbitone, 244
Percaine, 13, 118, 126
Perianal operations, 248
Pericarditis, constrictive, 252
Peridural segmental analgesia, 17, 31
Peridural space *see* Extradural space
Perineal operations, 247, 316
  bupivacaine and, 133
  extradural analgesia, 208
  gynaecological, 247
  intradural analgesia, 133, 189, 191, 200
Perineorrhaphy, sacral block and, 231
Peripheral blood flow, 105
Peristalsis, 110
Pervitin, **138**
Pethidine, 145, 244, 268, 309
  bupivacaine toxicity and, 131
pH of injected solution, meningitis and, 291
Phaeochromocytoma, 112
  surgery, 249
Phantom limb pain, 293
Pharmacology, **118-145**
Phenol
  5 per cent in glycerine, 302
  7.5 per cent in iophendylate, 302
Phenoperidine, 145
Phenoxybenzamine, 309
Phenylephrine hydrochloride BP, 108, **136-137, 139**
  intradural analgesia and, 202
  with lignocaine, 127
  obstetric use, 139
Phrenic nerve roots, extradural analgesia and, 210
Pia mater, 54, **57**
Physiology, **98-112**
Pilomotor fibres, 52, 98
Piperocaine, 18
Plain solutions, intradural analgesia and, 191, **199-200**
Planocaine, 124

Plasma
  esterases, 119
  intravenous infusion, 141
  protein fraction, intravenous infusion, 141
Plasma volume expanders, **141–142**, 244
Plastic disposable syringe, 214
Plastic gallipots, 155
Polygelatine, 262, 270
Polygeline, 142, 262, 270
Pontocaine, 125
Posterior inferior cerebellar arteries, 53
Posterior longitudinal ligament, 55
Posterior median septum, 51
Posterior primary division, spinal nerve trunk, 51
Posterior repair, 226
Posterior root ganglion, 52, 79, 98
Posterior spinal arteries, 53
Posterior subarachnoid septum, 64
Posterior superior iliac spines, 66
Postganglionic fibres, 52
  plexuses of origin, 52
Postganglionic sympathetic grey rami, 99
Post-lumbar puncture headache *see* Headache
Post-lumbar puncture pain in back, 285
Postoperative atelectasis, 250
Postoperative pain, 125, 236, 309
  bupivacaine and, 134
  catheters, extradural analgesia and, 220, 222
  caudal analgesia in infants/children, 232 lignocaine, 127
  narcotic analgesics and, 310
Postoperative pulmonary complications, 104
Postoperative urinary retention, 309
Post-traumatic analgesia, 134
Pre-anaesthetic clinic, 209
Pre-aortic plexuses, 78
Pre-eclampsia, 144
Preganglionic fibres, 52
Pressor drugs, 244, 270, 289
  obstetrics, 262
Prilocaine hydrochloride, 119, **128–129**
  carbonated salts, 220
  patchy analgesia, 220
  methaemoglobinaemia and, 129, 264
  obstetric use, 264
  oxygen dissociation curve and, 129
  5 per cent, intradural analgesia, 199
  placental transfer, 264

Prinzmetal's variant angina, 289
Procaine hydrochloride BP, 118, **124**, 200, 220, 257
  extradural analgesia, 17
  intradural analgesia, 13, 199, 200
  intravenous analgesia, 25
  powder, 32
Prolapse, repair of, 226
Propitocaine, 128
Prostatectomy, 133, 248
  suprapubic, 225
Protein binding
  bupivacaine, 131
  etidocaine, 130
Pulmonary arterial pressure, 103
Pulmonary blood volume, 103
Pulmonary embolism, 290
Pulmonary hypertension, **109**
Pulmonary sympathetic innervation, 109
Pyriformis muscle, 66

Queckenstedt's test, 96, 185
Quincke needle, 156

Rate pressure product, 107
Rectal operations, 242
  abdomino-perineal resection, 249
Regurgitation of gastric contents, 233
Renal blood flow, 140
Renal complications, 248
Respiration, **102–104**
  assisted, 26
  during operation, 243
    spontaneous, 247
  functional residual capacity (FRC), 104, 251
Respiratory acidosis, CSF formation and, 89
Respiratory arrest, 77, 233, 278, 289–290
  apnoea, 290
  hypoventilation, 289
  positive pressure respiration and, 290
Respiratory centre, 77
Respiratory depression, 278, 309
  extradural analgesia and, 216
  narcotic analgesics and, 307, 309, 310
Respiratory minute volume, 103
Retching, 288
Retention of urine, 110, 291
  obstetric analgesia and, 266
  postoperative, 309

INDEX 333

Retrobulbar neuritis, 294
Retroperitoneal preaortic plexuses, 98
Right atrial pressure, 105
Rubber gloves, 28
Rubber-stoppered stock bottle, sepsis prevention and, 153

Sacral block
 breakage of needle/catheter and, 232
 historical aspects, 30
 obstetrics, **268–269**
 sepsis and, 231
 see also Sacral injection
Sacral canal, 66, 69, 227, 228
Sacral hiatus, 59, 66, 69, 228
Sacral injection, 227–232
 blood on aspiration, 230
 depth of intergluteal cleft and, 228
 failure rate, 231
 lumbo-sacral angle and, 231
 in negroes, 231
 prone position, 227
Sacral nerves, intradural analgesia and, 191
Sacral outflow, 79
Sacral parasympathetic fibres, 79, 110
Sacral plexus, 66
Sacral sympathetic fibres, 101
Sacro-coccygeal membrane, 66, 227
 extradural analgesia and, 211
Sacrum, **66**
Saddle block, 101
 obstetrics, 257, 270
Scandicaine, 130
Sciatica treatment, extradural sacral cocaine injection, 29
Scurocaine, 124
Sedative drugs in central neural blockade, 142–145
Segmental nerves, 58
Sensory analgesia, post spinal, 292
Sensory fibres, spinal nerves, 51
Sepsis, 151
Sequelae, **278–295**
 neurological *see* Neurological sequelae
Servocaine, 124
Shock, 12, 316
Short duration of action, agents of, 121
Silicone oil, 215
Single-handed doctors, 249
Sise introducer, 154
Sixth cranial nerve paralysis, 25, 299
 bilateral, 290
Skin
 preparation, 151–152
 addition of dye to antiseptic solution and, 152
 sepsis, 253
 temperature, 105
Sodium metabisulphite, addition to bupivacaine, 132
Sodium salicylate, 30
Sovcaine, 126
Spermatorrhoea, 110
Sphincter control, post-spinal loss, 292
Sphincter of Oddi, 111
Spina bifida occulta, 219, 252
Spinal block
 fall in blood pressure and, 106–107, 108
 myocardium, effects on, 105
 vascular bed, effects on, 107
Spinal cord
 anatomy, 51–52
 damage, 291–295
 ischaemia, 53
Spinal ganglion, 52
Spinal needle director *see* Needle director
Spinal needles *see* Needles
Spinal nerve trunks, 51
Spinal nerves, 51
Spinal subarachnoid space, 76
Spinocaine, 13
Spironolactone, CSF formation and, 89
Splanchnic nerves, 78–79, 98
 intradural analgesia for abdominal operations and, 192
Spleen, 111
Status epilepticus, 144
Steep head-down position, 242
'Sterile distilled water', sepsis prevention and, 153
Sterilisation methods, 151
 'in the field', 155
Stomach handling, hiccups and, 288
Stovaine, 9, 10, 26, 28, 118
Stress, postoperative, 112
Stretch reflex, 100
Subarachnoid block *see* Intradural analgesia
Subarachnoid haematoma, 292
Subarachnoid haemorrhage, 252
Subarachnoid space *see* Intradural space
Subdural extra-arachnoid injection, 218
Subdural haematoma, 293
Subdural space, **57**, 218, 225, 244
Substantia gelatinosa, 306
Sudomotor fibres, 52, 98
Superior articular processes, 73–74

Superior mesenteric plexus, 52
Supraspinous ligaments, 46, 49, 73
Supratentorial region, CSF circulation and, 91
Surface markings, 38
Surgical emphysema, 215, 287–288
Surgical shock, 12
Sympathetic cardiac accelerator fibres, 80
Sympathetic preganglionic axons, 52, 78
Sympathetic trunk, 66
Sympathomimetic agents
  acting on alpha receptors, **139–140**
Sympathomimetic amines, **137–139**
  acting on beta receptors, **140–142**
Syncaine, 124
Synthetic beta-endorphins, 303
Syringes, **153–155**
Syringomyelia, 315

Tabes dorsalis, 315
  extradural sacral cocaine injection, 29
Tachyphylaxis, 122, 123, 264
  ephedrine, 138
  'interanalgesic interval' and, 123
  lignocaine, 127, 264
Tactile sensibility of the trunk, 77
Tentorium cerebelli, 54, 76, 280
  CSF circulation, 91
'Test dose', 100, 215
  bupivacaine with adrenaline, 313
Tetanus, 8
Tetracaine, 125
Thalamonal, 204, 243, 244
Theca, 54
Third ventricle, 76
  CSF circulation, 89
Thoracic concavity, 192
Thoracic enlargement, blood supply, 53
Thoracic operations, 208, 248, 252
Thoracic trauma, 310
Thoraco-abdominal splanchnicectomy, 15
Thrombophlebitis, postoperative, 292
Thyroid operations, 210
Tight mitral stenosis, 253
Tinnitus, 290
Total central neural blockade, 217, 233
Total spinal block, 14–15, 215, 217
  apnoea and, 244
Toxic effects of local analgesic agents, 121, 132, 216, 218
  acid-base status and, 122
Tracheal intubation, 16, 242, 245, 247
Traction on mesentery, 79

Transcutaneous stimulation, 304
Trans-sacral block, 19
Transtracheal analgesia, 246
Transurethral resection of prostate, sacral block and, 231
Transverse myelitis, 292, 294
Trauma, acute, narcotic analgesics and, 310
Trendelenburg position, 12, 107
Trichloroethylene, 242
Tricyclic antidepressants, 136, 139
Trigeminal nerve paralysis, 290
Tropocaine, 118
Tuffier's line, 162
Tuohy needle, 156, 212, 259, 265

Uncooperative patient, 208, 252
Unilateral block, 200, 316
Unsuccessful spinal analgesia, **287**
Upper abdominal pain, 308
Upper abdominal operations, 79, 84, 252
  blockage of vagal impulses and, 198–199, 252
  bucking, 199
  extradural analgesia, 209
  hypotension and, 252
  spinal puncture in thoracic region and, 189
  spread of local analgesic solution, 189
  in very ill patient, 248
Ureters, 110
Urinary catheterisation, 110, 266
Urinary retention *see* Retention of urine
Urokinase release, 249

Vagotomy, 79
Vagus, 52, 80, 110
  blockade of impulses, 198–199, 252, 288
  intradural analgesia and, 198–199
Valium, **143**
Vasoconstrictor drugs, **135–137**
  intradural analgesia, **202**
Vasomotor fibres, 52, 98
Vasomotor paralysis, collapse and, 288
Vasopressin, CSF formation and, 89
Vasopressor drugs, **316**
  in hypotension, 137
Vasoxine, **139–140**
Vena cava, inferior, 53–54
  compression
    dosage and, 226
    in obstetrics, 261, 262
  obstruction, 54, 252
Venous air embolism, 215, 288

Venous plexus, 60
Venous return, 105
Vertebra, 39
  bodies of, 46
Vertebra prominens, 163
Vertebral arches, 46
Vertebral canal, **43–45**, 54
Verterbral column, **38**
Virchow-Robin spaces, 102
Visceral afferent fibre, 52
Visceral afferent impulses, 78
Visceral motor nerve supply, 78
Visceral parasympathetic nerves, 79

Vomiting, 288

W–19053, 134
Wertheim's hysterectomy, 249
Wheeze, 250
Whitacre needle, 156
White rami communicantes, 52, 98, 99
Wright's anemometer, 103
Wyamine, **139**

Xylocaine, 127
Xylonest, 128